Nursing Care in an Aging Society

Donna M. Corr, R.N., M.S.N., is Assistant Professor of Nursing, St. Louis Community College at Forest Park, St. Louis, Missouri. With her husband, she is coeditor of *Hospice Care: Principles and Practice* (Springer Publishing Company, 1983) and *Hospice Approaches to Pediatric Care* (Springer Publishing Company, 1985).

Charles A. Corr, Ph.D., is Professor in the School of Humanities, Southern Illinois University at Edwardsville, and Chairperson, International Work Group on Death, Dying, and Bereavement. Previous volumes he has coedited include: *Helping Children Cope with Death: Guidelines and Resources* (2nd ed.; Hemisphere Publishing Corporation, 1984); *Childhood and Death* (Hemisphere Publishing Corporation, 1984); and *Adolescence and Death* (Springer Publishing Company, 1986).

Nursing Care in an Aging Society

Donna M. Corr
Charles A. Corr

Editors

SPRINGER PUBLISHING COMPANY
New York

Copyright © 1990 by Springer Publishing Company, Inc.

Springer Publishing Company, Inc.
536 Broadway
New York, NY 10012

90 91 92 93 94 / 5 4 3 2 1

Library of Congress Cataloging-in-Publication Data

Nursing care in an aging society / Donna M. Corr, Charles A. Corr, editors.
    p.   cm.
   Includes bibliographical references.
   ISBN 0-8261-6630-X
   1. Geriatric nursing. I. Corr, Donna M. II. Corr, Charles A.
   [DNLM: 1. Geriatric Nursing. WY 152 N97435]
   RC954.N882 1990
   610.73'65—dc20
DNLM/DLC
for Library of Congress   90-9601
                                              CIP

Printed in the United States of America

Dedication:

To Our Mothers Who Taught Us to Care:

Sadie

Elizabeth

To Special Persons Who Taught Us About Living:

James Sands

Yvonne Collins

To Special Persons Who Taught Us About Nursing Care for Aging Persons:

Mrs. Gertrude Holmes (U.S.A.)

Mrs. South (Sheffield, U.K.)

Mr. and Mrs. William Clayton (Sheffield, U.K.)

To Our Special Gerontological Person:

Karen M. Corr

Contents

Preface

This book is intended as a contribution to the development of gerontological nursing. It has been designed to be useful in three primary ways: (1) as a guide to direct, hands-on care of the elderly, whether in the community, in acute care institutions, or in long-term care facilities; (2) as a textbook for nursing students and others involved in education concerning care for older adults; and (3) as a resource for reference that might be utilized by nurses and a wide variety of others concerned about this field of interest.

Our aim has been to address the full and rich scope in nursing care of the elderly through promotion of wellness or optimal health status, anticipation and prevention of potential health problems, and resolution of actual health problems or rehabilitation and restoration to the highest achievable level of health status. To attain these goals, we sought contributors who could call upon extensive clinical experience and the latest nursing research in their respective fields. Also for that reason, we have attempted to create something more substantial than a slim handbook of care in this field.

At the same time, we have not intended to duplicate the encyclopedic tomes currently available in gerontological nursing. Such volumes are essential for reference, but they are impractical for daily use. More to the point, such volumes are usually organized around biochemical organ systems. Our interest has been to recapture a sense of living persons, with dignity and individuality, among the older adult population. We believe nursing has moved away from narrow training, intuitive behavior, and rote practice to an impressive professionalism which emphasizes caring for human beings and which rejects impersonal, uncoordinated, and discontinuous approaches to care.

The heart of this book lies in its emphasis on the nursing process and specified nursing diagnoses. The nursing process is the single, indispensable, problem-solving method of organizing responsible, autonomous, and professional nursing care. This method guides nurses in anticipating potential problems and promoting wellness, and in minimizing or resolving actual problems. From the perspective of the nursing process, this book examines a set of fundamental and common needs in older adults which will be well known to practicing nurses. These needs or issues do not apply to all elderly persons as existing problems, but their recognized potential enables nurses to maintain positive outcomes and thus contributes to independence, health, self-esteem, and quality of life for every older adult.

The list of topics addressed in this book has affinities with Maslow's basic needs and Gordon's functional health patterns, as well as with broad theoretical frameworks or conceptual models in nursing which emphasize self-care, adaptation, etc. Even as we recognize the value of these theories, frameworks, and models, we have not chosen among or made much specific reference to them in this book. Rather, we have designed this book around the nursing process as the primary, common, structuring principle which all nurses can implement, which can be the linchpin for continuity of care—especially for chronic problems—in any setting, and which requires the least need for adjustment and energy on the part of elderly persons being served. The first challenge for each professional nurse, educator, or researcher is to insure that care of the elderly is energized through this approach. Subsequently, that newly invigorated care can be linked to larger theories, frameworks, and models—as they may be relevant to and valuable for the actual work at hand.

In the preparation of this book, we have incurred many personal and professional debts, only some of which can be acknowledged here. Above all, an impressive cadre of contributors worked diligently with us to shape the result presented in this volume. Before that and throughout the entire process, a large number of nursing consultants, the staff at our publisher, and three anonymous reviewers provided essential guidance on a wide range of issues from broad plan to fine detail. Special thanks are owed to Florence S. Downs, Marjory Gordon, Neville Strumpf, and Anthony J. Traxler for early encouragement in this endeavor. St. Louis Community College at Forest Park and Southern Illinois University at Edwardsville have graciously supported our work over a long period of time. Much of what is good in this book is owed to those who guided and assisted our work; the inevitable imperfections that must remain are our own responsibility.

DONNA M. CORR, R.N., M.S.N.
CHARLES A. CORR, PH.D.

Contributors

Jane Ashley, R.N., M.S., is Assistant Professor, Department of Nursing, Boston College, Chestnut Hill, Massachusetts.

Barbara A. Brant, M.S., R.N., C., is Instructor, Graduate Program in Gerontologic Nursing, Gerontologic Nurse Specialist, and Executive Council Member, Geriatric Education Center, School of Nursing, Medical College of Virginia, Virginia Commonwealth University, Richmond, Virginia.

Kathleen Coen Buckwalter, R.N., Ph.D., is Associate Professor, College of Nursing, University of Iowa, Iowa City, Iowa.

James P. Curry, Ph.D., is Assistant Professor, Center for Health Services Research, Graduate Program in Health and Hospital Administration, University of Iowa, Iowa City, Iowa.

Lesley F. Degner, R.N., Ph.D., is Director, Manitoba Nursing Research Institute, and Professor, School of Nursing, University of Manitoba, Winnipeg, Manitoba, Canada.

Pamela Muhm Duchene, R.N., D.N.Sc., is Associate Chairperson, Geriatric/Gerontological Nursing, Johnston R. Bowman Health Center for the Elderly, Rush-Presbyterian-St. Luke's Medical Center, Chicago, Illinois.

Sister Karin Dufault, S.P., R.N., Ph.D., is Administrator, St. Elizabeth Medical Center, Yakima, Washington, and formerly clinical nurse specialist in oncology and gerontology at Providence Medical Center, Portland, Oregon.

Betty R. Ferrell, R.N., Ph.D., F.A.A.N., is Research Scientist, Department of Nursing Research, City of Hope National Medical Center, Duarte, California.

Bruce A. Ferrell, M.D., is Assistant Professor, School of Medicine, University of California at Los Angeles, and Staff Physician, Sepulveda Veterans Administration Hospital, Sepulveda, California.

Terry T. Fulmer, R.N., Ph.D., C., is Associate Professor, School of Nursing, Yale University, and Geriatric Clinical Nurse Specialist, Yale-New Haven Hospital, New Haven, Connecticut.

Lorna W. Guse, R.N., M.A., is Associate Professor, School of Nursing, and a doctoral candidate at the University of Manitoba, Winnipeg, Manitoba, Canada.

Mary Marmoll Jirovec, R.N., Ph.D., is Assistant Professor, College of Nursing, Wayne State University, Detroit, Michigan.

Joan LeSage, R.N., Ph.D., is Chairperson, Geriatric/Gerontological Nursing, Johnston R. Bowman Health Center for the Elderly, Rush-Presbyterian-St. Luke's Medical Center, Chicago, Illinois.

Joan G. Magit, R.N., M.N., C-G.N.P., is a doctoral candidate in the School of Nursing, University of California at San Francisco, San Francisco, California, and a consultant to the Senior Health and Peer Counseling Center in Santa Monica, California.

Stephanie J. Nagley, R.N., Ph.D., is Assistant Professor, Gerontological Nursing, Frances Payne Bolton School of Nursing, Case Western Reserve University, Cleveland, Ohio.

Linda R. F. Phillips, R.N., Ph.D., F.A.A.N., is Professor and Associate Dean for Research, College of Nursing, University of Arizona, Tucson, Arizona.

Eileen Quinlan, M.S., R.N., is Assistant Professor of Clinical Nursing and Director, Graduate Program, School of Nursing, Columbia University, New York, New York.

Joan Rifkin Sellers, M.S.S.W., L.C.S.W., A.C.S.W., is a substance abuse consultant in private practice in Beverly Hills, California.

Eleanor Taggart, R.N., M.S.N., M.A., is Assistant Professor, School of Nursing, The University of North Carolina at Chapel Hill, Chapel Hill, North Carolina.

Sharon M. Valente, R.N., M.N., C.S., F.A.A.N., is Adjunct Assistant Professor, Department of Nursing, University of Southern California, and a clinical specialist in mental health in private practice in Los Angeles, California.

Kay Weiler, R.N., M.A., J.D., is Assistant Professor, College of Nursing, University of Iowa, Iowa City, Iowa.

Jean F. Wyman, Ph.D., R.N., C., is Assistant Professor and Director, Graduate Program in Gerontologic Nursing, School of Nursing, Medical College of Virginia, Virginia Commonwealth University, Richmond, Virginia.

Stephanie Zeman, R.N.C., M.S.N., is President, Geriatric Educational Resources, Inc., Fairfax Station, Virginia.

Part I

Nursing Approaches to the Elderly

Two key elements to effective gerontological nursing practice are a thorough knowledge base concerning human processes and functional responses in the elderly, and the way in which nurses approach and communicate with older adults and the significant persons in their lives. In Chapter 1, Linda Phillips outlines a philosophy of care to help those elders who need the assistance of nursing to achieve wellness and to maintain the highest level of functional well-being possible for each individual. The emphasis is on challenges presented to nursing in achieving health promotion and wellness, as well as on satisfactions and rewards for those who undertake a commitment to care of the elderly. Phillips identifies elderly persons as a growing segment of the population in North America composed of differing groups and unique individuals, and she indicates how developments in gerontological nursing can contribute to a new view of general nursing practice and roles.

Chapter 2 stresses the crucial role of the nursing process and the formation of nursing diagnoses as indispensable means to provide expert and professional nursing care in an orderly and consistent way for elderly persons. As Jane Ashley notes, the nursing process is widely recognized by the profession as its mechanism for exercising autonomy and accountability. Thus, the five steps of the nursing process and appropriate nursing diagnoses define the structure of the central chapters in this book.

Finally, in Chapter 3 Terry Fulmer and Eileen Quinlan demonstrate that within the nursing process assessment of the elderly person is the main prerequisite upon which all other elements of nursing care depend. The chapter describes essential elements of a comprehensive nursing assessment for older adults, offers guidelines for carrying out such assessment, and shows how nursing assessments direct gerontological nursing care.

Chapter 1

The Elderly, the Nurse, and the Challenge

Linda R. F. Phillips

CHALLENGES OF OUR AGING SOCIETY

Regardless of the area of specialization chosen, virtually all nurses in North America are gerontological nurses. In light of demographic trends and health care service utilization patterns, nurses working in critical care units, general medical-surgical units, ambulatory care units, and home care are unavoidably gerontological nurses. Based on the nature of family relationships and the intense involvement that many elders have with their children and grandchildren, even nurses working in settings that seem remote from gerontology (e.g., maternity and pediatrics) are quite likely to be providing some care to elders. The purpose of this chapter is to explore the challenges that caring for the elderly in our aging society pose to nurses and to outline approaches to aging clients that promote health and create mutual rewards and satisfactions for elders and nurses.

To illustrate the need, one can note that the number of aging individuals in the United States increases exponentially each year. Because of the reduction in infant mortality and the biomedical and health care advances that have significantly reduced the number of early deaths, the percentage of Americans over age 65 has more than tripled since 1900 (from 4.1% in 1900 to 12.7% in 1990). In actual numbers, there has been a ninefold increase to the over-65 age group since 1900 (from 3.1 million in 1900 to 28 million in 1984). If current fertility and immigration levels remain stable, the only age groups to experience significant growth in the next century will be those past age 55. In addition, the demographic composition of the older population is changing, with the 16.7 million individuals in the 65–74 age group representing a group seven times larger, the 8.6 million in the 75–84 age group representing a group 11 times larger, and the 2.7 million in the 85+ age group representing a group 21 times larger than in 1900. The fastest growing age group in the United States consists of individuals over the age of 85. By 2050, this group will likely consist of 15 million individuals (Seigel & Taeuber, 1986).

These demographic trends suggest that the United States is facing a social and health care challenge of unparalleled proportions that is unlike any previous challenge in the history of this country. To explore the implications of these demographic trends and the challenges that they present to nurses, several issues must be addressed, including: (1) ways in which these trends are influencing health care delivery; (2) ways that these trends are influencing the practice of nursing; and (3) factors that make caring for the elderly unique and different from any other kind of nursing.

HEALTH CARE DELIVERY AND THE ELDERLY

Although the elderly constitute approximately 12% of the total population in the United States, the health care services they use account for more than 30% of the total cost of health care (Sundwall, 1988). Elders constitute a majority of the consumers in almost every health care setting. While the majority of elderly individuals live independently in the community, those over the age of 65 are more likely than others to require the services of the health care delivery system for a number of reasons.

First, although mortality rates among the elderly have decreased more than 15% nationally since 1970, *chronic illness and functional disability* are not unusual among this age group. Rice and Feldman (1983) suggested that over 80% of the people 65 years and older have one or more chronic conditions. Activity limitations are more common among those over the age of 75 than those under the age of 75. In total, about 10% (2.5 million) of noninstitutionalized, elderly Americans are functionally limited as measured by their need for assistance with personal care activities. About 22% (5.9 million) of noninstitutionalized, elderly Americans receive assistance with performing home management activities (Dawson, Hendershot, & Fulton, 1987). Common chronic conditions affecting the elderly are arthritis (44%), hypertension (39%), hearing impairments (28%), heart disease (27%), visual impairments (12%), and arteriosclerosis (12%) (Brotman, 1982). Three-fourths of all deaths among the elderly are caused by the chronic conditions of heart disease, cancer, and stroke. Rice and Feldman (1983), Myers and Manton (1984), and Koshland (1985) have suggested that increased longevity, which is the likely result of scientific advancements, will be accompanied in the future by increased chronic disease, functional disability, and mental disorders. It has even been suggested that by the year 2000, Alzheimer's disease will be the single-most prevalent health problem in the United States (Koshland, 1985).

The second reason for elders frequently requiring the services of the health care delivery system relates to the incidence of *acute illnesses* among members of this group. In 1986, individuals 65 years and over accounted for 40% of the short-stay hospitalizations in this country (National Center for Health Statistics [NCHS], 1987). The higher rate of hospital utilization is directly related to the number of surgical procedures experienced by this group. Those over the age of 65 experience three times the rate of surgery involving the respiratory, cardiovascular, digestive, and urinary systems as compared to the total population. The rate of eye surgery among the elderly is five times the rate for the total population (Haupt, 1982).

The higher rate of hospital utilization among the elderly is also related to the increased vulnerability of this group to: infection (Pesanti, 1977); adverse drug reactions (Pulliam, Hanlon, & Moore, 1988), injuries caused by falls and motor vehicle accidents (Sattin, et al., 1988), mental manifestations accompanying physical illness (Sakauye, 1986); and the frequency of acute exacerbations of chronic conditions, such as arteriosclerotic heart disease, diabetes, and chornic lung disease (Kovar, 1986). With high rates of short-stay hospital use among the elderly, it is no surprise that the elderly use about 70% of the home health services in this country (Schewenger, 1977). It is also interesting that the majority of an individual's lifetime expenditures for health care services in hospital settings occurs during the last two years of his or her life (Emergency Medicine Symposium, 1985).

The third reason for elders frequently requiring the services of the health care delivery system is that in comparison to the young, the elderly require *longer periods of skilled and semi-skilled care* for acute illnesses and acute exacerbations of chronic conditions before the level of pre-illness functioning returns. Because the illnesses of the elderly are usually complicated by multiple medical and nursing diagnoses, protracted recovery periods are required which make the elderly's utilization of extended care facilities higher than the young. In 1985, individuals over age 65 occupied 88% of the available beds in long-term care facilities (Hing, 1987). Further, whereas 4.8% of the elderly are institutionalized at any point in time, an elderly person has one chance in four of dying in an extended care facility (Palmore, 1976). In addition to simply having more elderly in extended care facilities than any other age group, the average length of stay (bed-days) in long-term care facilities is 6.2 times longer for the elderly than for the total population (Haupt, 1982).

The fourth reason for elders frequently requiring services of the health care system is related to the *incidence of mental health problems* among this group. There are estimates that between 12 and 40% of all people 65 years or older experience psychological difficulties (Reifler & Eisdorfer, 1980). The incidence of functional mental disorders, such as depression and paranoid states, is disproportionally high among the elderly (Pardes, 1981), and approximately 17% of all suicides occur among the over-65 population (McIntosh, 1985). Although teenage suicides have received a great deal of public attention recently, the suicide rate among the elderly (particularly elderly men) actually exceeds that of teenagers.

More than half of the elderly in long-term care facilities have some form of emotional distress that interferes with their daily functioning—one out of five nursing home residents has a mental disorder as a primary medical diagnosis, and about 30% of nursing home residents have a medical diagnosis of senility without psychosis (Harper, 1986). Sixty-six percent of nursing home residents have a specific behavioral problem including depressed or withdrawn behavior (35%), nervous or hyperactive behavior (34%), abusive or disruptive behavior (17%), and wandering (11%) (Hing, 1981). Among those in mental health institutions, 30% are estimated to be elderly (Gatz, Smyer, & Lawton, 1980).

The fifth reason for elders frequently requiring services within the health care system is related to the *need for ongoing supervision in the community* for the management and prevention of acute and chronic conditions. According to a recent national survey, although the majority of community-dwelling elders viewed their health as good to excellent, most (82%) had seen a physician during the year previous to the study (Kovar, 1986). Of the elders who had seen a physician, 27.8% had one or two contacts with the physician, 31.7% had three to six contacts, and 13.2 percent had seven to 12 contacts. In total, individuals 65 years or older accounted for 20.5% of physician office visits in 1985 (Koch & Knapp, 1987). In addition to physician visits, a large number of elders are seen regularly by gerontological nurse practitioners and by nurses in nurse-run, community-based clinics for health promotion and disease management services.

The need of elders for health care services is influencing health care delivery in the following ways. First, *the provision of hospital care for the elderly continues to become more complex.* Compared with the past, there is a larger array of hospital services available to the elderly because of scientific advancement. More elders survive acute illnesses than ever before. The focus on curing that has resulted from scientific advancement has exacted a large cost, however, because highly technical care has changed the relationship between individual providers and the client. This change has been sorely felt by the elderly. Technological and scientific advancement has also influenced provider specialization. As knowledge in one area becomes greater, the ability of an individual provider to "know it all" has been significantly reduced. Consequently, health care is becoming increasingly fragmented with fewer and fewer providers who are able to see the "whole" rather than the "parts." In addition, the implementation of prospective payment in the United States in 1983 based on Diagnostic Related Groups (DRGs) has resulted in shorter hospital stays and in a great emphasis on the medical aspects of illness to the exclusion of the personal/social aspects.

With the advent of DRGs, hospital stays have been shortened on the "back end" and, as a consequence, there is now little time to attend to the older adult's needs for education and counseling, to assess the degree to which the hospitalization has influenced the elder and his or her family, or to do discharge planning. Hospital stays have also been shortened on the "front end," which means that patients receive less education and preparation for surgery than before and that patients are admitted more acutely ill than before. Prior to this decade, the majority of acute care was provided in the hospital. Now health care providers have significant incentives to provide as much acute care as possible outside of the hospital setting. Whereas elders used to have surgeries, such as cataract surgery, in the hospital, now most such surgery is done on an outpatient basis. As a consequence, the contact that many elders have with health professionals other than physicians has been reduced and the burden of post-surgical monitoring and care has shifted from health professionals in institutions to the family.

Second, as a result of these trends, *long-term care of the elderly has become a major crisis.* Most secondary and tertiary care provided to elders now occurs outside of the hospital setting and the most significant and involved care providers for the elderly are family members and friends (informal caregivers), rather than health care providers. Home care has grown significantly. In 1980, for example, home care accounted for 2% of all Medicare expenditures; in 1987, it accounted for 3.7%. Whereas $37 billion was spent in 1987 for home care, $129 billion is expected to be spent in the year 2000 (Davis, 1987). Despite these growth patterns, however, the majority of elderly individuals still receive most in-home service from informal caregivers.

Medicare only pays for home care services for individuals who are homebound and who require skilled nursing care. The majority of the care needed by the community-dwelling elderly does not fit these categories, and the response of the health care system to provide appropriate, accessible, and affordable maintenance services has been slow. Similarly, services provided under Medicare by long-term care facilities are limited. Since Medicare covers the costs of post-hospital institutional care only if skilled nursing services are required, and because most elderly who require institutionalization need supervisory and maintenance rather than skilled nursing services, Medicare covers less than 2% of the total nursing home costs in this country. Elderly persons and their families spend about $18 billion yearly on nursing home care, which is about one-half of the cost (Harrington, 1987).

The consequences of this crisis are that elders who receive hospital care are very likely to return home to receive highly technical, complex care from unassisted, unprepared, and untrained family caregivers. In light of demographic patterns, it is quite likely that the family members providing the care are spouses or adult children who are themselves over the age of 65. Although some portion of the elders who are discharged to home care are likely to have some home health visits early in their recovery—the national average is 30 visits (Harrington, 1987)—if their recuperation is prolonged or if their disease is chronic, the only help likely to be available to them and their caregivers is that which is paid for out-of-pocket.

If home care is not an option, nursing home placements are of course possible. Aside from the psychological and social complications of nursing home placement, however, the financial burdens associated with nursing home placement are profound. It is, for example, estimated that 63% of unmarried elders in nursing homes totally exhaust their savings within 13 weeks and that 83% do so within one year (Harrington, 1987).

The third way that the need of elders for health care services is influencing health care delivery is that *alternative methods of providing care for the elderly are beginning to develop.* The vast majority of elderly individuals live at home regardless of health and functional status. Most in-home care is provided by family members regardless of the elder's health status or intensity of needs (Archbold, 1983), the family member's other responsibilities (Brody, 1985), whether or not the elder lives alone (Shanas, 1979), extreme geographic distance of family members (Moss, Moos, & Moles, 1985), whether or not there are female relatives to assist with care (Horowitz, 1985), and the family's ethnicity (Chatters, Taylor, & Jackson, 1986; Guttman, 1979; Jackson, 1980; Maldonado, 1979; Markides & Mindel, 1987; Taylor, 1985). The caregiving research shows that family care can be provided over many years with the complexity of care generally increasing over time.

In response to the needs of elders and families, creative methods for providing secondary and tertiary care are beginning to be seen. For example, day care facilities are being created to meet the needs of working caregivers. Respite services are becoming available to assist family members with the intense burden of 24-hour-a-day care. In addition, attention is now being paid to the "leveling" of care. In the past, a major difficulty with providing care for the elderly was that the services available were designed based on the "all or none" principle. Therefore, any elders with any needs were likely to receive all services rather than only the ones they needed. For example, an elder living at home who had no informal care providers and who required only assistance with a bath and medications might be institutionalized because there were no resources available that provided only the supervisory care required. "Leveling" of care assures that an elder receives only the care required from the most cost-effective care alternative.

The concept of care "leveling" has been the impetus for the development of a continuum of services that range from the simple services provided by Socialization and Nutrition Sites to the extremely complex services provided by a Skilled Nursing Facility or Hospice. The most important requisite of alternative care services is health care providers who are equipped with the *complex assessment skills* needed to assure that each individual elder receives the appropriate level of care based on his or her physical, functional, emotional, social, and financial needs.

The last way that the need of elders for health care services is influencing health care delivery is in *the new emphasis on primary prevention for the elderly*. Fatalism and pessimism have been the driving force of health care for the elderly for the past century. Since the focus of health care has historically been on cure, and death, which marks the end period of life, defies cure, most health care for the elderly has been based on the premises that: (1) illness and decline in older age are inevitable and not preventable; and (2) the end years of life are entirely shaped by the health behaviors that characterized the beginning of life. Recent research as outlined during the Surgeon General's Conference on Health Promotion and Aging in 1988 (Abdellah & Moore, 1988a) identifies the fallacy in these beliefs.

Aging is not a disease. Disability and dysfunction are not normal or inevitable outgrowths of aging. Research shows that preventive health services, preventive mental health programs, exercise programs, injury prevention programs, and dental health programs can have a significant impact on morbidity and mortality even late in life. Changes in patterns of nutrition, alcohol use, smoking, and medication use can increase both the quality and length of life (Abdellah & Moore, 1988b). As a consequence, now and in the future, while the emphasis in health care is likely to continue to include attention to secondary and tertiary prevention, primary prevention is also going to assume a more and more important place in the services provided to community-dwelling elders and their caregivers.

NURSING PRACTICE AND THE ELDERLY

Demographic trends and changes in the health care delivery system have profound implications for nursing practice if nurses are to be responsive to the needs of elderly persons. These trends suggest that nursing is required to expand its vision of the scope of nursing practice if the needs of the elderly are to be met. The needs of the elderly are complex. It is the rare elder who presents with a single medical or nursing diagnosis. Needs for highly technical, curative services are minimal compared to needs for support, education, maintenance, counseling, and care. In short, gerontological nursing requires a new and enlightened view of the scope of nursing practice that goes beyond simply assisting physicians to perform curative services (Redfern, 1988). It requires a view of nursing in which the nurse is an autonomous health care professional who prescribes and coordinates complex care to elders and their families, and who assumes a leadership role on the multidisciplinary team.

These trends also suggest that the time is now ripe for expansion and refinement of a nursing model as the basis for health care delivery to the elderly. It is clear that the emphasis of the disease-focused medical model is largely ineffective for meeting the needs of most elders. For the past century, health care for individuals in all age groups has been disease-focused with individuals seeking curative services only when they are acutely ill. Yet, the majority of problems experienced by the elderly involve chronic, ongoing conditions that are, though manageable, not resolvable. It is estimated (Fagin, 1982) that 90% of the problems for which the community-dwelling elderly seek health care in ambulatory settings are best handled (economically and philosophically) by nurses. Similarly, in long-term care, the majority of client problems are associated with daily functioning and the management of chronic conditions, problems that are most responsive to nursing rather than medical management.

Nursing and the models for nursing practice are based largely on the principles that: (1) clients have the right to self-determination and independent decision making; (2) clients are holistic in nature and their health and well-being are affected by the interaction of physiological, pathological, psychological, social, financial, and environmental factors; and (3) nursing has a role in assisting clients to optimize health, to improve the quality of life, to achieve comfort, and to facilitate personal growth. These are the principles on which quality health care for the elderly is dependent.

In addition, because of these trends, nursing is being challenged for the first time to focus its practice in the settings where the majority of elders receive care. In 1980, for example, 65% of all nurses practiced in the hospital (Anonymous, 1982), but health statistics indicate that the majority of the elderly now live in the community and receive their health care services in the community. The shortage of well-educated nurses to direct, coordinate, and prescribe care in ambulatory care settings, home care agencies, day care facilities, and community-based maintenance agencies is profound. The need for nurses to provide primary care for the community-dwelling elderly and educational and support services for family caregivers is equally acute. Although only a small percentage of elders are ever institutionalized at any given time, the dearth of well-educated nurses in long-term care settings is appalling. Therefore, a major change likely to occur in nursing as a result of current demographic and health care trends is the redistribution of nurses from acute-care facilities to community-based practice settings.

UNIQUENESS OF GERONTOLOGICAL NURSING

Gerontological nursing is different from every other field of specialization within nursing in a number of ways. The central focus of gerontological nursing is the aging client. Although there is nothing particularly unusual about aging (all individuals do it all the time), and there is nothing magic about the age of 65 that sets those at that age apart from the rest of the population, as individuals age there are certain changes that occur that increase their risk status for certain problems as compared to their middle-aged counterparts. Admittedly, many of these changes are directly related to elderly people being required to function in a world that is designed for the convenience and optimal functioning of middle-class, young- to middle-aged people, and our perceptions of the degree of change are related to using only middle-aged individuals as standards of measurement. We do not know how well individuals would function in old age if the world were designed to optimize their function. Nevertheless, in the world as currently designed, aging individuals are more vulnerable to many problems than are younger people.

These vulnerabilities affect every facet of life. Physiologically, for example, changes in the cardiovascular and pulmonary systems make it difficult for elderly individuals to maintain and to regain a homeostatic state when presented with physiological stressors. Changes in the musculoskeletal system and the visual apparatus make ambulation in an uncompromising world more dangerous. Psychologically, patterns of social reinforcement, a socially-imposed preoccupation with memory deficit possibilities, and the information processing requirements of a lifetime of memories alter perceptions of cognitive function and memory. External cues and life circumstances alter the view that elders have of themselves and increase the possibility of depression. Sociologically, life events serve to decrease the number of individuals available in the social network of elders. They also alter the types and amount of social support available and the relationship that elders have with significant others, making older adults more vulnerable to loneliness. Economically, the decreases in liquid assets imposed by retirement coupled with the cost of health care, make it possible for elders to face, often for the first time, the possibility of impoverishment.

Nursing the elderly makes an appreciation of these complex, interrelated vulnerabilities more important than it is with any other group. These vulnerabilities require that the nurse use a broad range of assessment skills that include consideration of every single interrelated aspect of the elder's life. Assessment of the elderly requires that the nurse be able to take information about parts and to integrate it into a coherent, sensitive view of the whole. The assessment skills of well-prepared gerontological nurses make it possible for these nurses to assume a primary role as the determinant of the level and type of care required, the coordinator and director of service provision, and the spokesperson who protects the rights and prerogatives of elderly individuals.

These vulnerabilities also require that the view of the client in gerontological nursing is different than it is in most other types of nursing. They demand an expansion of the definition of client from the view of client as one system or one person to the view of client as the person, his or her environment, and his or her network of intimates. It is the rare elderly individual who is totally alone. In fact, only rarely is the elderly individual the sole client who requires nursing care. In most situations, there are *at least* two individuals who are the nurse's clients: the elder and his or her significant other. With one particular elder, there may be a number of individuals who qualify as clients based on age, health status, and the psychological and physical demands of being responsible for care management activities. The older the elder is, the more likely the elder is to have an old spouse, old children, and old grandchildren who require the nurse's special skills.

In addition, these vulnerabilities make the nursing intervention needed by elders more complex and intense than interventions with almost any other group. Carter (1988, p. 9) noted four interventions that are unique to gerontological nursing practice: (1) taking charge; (2) being with the patient; (3) empowering the patient to make decisions; and (4) understanding and experiencing life's momentary meanings. These are all highly complex activities that require nurses to interact with clients at an intense level of intimacy. Each requires the nurse to become a part of the client and to take the risks involved with the investment of self.

In nursing models, it is common for theorists to identify that the relationship between nurse and client results in a permanent change in the client that enhances the client's self-understanding and facilitates the client's personal growth. The permanent changes and personal growth experienced by the nurse as a result of these intimate interactions are frequently ignored. Nursing of the aged and the vulnerabilities experienced by older clients force the nurse to experience his or her own personal vulnerabilities and to be permanently changed in the process.

The vulnerabilities of the elderly add one other complicating dimension to designing nursing interventions. Extreme creativity and resourcefulness are often required to implement a plan of care based on deficits that the elderly may be experiencing. For example, implementing an educational intervention with an elder who is experiencing visual or hearing deficits requires that nurses design the intervention in a way that capitalizes on the elder's existing sensory capabilities. Although "senility" is not a normal consequence of aging and is experienced by relatively few elders, many elders do experience what is called benign senescent forgetfulness. This is characterized by mild, short-term memory lapses that are often associated with everyday activities. For example, individuals may be unable to retrieve the names of persons or things, or may not remember if they have taken their medicine. Memory cuing activities or the use of mnemonics may need to be included in a teaching program for individuals experiencing this problem.

Although intelligence is not affected by aging, the ways in which elderly individuals learn may be different from the ways in which younger people learn. Elders are much more capable of using their previous experiences in solving problems and learning new content than are younger people. Designing an educational program that capitalizes on this ability requires a different approach than one would use with younger clients. Therefore, another unique aspect of gerontological nursing is that the body of knowledge necessary for effective practice is extremely specialized and, in many ways, more complex than that used in other areas of specialization.

Another uniqueness that sets gerontological nursing apart from all other types of nursing is the diversity of the clients encountered. Up to this point in this chapter the elderly have been referred to as if they compose one, homogeneous group who are all similar in their experiences, their views of the world, and the problems they encounter. Nothing could be farther from the truth. Elders are of both genders (although the older they are the more likely they are to be women based on the different mortality rates of older men and older women) and all races (although the life expectancy of individuals in minority groups tends to be lower than for whites). While there are life experiences that many people share, such as parenthood, marriage, widowhood, and retirement, not all elders are married or parents or retired. There are many elders who have never married. Just like individuals in younger age groups, many elders have living arrangements or sexual preferences that are different from the "norm."

In addition, the degree of diversity among the elderly population is intensified by the large age span involved. Whereas no intelligent person would claim that a newborn infant has the same needs and preferences as a 20-year-old, assuming that a 60-year-old and an 80-year-old are just alike is an error that is commonly committed. The diversity among the elderly population is affected by differential genetic endowments, cohort experiences, and health habits of the individuals in the group. Thus, while many elderly people have visual and hearing problems, a larger number do not, and while a large number of elderly people have functional deficits, the majority are able to care for themselves just as effectively as do individuals who are younger. Recent social trends also enhance the diversity of this group. For example, divorce in the later years is becoming an increasingly frequent phenomenon, and more elders than ever before are insisting on maintaining their own places of residence rather than moving in with family members.

Gerontological nursing is also unique in the way in which most care for the elderly is accomplished. Although the skills of professional nurses are *required* for quality nursing care of the aged, nurses actually only do a small percentage of the care activities. In long-term care settings, for example, 80 to 90% of actual care is provided by nonprofessionals (Harper, 1986). In the home, the situation is similar. To provide excellent nursing care to the aged, nurses must be able to perform care and to educate and inspire others to perform care. In no other field of nursing is the need more acute to develop strategies for accomplishing care goals by working through others.

In summary, gerontological nursing is among the most specialized areas of nursing practice that exist. Gerontological nursing demands that nurses are able to practice autonomously in a wide variety of settings. It requires a specialized body of knowledge that is derived from nursing and other kinds of research, a broad definition of "client," and a view of nursing that emphasizes the interaction of biopsychosocial factors and deemphasizes pathology. It requires sophisticated assessment and intervention skills that are specialized, complex, and unique. Gerontological nursing, more than any other type of nursing, requires coordination and case management skills, as well as the ability to work through other providers in order to provide quality care. It requires the establishment of long-term intimate relationships between the nurse and the elder through which both the elder and the nurse experience personal growth and intense satisfaction.

A PHILOSOPHY OF NURSING CARE FOR THE ELDERLY

Gerontological nurses have always believed that caring for the elderly is special and unique, but this belief has not been universally espoused by others in the health professions. Gerontological nursing, historically, has been accorded low status. The reasons for this are many, but the most important reason has been the prevalence of the decremental model as the predominant view of aging in our society.

The *decremental model* basically states that aging is an event that is characterized by personal decline. Within this model, the changes that occur as a result of aging (e.g., the changes seen in the cardiovascular system) are viewed as evidence that aging involves deterioration and decay since the various body systems obviously do not work as well as they once did. As a result, aging is seen as a negative, undesirable event that is to be avoided and forestalled as long as possible. If evidence is required that the decremental model is dominant in our society, one only needs to look at advertisements for cosmetics, jokes on birthday cards, and the popularity of plastic surgeons and hair dye manufacturers.

Those in the health professions have not been immune to the effects of the decremental model. The most-rewarded professions are those that can cure (as evidence, examine the annual salaries of surgeons who perform heart transplants as compared with those of internists) and those who assist in cures (as evidence, think of the status afforded nurses in critical care as compared with those in long-term care). The behavioral sciences have also been profoundly affected by the decremental model. Psychiatry, for example, is founded on the "principle of primacy" (Birren & Renner, 1981), which states that personality formation occurs during the formative years (0 to 20 years) and that no further growth or development occurs after that time. Evidence for the effect of the decremental model on the behavioral sciences is found in the works of theorists such as Sigmund Freud (1949) and the well-documented (e.g., Kermis, 1986) inability of older clients to receive anything other than cursory mental health services. Even the idea behind gerontological and geriatric medicine was originally to "fix" aging so that the human life span could be significantly lengthened.

The decremental model has also had a profound impact on the ways in which aging individuals view themselves. Self-deprecation and lamentations about increasing age are extremely common even among 30-year-olds. Mid-life crisis is a tangible manifestation of the ways in which many individuals cope with advancing age and the realization of mortality. So profound are the effects of the decremental model on individuals that after observing how aging individuals respond to aging, sociologists Kuyers and Bengston (1973) proposed the Social Breakdown Model. This model asserts that internalization of the view of aging as personal decline leads to a cycle in which individuals first expect that they will be incompetent and then take every small deficit or failure as evidence of incompetence. Over time, this process is repeated many times until the individual is so lacking in self-worth and self-confidence that being anything but incompetent is impossible.

Viewed from the decremental model, gerontological nursing is an extremely dismal area of specialization. Not only is the nurse performing meaningless tasks for individuals who are going to die anyway (sort of like a warehouse attendant), but also the individuals being cared for are profoundly depressed and so incapacitated by their depression that rewards and personal satisfactions for the nurse are few. Successful gerontological nurses, however, realize that the decremental model is only one way of interpreting the aging process and it is actually a very biased and limited view of aging.

The *negentropic model* (Katch, 1983) is an alternative model that forms the philosophical base for successful gerontological nurses. The negentropic model is based on a lifespan view of aging which seeks to set aging within the context of living. According to this model, aging is a normal developmental process that begins with conception. Aging is inevitable and irreversible. Within the negentropic model, the concept of regression or going back to a former stage of development is meaningless. Therefore, the idea that old people are having a second childhood or are anything like children is, at best, silly and, at worst, destructive. Aging is viewed as the thread that provides coherence and meaning to life. Development and personal growth begin at conception and are progressive throughout life. Death, therefore, is viewed as a developmental task rather than as a treatment failure.

Differences between the decremental and the negentropic model are evident in a comparison of their views of various age-related changes. For example, benign senescent forgetfulness viewed from the decremental model is interpreted as evidence of cellular loss in the central nervous system. From the negentropic model, it is viewed as evidence that older individuals have many more events to remember than do younger people, and that the complexity of their thought patterns is greater than those of the young. Interestingly, there is physiological evidence to support both these views. Admittedly, there is some cell loss in the central nervous system that accompanies normal aging. This supports the decremental model. However, recent evidence suggests that the axions of the neural cells lying next to lost cells become increasingly complex and interrelated with aging, suggesting better and more complex functioning. This supports the negentropic model. Similarly, the sensory changes associated with aging can be viewed as losses (decremental model) or as a natural method for facilitating the introspection needed for advanced personal growth (negentropic model).

Levine and Levine (1980) have suggested two important ideas relevant to a discussion of views of aging and philosophies of working with aging people. First, they observed that the measurement standards that are used for effective functioning are those derived from observation of and research with young to middle-aged people. For example, early studies of the intelligence of the elderly suggested that there were significant declines with aging. However, the standards of comparison being used were young college students who were better educated and more acquainted with testing procedures than the elderly. More recent studies have been longitudinal (meaning data were collected on the same individuals over time) and some have involved the use of elderly college students as one of the standards of comparison. With these factors taken into consideration, studies have shown that when an individual's performance is repeatedly measured over time, there is no decline in performance. In addition, when elderly college students are compared to young college students, there is no difference in intelligence.

Second, Levine and Levine (1980) observed that the world as designed is basically unsympathetic to needs of anyone other than the healthy young. For example, public transportation and grocery stores are designed for the convenience of the young. As a result, elders who use them who have any kind of visual or ambulatory change appear slower and more disabled than they actually are. These two observations raise questions about how aging would be experienced and would be viewed in a society that was designed to accommodate the needs of the elderly rather than the needs of the young.

Gerontological nursing requires a philosophy that is different from the philosophy that drives other kinds of nursing. In addition, it requires a philosophy that is contrary to the predominant view of aging in our society. On the one hand, developing the philosophy needed is difficult because there are few reinforcements for changing one's view of the world and few role models that can assist in the process. On the other hand, seeking to develop a growth-oriented view of aging is worth the effort. Not only does it permit nurses to realize the rewards in serving a large proportion of our population, but it allows the nurse's own aging to become an exciting prospect that can be assisted by the elders whom he or she serves.

CONCLUSION

As Yarling (1977, p. 42) has stated, nursing is the "last and best hope of the aged for decent health care." Because of their employment settings, nurses are the most likely of all health care providers to encounter elderly people in their daily practices. Nursing professionals currently provide more health care to the elderly than any other group of health professionals. Not only is nursing the largest of the health professions and as a result has the potential for more contact with the elderly, but studies have shown that nurses are the only health professionals that are in contact with the institutionalized elderly a statistically significant amount of time (Barney, 1972). Of total nursing time available to care for all age groups, the percentage of nursing time devoted to the elderly is larger than for any other single age group. Elderly patients require more care than younger patients. Oakley (1986) estimated that in hospitals alone, in 1980, just over 40% of the direct care Registered Nurse Full-Time Equivalents (RN FTEs) were required to care for people 65 years and older. Further, Oakley estimated that by the year 2000, 47% of the RN FTEs, and by the year 2050, 80% of the RN FTEs will be required by elderly patients in hospitals.

In short, although no health profession has yet claimed care of the elderly as its unique responsibility, nurses are in the most advantageous position to do so (Strumpf, 1988). Nurses have the assessment, counseling, support, education, and coordination skills needed by the elderly, an interest in caring for and about individuals, and a commitment to improving quality of life and assisting individuals to reach their greatest potential. Over 90% of the health care needs of elders and their caregivers fall squarely within the domain of independent nursing practice. Since nurses are currently providing the majority of care to the elderly, taking the lead in health care delivery for the elderly is both a professional imperative and a moral obligation.

REFERENCES

Abdellah, F. G., & Moore, S. R. (Eds.). (1988a). *Surgeon General's workshop: Health promotion and aging—Proceedings.* Menlo Park, CA: Henry J. Kaiser Family Foundation.

Abdellah, F. G., & Moore, S. R. (Eds.). (1988b). *Surgeon General's workshop: Health promotion and aging—Background papers.* Menlo Park, CA: Henry J. Kaiser Family Foundation.

Anonymous. (1982). Nurses today—A statistical portrait. *American Journal of Nursing, 82,* 448–451.

Archbold, P. G. (1983). Impact of parent-caring on women. *Family Relations, 32,* 39–45.

Barney, J. (1972). Community presence as a key to quality of life in nursing homes. Speech at the 100th Annual Meeting of the American Public Health Association, Atlantic City, NJ.

Birren, J. E., & Renner, V. J. (1981). Concepts and criteria of mental health and aging. *American Journal of Orthopsychiatry, 51,* 242–254.

Brody, E. (1985). Parent care as a normative family stress. *The Gerontologist, 25,* 19–29.

Brotman, H. B. (1982). *Every ninth American: An analysis for the chairman of the Select Committee on Aging, House of Representatives.* Comm. Pub. No. 97–332. Washington, DC: U.S. Government Printing Office.

Carter, M. A. (1988). Reflections on professional practice. *Journal of Professional Nursing, 4*(1), 9.

Chatters, L., Taylor, R., & Jackson, J. (1986). Aged Blacks' choices for an informal helper network. *Journal of Gerontology, 41,* 94–100.

Davis, C. (1987). Home care and its financial support: Future directions and present policies—Impact on care (Keynote Address). *Home health care: Report of a conference.* Rockville, MD: DHHS, Health Resources and Services Administration, Public Health Service.

Dawson, D., Hendershot, G., & Fulton, J. (1987). Aging in the eighties: Functional limitations of individuals age 65 years and over. *National Center for Health Statistics Advance Data, 133,* 1–12.

Emergency Medicine Symposium. (1985). The emergencies of old age: The patient. *Emergency Medicine, 17*(10), 21–28.

Fagin, C. M. (1982). Nursing as an alternative to high-cost care. *American Journal of Nursing, 82,* 56–60.

Freud, S. (1949). *Collected papers,* Vol. 4. E. Jones (Ed.). London: Hogarth.

Gatz, M., Smyer, M. A., & Lawton, M. P. (1980). The mental health system and the older adult. In L. W. Poon (Ed.), *Aging in the 1980s: Psychological issues* (pp. 5–18). Washington, DC: American Psychological Association.

Guttman, D. (1979). Use of informal and formal supports by white ethnic aged. In D. Gelfand & A. Kutzik (Eds.), *Ethnicity and aging* (pp. 246–262). New York: Springer Publishing Co.

Harper, M. S. (1986). Introduction. In M. S. Harper & B. D. Lebowitz (Eds.), *Mental illness in nursing homes: Agenda for research* (pp. 1–6). DHHS Publication No. (ADM) 86-1459. Rockville, MD: National Institute of Mental Health.

Harrington, C. (1987). Catastrophic health insurance: What is needed? *Nursing Outlook, 36,* 254–255.

Haupt, B. J. (1982). *Utilization of short-stay hospitals: Annual summary for the United States, 1980.* Vital and Health Statistics, Series 13, No. 64. DHHS Pub. No. (PHS) 82-1725. Washington, DC: Public Health Service.

Hing, E. (1981). *Characteristics of nursing home residents, health status, and care received.* Vital and Health Statistics, Series 13, No. 51. DHHS Pub. No. (PHS) 81-1712. Washington, DC: U.S. Government Printing Office.

Hing, E. (1987). Use of nursing homes by the elderly: Preliminary data from the 1985 National Nursing Home Survey. *Advance data from vital and health statistics.* No. 135. DHHS Pub. No. (PHS) 87-1250. Hyattsville, MD: Public Health Service.

Horowitz, A. (1985). Sons and daughters as caregivers to older parents: Differences in role performance and consequences. *The Gerontologist, 25,* 612–617.

Jackson, J. (1980). *Minorities and aging.* Belmont, CA: Wadsworth.

Katch, M. P. (1983). A negentropic view of the aged. *Journal of Gerontological Nursing, 9*(12), 656–660.

Kermis, M. D. (1986). The epidemiology of mental disorder in the elderly: A response to the Senate/AARP report. *The Gerontologist, 26,* 482–487.

Koch, H., & Knapp, D. E. (1987). Highlights of drug utilization in office practice, National Ambulatory Medical Care Survey, 1985. *Advance data from vital and health statistics,* No. 134. DHHS Pub. No. (PHS) 87-1250. Hyattsville, MD: Public Health Service.

Koshland, D. (1985). Health, wealth and unhappiness. *Science, 227,* 1419.

Kovar, M. G. (1986). Aging in the eighties: Preliminary data from the Supplement on Aging to the National Health Interview Survey, United States, January–June 1984. *Advance data from vital and health statistics*, No. 115. DHHS Pub. No. (PHS) 86-1250. Hyattsville, MD: Public Health Service.

Kuyers, J. A., & Bengston, V. L. (1973). Competence and social breakdown: A social-psychological view of aging. *Human Development, 2,* 37–49.

Levine, J., & Levine, W. C. (1980). *Ageism: Prejudice and discrimination against the elderly.* Belmont, CA: Wadsworth.

Maldonado, D. (1979). Aging in the Chicano context. In D. Gelfand & A. Kutzik (Eds.), *Ethnicity and aging* (pp. 175-83). New York: Springer Publishing Co.

Markides, K., & Mindel, C. (1987). *Ethnicity and aging.* Beverly Hills, CA: Sage.

McIntosh, J. L. (1985). Suicide among the elderly: Levels and trends. *American Journal of Orthopsychiatry, 55,* 288–293.

Moss, M., Moos, S., & Moles, E. (1985). The quality of relationships between elderly parents and their out-of-town children. *The Gerontologist, 25,* 134–140.

Myers, C. G., & Manton, K. G. (1984). Compression of mortality: Myth or reality? *The Gerontologist, 24,* 346–353.

National Center for Health Statistics [NCHS]. (1987). 1986 summary: National hospital discharge survey. *Advance data from vital and health statistics,* No. 145. DHHS Pub. No. (PHS) 87-1250. Hyattsville, MD: Public Health Service.

Oakley, D. (1986). Projecting the number of professional nurses required for in-hospital, direct care of older people, 1970-2050. *Western Journal of Nursing Research, 8,* 343–349.

Palmore, E. (1976). Total chance of institutionalization among the aged. *The Gerontologist, 16,* 504–507.

Pardes, H. (1981). The aging: Mental problems. *New York State Journal of Medicine, 81,* 798–804.

Pesanti, E. L. (1977). When phagocytic dysfunction increases susceptibility to infectious diseases. *Geriatrics, 32*(3), 110–113.

Pulliam, C. C., Hanlon, J. T., & Moore, S. R. (1988). Health promotion and aging: Medications and geriatrics. In F. G. Abdellah & S. R. Moore (Eds.), *Surgeon General's workshop: Health promotion and aging—Background papers* (pp. E1–E20). Menlo Park, CA: Henry J. Kaiser Family Foundation.

Redfern, S. J. (1988). Services for elderly people by the year 2000: Education and training issues—Preparation of new entrants to the nursing profession. *Journal of Advanced Nursing, 13,* 418–419.

Reifler, B. V., & Eisdorfer, C. (1980). A clinic for the impaired elderly and their families. *American Journal of Psychiatry, 127,* 1399–1403.

Rice, D., & Feldman, J. (1983). Living longer in the United States: Demographic changes and health needs of the elderly. *Millbank Memorial Fund Quarterly—Health and Society, 61,* 362–396.

Sakauye, K. (1986). Interface of emotional and behavioral conditions with physical disorders in nursing homes. In M. S. Harper & B. D. Lebowitz (Eds.), *Mental illness in nursing homes: Agenda for research* (pp. 65–82). DHHS Publication No. (ADM) 86-1459. Rockville, MD: National Institute of Mental Health.

Sattin, R. W., Nevitt, M. C., Waller, P. R., & Seiden, R. H. (1988). Health promotion and aging: Injury prevention. In F. G. Abdellah & S. R. Moore

(Eds.), *Surgeon General's workshop: Health promotion and aging—Background papers* (pp. D1–D20). Menlo Park, CA: Henry J. Kaiser Family Foundation.

Schewenger, C. W. (1977). Health care for aging Canadians. *Canadian Welfare, 59,* 9–12.

Seigel, J. S., & Taeuber, C. M. (1986). Demographic perspectives of the long-lived society. *Daedalus, 115,* 72–117.

Shanas, E. (1979). The family as a social support system in old age. *The Gerontologist, 19,* 169–174.

Strumpf, N. E. (1988). A new age for elderly care. *Nursing and Health Care, 8,* 445–448.

Sundwall, D. (1988). Health promotion and Surgeon General's workshop. In F. G. Abdellah & S. R. Moore (Eds.), *Surgeon General's workshop: Health promotion and aging—Proceedings* (pp. 14–19). Menlo Park, CA: Henry J. Kaiser Family Foundation.

Taylor, R. (1985). The extended family as a source of support to elderly blacks. *The Gerontologist, 25,* 488–495.

Yarling, R. (1977). The sick aged, the nursing profession, and the large society. *Journal of Gerontological Nursing, 3*(2), 42–51.

Chapter 2

The Nursing Process in Care of the Elderly

Jane Ashley

OVERVIEW OF THE NURSING PROCESS

The nursing process is the method used by nurses to assist clients in promoting wellness and solving health problems. It is an elegant process because it is simple and straightforward, and because it is applicable to any clinical specialty within the nursing discipline. Five steps comprise the process: assessment, diagnosis, planning, intervention, and evaluation.

The focus of these steps is on those potential or actual health problems which nurses are both able and licensed to treat (Gordon, 1987b). In order to use the nursing process effectively, the nurse needs an understanding of those activities that fall within the realm of nursing. Nurses care for people, and because each person is unique and infinitely complex, the activities of nursing are multiple and complex. The scope of nursing activities can be summarized as those activities which serve to maintain physical and mental health, prevent the development of health problems, and assist the individual to recover from illness and trauma and to minimize functional loss. The focus of nursing is not on the treatment of biological, physiological, and pathophysiological processes, but on human processes and functional responses (Carnevali, 1986).

Perhaps this can best be illustrated with an example. Arthritis, a common disease in the elderly, is a medical problem that can be treated in a number of ways, including the use of analgesics, anti-inflammatory agents, traction, and sometimes surgery (Grob, 1983). The prescription of these treatments is focused on the disease and is, appropriately, within the realm of medicine. In this same situation, the focus of nursing is on determining how the disease has affected the life and daily activities of the individual. Nursing questions that might arise include: Has the disease caused any problems with mobility? Is the elder able to perform self-care activities? Has the arthritis affected the person's ability to participate in work or leisure activities? Has the impairment affected the elder's self-concept? These are only a sample of the areas with which nurses are concerned and that they are capable of treating. In gerontological nursing the realities of the full scope of nursing practice come alive.

The purpose of the nursing process is to provide a systematic approach to identifying and solving those problems within the scope of nursing. The nursing process provides an approach to nursing care which is thoughtful, organized, and deliberate (Gordon, 1987b; Pinnell & de Meneses, 1986). This is especially critical in planning care for the older client. Each elder comes to the nursing relationship with a long history of health behaviors, social patterns, coping strategies, and personal strengths and limitations. The aging process, as well as the likelihood of chronic disease, further contributes to the complexity of an elder's health concerns and problems. The nursing process provides a step-wise plan to facilitate problem resolution in an orderly and comprehensive fashion. Without this mechanism, interventions and thus problem solving would occur in a haphazard and unpredictable way.

Suppose, for example, that a nurse is working with an 85-year-old woman who is concerned because she is experiencing difficulty sleeping. There may be a number of interventions that could be suggested: increase exercise, take fewer daytime naps, follow a bedtime ritual, eliminate caffeine from the diet, or reduce fluids after 6:00 P.M. Which of these interventions should the nurse suggest? If one considers the steps of the nursing process before answering this question, it should be clear that any intervention suggested at this point would be pure guesswork and unlikely to resolve the problems except through chance. If, for example, in further discussion with this client, she mentions that she walks five miles a day, then the suggestion to increase exercise would be of no value in helping this woman sleep better. The difficulty in selecting any of the interventions listed above is that they were developed before the nature of the problem and possible causes of the problem were identified.

The nursing process is sequential. The initial step is the collection of data relevant to the problem. Once data have been collected, they can be categorized so that one or more specific nursing diagnoses can be recognized and the possible causes of the problem identified. Nursing diagnoses and etiologies provide guidance for the development of patient outcomes and the selection of interventions. The orderliness of this process increases the probability that problem resolution will occur since the nursing actions are selected specifically for each nursing diagnosis.

VALUE OF USING THE NURSING PROCESS

The value of the nursing process in providing a systematic and sequential method for understanding complex problems and planning treatments has already been addressed. There are several other reasons that the nursing process is of importance.

The American Nurses' Association has established *Standards and Scope of Gerontological Nursing Practice* (ANA, 1987). A standard serves as a model of expected level of nursing practice. Standards generally represent the minimal performance necessary to meet the accountability requirements of the practice discipline. The *Standards and Scope of Gerontological Nursing Practice* recognize the validity of the nursing process. The standards address each component of the nursing process and its appropriate use in providing nursing care for the older adult. One might wonder why the nursing process has taken such a prominent position in the standards of the profession? The answer is simple. It is through the nursing process that nurses exercise their ability to make clinical judgments and prescribe treatments independently of other disciplines. Nurses have many opportunities to demonstrate a collaborative spirit and an ability to work interdependently. The nursing process provides the mechanism for nurses to contribute their own specialized knowledge and skills to the health of others in a totally autonomous manner.

The nursing process is also important in improving the overall quality of patient care. One characteristic of nursing care which distinguishes it from other health-related disciplines is its tradition of continuity in time (Beth Israel Hospital, 1985). This concept describes the element of time as it exists in most client-nurse relationships. Nurses provide care over time. In acute-care hospitals, long-term care facilities, and nursing homes, nursing care is provided continuously (24 hours per day) for the duration of the client's stay. In community settings, nursing care is typically provided over an extended period of time (weeks to years). It is this continuity of time which adds a richness to the client-nurse relationship and which is not usually possible in episodic encounters. Because nursing does occur over time, nurses other than the primary nurse will occasionally be responsible for implementing the plan of care. The nursing process and the written nursing care plan derived from the process are the best mechanisms to ensure continuity of patient care in the absence of the primary nurse. In this way, the nursing process improves the delivery of nursing care by facilitating communication among nurses.

A final importance of the nursing process is its use in justifying the need for care and validating the role of nursing (Gordon, 1987a; Turkoski, 1988). Current systems of reimbursement to health care providers and agencies are typically based on treatments performed and care associated with specific medical diagnoses. In this type of reimbursement equation, the many services performed by nurses through the utilization of nursing diagnoses remain unrecognized. The nursing process provides nurses with the opportunity to document in a systematic manner the nursing care being provided to clients. This not only serves to validate the independent role and functions of the nurse, but it may be important in the future in securing compensation for professional services rendered.

SPECIAL CONSIDERATIONS IN USING THE NURSING PROCESS WITH THE ELDERLY

Is the nursing process different when implemented with the elderly? The answer is both "yes" and "no." The components of the process and the sequence in which they are carried out remain the same regardless of whether they are being used to plan nursing care for a toddler, a teenager, an adult, or an elder. There are, however, special knowledge and skills which are critical to using the nursing process with different age groups. It would be outside the scope of this chapter to outline the full range of knowledge and skills in gerontological nursing, but a few aspects warrant a brief mention. First, nurses working with the elderly need a basic knowledge of normal aging processes and the kind of changes these can create in human functioning. Second, an understanding of the common problems, both pathological and functional, that can occur in the aged is important. Third, there are special life concerns, such as retirement, losses, and approaching death, with which gerontological nurses should be familiar. Developing a knowledge base in these areas is essential to the establishment of a comprehensive data base, the skill in making diagnostic judgments, and the formation of goal-directed interventions.

There are also some special considerations which should be kept in mind when implementing the nursing process with the elderly.

1. Search for the elder's areas of strengths. By virtue of longevity alone, elders have demonstrated resiliency and the ability to cope with life's stressors. The plan of care should always build on the strengths and abilities of the elder (Burnside, 1988).

2. Recognize that the difference between normal aging and pathology is always being redefined. Current understanding of the normal aging process is limited (Rowe & Kahn, 1987). It is possible that as more studies are conducted, problems which were once accepted as part of the normal aging process (such as osteoporosis) will be determined to be modifiable and, as such, will be identified as pathological rather than normal.

3. Recognize the lowered threshold for stress of the elder. The most significant physiological change of aging is the reduction in physical reserves. While elderly individuals may be able to make normative adaptations to both the aging process and the presence of chronic illness, sudden or prolonged stress can severely compromise their physiological status (Fulmer, Ashley, & Reilly, 1986).

4. Consider the fact that the elderly may respond to stress and illness in atypical ways. Research has demonstrated, for example, that normal body temperature in the elderly runs well below (at 97.9° F) the usual standard body temperature (98.6° F) (Thatcher, 1983; Higgins, 1983). A "normal" body temperature of 98.6° F may actually indicate fever in elders.

5. Expect the presence of multiple problems. Chronic illness is generally present by age 60, and it is estimated that at least 85% of those over age 65 have at least one chronic condition (Bowles, Portnoi, & Kenney, 1981; Ebersole & Hess, 1985). Chronic disease does not always create functional health problems with consequent nursing diagnoses, but it is likely that chronic illness will increase the vulnerability of elders.

6. Recognize the complexity of the health problems of the elder. It is not unusual for a nursing diagnosis to have multiple etiologies. Consider the situation of a 93-year-old praticing attorney who developed acute confusion (impaired thought processes) five days after admission to an acute-care facility. Data collection on this gentleman revealed a number of possible causes including: hypothyroidism, electrolyte imbalance, fever, sensory impairment (his hearing aid and glasses had been left at home), the presence of a new and unfamiliar environment (over the five-day course, he had been transferred to two hospitals and three hospital floors), sleep disturbances (his primary nurse reported that he was awake most of the night, but slept during the day), and lack of orienting cues (he usually read the papers and watched the morning and evening television news shows as part of his daily routine, neither of which he did in the hospital).

7. Recognize the theme of loss in the lives of the elderly. Learning to live with losses is a continuous process for the aged (Burnside, 1988).

The presence of multiple losses and sustained losses can be a serious source of stress for the elder.

STEPS OF THE NURSING PROCESS

Step 1: Assessment

Assessment is the process of collecting information relevant to the health status of the client (Leddy & Pepper, 1985). The focus of the data should be on that information which is needed to plan and implement nursing care. The emphasis in a nursing assessment is therefore on such areas as the client's functional abilities, life style, knowledge, and beliefs and values concerning health. The nursing assessment may include data collected by other health providers, but it should not merely be a duplicate of these assessments. The medical history, for example, focuses on the structural, biological, physiological, and pathophysiological functioning of the elder. This is *not* the focus of nursing. While some of the medical history will be of relevance to nursing care, the nursing assessment provides a fuller picture of how the elder functions in life activities. A full discussion concerning nursing assessment of the elderly can be found in Chapter 3.

Assessment is the first step in the nursing process, and it is of key importance for three reasons: (1) it establishes baseline information on usual behaviors and functional abilities; (2) it documents current behaviors and functional abilities; and (3) it provides the data from which nursing diagnoses will be identified. In order for an assessment to accomplish these purposes, it must be comprehensive and presented in a format that is easily communicated to others. There are a number of nursing models which can be used to guide the collection of assessment data and facilitate the emergence and recognition of meaningful patterns. Gordon (1987b) suggested the use of Functional Health Patterns for organizing nursing assessment data. This framework (see Table 2.1) identifies 11 patterns which represent important areas for life functioning. Carnevali (1986) recommended that data be collected around two domains: daily living (e.g., activities of daily living, demands of daily living), and functional health status (e.g., eating, sleeping, grooming). Matteson and McConnell (1988) used patterns of self-care (e.g., fluid, activity-rest, social interaction) as a model for structuring data collection. These represent only a sample of the nursing models available. The important point is that use of a model will help to direct the collection of relevant data, will provide a framework for understanding the data, and will increase the likelihood of collecting comprehensive data.

As indicated earlier, knowledge of gerontology is essential to all steps of the nursing process. In the assessment phase, it will heighten

TABLE 2.1 Typology of Eleven Functional Health Patterns

Health-perception-health-management pattern. Describes client's perceived pattern of health and well-being and how health is managed.

Nutritional-metabolic pattern. Describes pattern of food and fluid consumption relative to metabolic need and pattern indicators of local nutrient supply.

Elimination pattern. Describes patterns of excretory function (bowel, bladder, and skin).

Activity-exercise pattern. Describes pattern of exercise, activity, leisure, and recreation.

Cognitive-perceptual pattern. Describes sensory-perceptual and cognitive pattern.

Sleep-rest pattern. Describes patterns of sleep, rest, and relaxation.

Self-perception-self-concept pattern. Describes self-concept pattern and perceptions of self (e.g., body comfort, body image, feeling state).

Role-relationship pattern. Describes pattern of role-engagements and relationships.

Sexuality-reproductive pattern. Describes client's patterns of satisfaction and dissatisfaction with sexuality pattern; describes reproductive patterns.

Coping-stress-tolerance pattern. Describes general coping pattern and effectiveness of the pattern in terms of stress tolerance.

Value-belief pattern. Describes patterns of values, belief (including spiritual), or goals that guide choices or decisions.

Reproduced by permission from M. Gordon (1987). *Nursing diagnosis: Process and application* (2nd ed.). New York: McGraw-Hill, p. 93. Copyrighted by The C. V. Mosby Co., St. Louis.

the sensitivity and skill of the nurse in collecting data relevant to the elderly. Important data may be missed or minimized without this knowledge. Two examples will illustrate this point.

- A complete and well-documented assessment of cognitive function should be routinely performed with all elderly admitted to acute-care hospitals. A number of studies document the incidence of hospital-induced confusion among previously mentally intact and independent elders (Chisholm, et al., 1982; Liston, 1982; Roslaniec & Fitzpatrick, 1979; and Williams, et al., 1985).

- Descriptions of recent moves (relocations to new environments such as to the homes of relatives, to senior housing, to long-term care facilities, or to nursing homes) are important to document. Some studies have reported on the physical and mental deterioration of the elderly associated with forced relocation (Amenta, Weiner, & Amenta, 1984).

The nursing assessment lays the foundation for the second step in the nursing process.

Step 2: Nursing Diagnosis

A nursing diagnosis is a statement describing an actual or potential health problem which nurses are qualified and licensed to treat (Carpenito, 1987b; Gordon, 1987b). In other words, a nursing diagnosis identifies a health problem which can be treated with nursing interventions. Health problems can be both actual and potential. Actual health problems are those which the client currently has. If, for example, the client has a two-inch open lesion on the heel of his or her left foot, then an actual impairment of skin integrity exists. Potential health problems are those which the client does not have, but is at high risk for developing. Suppose a nurse is caring for an 84-year-old frail and debilitated woman who is on bedrest and whose heels are reddened and painful. This woman's debilitated state, coupled with her inactivity, place her at risk for developing problems with skin integrity. The sign (redness) and the symptom (pain) provide further evidence of her level of risk. When all factors are considered together, this woman has a clear potential impairment of skin integrity.

Components of a Nursing Diagnosis

There are three components of a nursing diagnosis: a statement of the problem or diagnosis; a statement of the cause or etiology; and identification of the defining signs and symptoms (Gordon, 1987b). The statement of the diagnosis is a clear and concise description of the specific health problem. The North American Nursing Diagnosis Association (NANDA) is a national organization of theorists and practitioners concerned with developing a classification system of nursing diagnoses (McLane, 1987). NANDA has approved a list of recognized nursing diagnostic categories which are available in a variety of published forms (e.g., Carpenito, 1987a; Duespohl, 1986; Kim, McFarland, & McLane, 1984). There is value to using NANDA-accepted diagnoses. First, these diagnoses have been through a review process and have been acknowledged as valid areas for nursing interventions. Second, the use of these diagnoses can facilitate communication among nurses because the terminology involved is somewhat standardized. The classification of nursing diagnoses is an evolving process. It may be difficult, in some situations, to identify a NANDA diagnosis which specifies the problem of a particular patient. NANDA recognizes this difficulty and encourages nurses to identify and use diagnoses in their practice which have not been classified. These diagnoses can eventually be submitted to NANDA for study (Gordon, 1987b).

The second component of a nursing diagnosis is the statement which indicates the factors which are causing or are suspected of causing the health problem. This is a necessary part to include because nursing interventions will focus on both the diagnosis and the etiology (Gordon, 1987b). Consider the differences in treatments that occur when the causes of the problems are different:

Diagnosis 1: Social isolation related to limited physical mobility.

Diagnosis 2: Social isolation related to lack of community resources.

In the first example, the client has limited social interaction because of his or her restricted level of mobility. It can be anticipated that at least some nursing interventions will be directed toward improving the client's mobility perhaps through exercise, range of motion, or assistive devices. This focus is clearly not appropriate for the client in the second example. Social isolation in this latter case has possibly occurred because the community does not provide some resource, such as transportation, that is required by this individual. This calls for a very different focus for nursing intervention.

The third aspect of a nursing diagnosis is a listing of the critical defining signs and symptoms. These signs and symptoms are not part of the diagnostic statement. However, they are the specific data in the assessment which justify the selecting of a particular diagnosis. Defining characteristics are important because they provide others with the data needed to validate the diagnosis.

An example may be helpful to illustrate these three components of a nursing diagnosis. Consider the situation of a 78-year-old woman who is at home recovering from a cerebrovascular accident. The stroke has left her with a right-sided weakness in both extremities. She reports to the visiting nurse that she has been feeling depressed and alone. Prior to the illness, most of her social activity centered around the common patio area of the apartment building. She enjoyed spending the afternoons on the patio talking with the other residents. Since her stroke, she had not left her apartment, and she missed seeing her friends. She says that she does not feel "confident enough" to maneuver her walker out to the patio. Her friends in the building call and occasionally drop by to visit, but she states that the days seem very long and she is lonely.

Critical Cues	*Nursing Diagnosis*	*Etiology*
Client reports feeling depressed, alone, lonely, and missing her friends.	Social isolation related to	Impaired physical mobility
Client is unable to participate in her previous level of social activity.		

The nursing diagnosis of social isolation refers to a state of social participation that is less than the type or amount needed for an individual's sense of personal satisfaction (Gordon, 1987b). In the example, critical cues that social isolation is an appropriate nursing diagnosis can be found in the client's report of depression, loneliness, and missing her friends. The diagnosis gets further verification by the fact that this woman is not able to participate in the social activities she once enjoyed.

The etiology of impaired mobility is derived from the physical assessment indicating right-sided weakness and the client's report of feeling a lack of confidence in using the walker. Presumably, the nursing care plan developed for this client will include a number of interventions designed to improve both her mobility and her confidence in her mobility.

Setting Priorities

Once nursing diagnoses have been developed, priorities among the diagnoses need to be established. Not all diagnoses will be of equal importance to the health and well-being of the client. There are a few guidelines which can assist nurses in selecting priorities (Burnside, 1988; Gordon, 1987b). These include: (1) highest priority should be given to problems which are serious and life-threatening; (2) moderate priority should be given to problems which if untreated are likely to cause destructive changes; and (3) lowest priority is given to problems in which the client requires minimal assistance.

Common Nursing Diagnoses in the Elderly

Nursing has a tradition of recognizing the heterogeneity of groups and valuing the uniqueness of the individual. This philosophical view mandates the development of a plan of care which reflects the individual needs of the elder. There is value, however, in knowing which diagnoses are commonly found among particular client groups. This knowledge can increase sensitivity to these problems and motivate the search for better prevention and treatment strategies. McCourt (1987) demonstrated this benefit in a study which was conducted on patient falls in a 212-bed rehabilitation hospital. In this small, non-random sample, patient falls showed a consistent decline, over a 7-month period, following the implementation of nursing diagnoses. McCourt attributed this result to more accurate identification of patient risk factors and the development of more specific interventions to prevent falling.

A few studies have been designed for the purpose of identifying the most common nursing diagnoses in the geriatric population. Caution should be exercised in generalizing the results of these studies beyond the sample used because of various limitations in the research designs. Despite this cautionary note, there are some interesting findings.

Hallal (1985) studied the nursing diagnoses of 106 elderly clients hospitalized in an acute-care institution. She found that there were an average of 5.06 diagnoses per patient. Older patients (80 years or older) had more diagnoses than the younger group (age 65–79). The 10 most common diagnoses and the percentage of elderly having these diagnoses as found in this study are as follows:

Nursing diagnosis	*Percentage of sample with the diagnosis*
Impaired physical mobility	79.2
Alteration in comfort: pain	40.6
Alteration in nutrition: less than body requirements	40.6
Fear	30.2
Alteration in bowel elimination: constipation	26.4
Alteration in urinary elimination	26.4
Impaired skin integrity	24.5
Disturbance in self-concept	22.6
Sleep pattern disturbance	22.6
Self-care deficit: total	21.7

There were some differences in the specific diagnoses and the order of the most frequent diagnoses when this researcher compared the young-old to the old-old, patients with medical problems versus those with surgical problems, and male versus female (Hallal, 1985).

Common nursing diagnoses have also been studied in long-term care facilities where the majority of patients are elderly (Leslie, 1981; McCourt, 1987; Rantz & Miller, 1987; Specht & Drey, 1987). The diagnoses identified in these studies are remarkably similar to those found by Hallal (1985). Not surprisingly, the studies conducted in long-term care facilities indicate more problems with self-care deficits of all levels (bathing, dressing, toileting) and potential for injuries, specifically risk of falling. It is particularly noteworthy that all of the research studies cited included on their lists of common diagnoses problems with: mobility, self care, comfort, and skin integrity. The number of diagnoses per patients in these studies ranged from 4.25 to 7.25. This is a clear reflection of the complexity of caring for older individuals.

More studies need to be done which identify the diagnoses common to particular settings (acute-care hospitals, rehabilitation facilities, nursing homes, and the home environment) and which identify diagnoses common to specific age groups (young-old, middle-old, and old-old). These types of studies can serve to further enlighten gerontological nursing practice.

Step 3: Planning

The planning aspect of the nursing process involves the establishment of goals and objectives. Goals are statements concerning the desired health state to be achieved. Goals are usually broad statements concerned with the promotion, maintenance, or restoration of a particular health function (Leddy & Pepper, 1985). Goals establish the end-point of care. Once a goal is selected, outcomes or objectives are determined. Objectives are the *measurable* behaviors that move one toward a goal or indicate that a goal has been achieved (Gordon, 1987b). Because they are observable behaviors, objectives can be used to evaluate whether a client is making progress in attaining the desired health state. The distinction between goals and objectives can be understood in the following example.

Nursing diagnosis	*Goal*	*Objective*
Self-care deficit; total, related to activity intolerance	Patient will perform self-care activities with minimal energy expenditure	Patient will be able to put on or take off clothing, in one week, without a significant change in vital signs

In this example, the goal is a global statement on the ideal health state of the client. The objective is much more specific. It states the activity that is to be accomplished and the time frame in which it should occur. In order to attain the goal, however, other objectives need to be developed. The goal refers to all self-care activities, whereas the objective refers only to dressing. One would expect this care plan also to include objectives for other self-care activities, such as eating, bathing, and toileting.

There are four important points to consider when writing goals and objectives. First, they should be stated in terms of client behaviors. Goals and objectives describe a state of the client, not a state or action of the nurse or health team. Second, objectives must be measurable. This allows the nurse to reach a clear decision as to whether the objective has been met. Third, objectives need to be realistic with consideration given to normative data and what is possible in light of the client's strengths and weaknesses. Fourth, objectives must be developed collaboratively with the elder. It is an appropriate role for nurses to suggest objectives and to influence their adoption, but the ultimate decision on the selection of objectives rests with the client.

Step 4: Intervention

Nursing interventions are those actions which assist the client in moving toward the stated goals. Gordon (1987b) identified several factors which will influence the choice of interventions, including: the client's personal situation and perception; the acuity and severity of the problem; the effect of the intervention on others; and the likelihood of the intervention's success. There are seven key points to consider in choosing interventions for the elderly client:

1.   Efforts should be geared toward maximizing the strengths and abilities of the elder.

2.   Consideration must be given to the values of the client. While value positions are a result of an individual's ethnic, religious, and family structure, as well as inherent personality differences, there is some evidence that values shift with age (Christenson, 1977). For example, material comforts may become more important with advancing age.

3.   Assess the environment for possible changes. Goals can be accomplished in a number of ways and changing factors which are external to the elder can be a successful approach. Arthritis, for example, can be so crippling as to prevent the individual from being able to fasten buttons, hooks, or zippers. Rather than losing independence in self care, the elder can be encouraged to select clothes that pull on or have velcro fasteners.

4.   Recognize the importance of coordinating support people and services. Nurses need to act as advocates and integrators in mobilizing sources of support for the elder. The positive influence of support networks on the health of elders has been documented (Boettcher, 1985; Cole, 1985).

5.   Analyze both the benefits and drawbacks of interventions before implementation. Because the elderly often have multiple health concerns, interventions directed toward improving one problem may, inadvertently, create other problems.

6.   Select the least restrictive interventions first. There may be occasions when an intervention is called for which threatens the independence and autonomy of the elder. In these situations, initial interventions should be those which are the least restrictive. For example, in providing safety for a confused elder, a bed alarm should be tried before a vest restraint is used.

7.   Utilize research in selecting interventions. Research studies serve to enlighten practice and assist in the selection of those interventions which have demonstrated success.

Step 5: Evaluation

Evaluation is the process of comparing the desired health outcome, as stated in the objectives and goals, to the actual health outcome as demonstrated by the client. Evaluation is a continuous process. Once interventions are initiated, the nurse collects data continuously to determine the client's responses. It is the ongoing collection of evaluative data which allows the nurse to modify the care plan as needed.

Yura and Walsh (1983) have identified four possible outcomes to the evaluation process and the corresponding changes in the nursing care plan:

1. The problem has been resolved. A new plan would be developed to maintain the optimal state.

2. The problem remains unchanged. The care plan can either be continued with plans for further evaluation, or the client would be reassessed with some modifications in the care plan.

3. The problem has gotten worse. The client needs to be reassessed and a new plan developed.

4. A new problem has emerged. The nursing process is implemented in order to develop a plan to recognize and resolve this new problem.

Evaluating the health problems of elders can be a difficult endeavor. Very few normative standards have been established for this age group. As a result, there are no objective criteria to which individual progress can be compared. As our understanding of aging and the aging experience grows, expertise in the evaluation of health problems of the elderly will be advanced.

CONCLUSION

The nursing process provides nurses with a systematic method for promoting wellness and addressing health problems. It is through the use of this process that nurses demonstrate their unique contributions as professionals and provide accountability to the consumer.

REFERENCES

Amenta, M., Weiner, A., & Amenta, D. (1984). Successful relocation. *Geriatric Nursing, 5*, 230–233.

American Nurses' Association. (1987). *Standards and scope of gerontological nursing practice.* Kansas City: Author.

Beth Israel Hospital. (1985). *Professional nursing at Boston's Beth Israel Hospital.* Boston: Author.

Boettcher, E. G. (1985). Linking the aged to systems. *Journal of Gerontological Nursing, 11*(3), 27–33.

Bowles, L. T., Portnoi, V., & Kenney, R. (1981). Wear and tear: Common biologic changes of aging. *Geriatrics, 36*(4), 77–86.

Burnside, I. M. (1988). *Nursing and the aged: A self-care approach* (3rd ed.). New York: McGraw-Hill.

Carnevali, D. (1986). Domains for nursing and medical diagnosis and management. In D. Carnevali & M. Patrick (Eds.), *Nursing management for the elderly* (pp. 18–25). Philadelphia: Lippincott.

Carpenito, L. J. (1987a). *Handbook of nursing diagnosis* (2nd ed.). Philadelphia: Lippincott.

Carpenito, L. J. (1987b). *Nursing diagnosis; Application to clinical practice* (2nd ed.). Philadelphia: Lippincott.

Chisholm, S., Denniston, O., Igrisan, R., & Barbus, A. (1982). Prevalence of confusion in elderly hospitalized patients. *Journal of Gerontology, 8,* 87–96.

Christenson, J. (1977). Generational value differences. *The Gerontologist, 17,* 367–374.

Cole, E. (1985). Assessing needs for elder networks. *Journal of Gerontological Nursing, 11*(7), 31–34.

Duespohl, T. A. (1986). *Nursing diagnosis manual for the well and ill client.* Philadelphia: W. B. Saunders.

Ebersole, P., & Hess, P. (1985). *Towards health aging.* St. Louis: C. V. Mosby.

Fulmer, T., Ashley, J., & Reilly, C. (1986). Geriatric nursing in acute settings. *Annual Review of Gerontology and Geriatrics, 6,* 27–80.

Gordon, M. (1987a). Implementation of nursing diagnosis. *Nursing Clinics of North America, 22*(4), 875–879.

Gordon, M. (1987b). *Nursing diagnosis: Process and application* (2nd ed.). New York: McGraw-Hill.

Grob, D. (1983). Prevalent joint diseases in older persons. In W. Reichel (Ed.), *Clinical aspects of aging* (pp. 344–359). Baltimore: Williams & Wilkins.

Hallal, J. C. (1985). Nursing diagnosis: An essential step to quality care. *Journal of Gerontological Nursing, 11*(9), 35–38.

Higgins, P. (1983). Can 98.6 F be a fever in disguise? *Geriatric Nursing, 4,* 101–102.

Kim, M. J., McFarland, G. K., & McLane, A. M. (1984). *Pocket guide to nursing diagnoses.* St. Louis: C. V. Mosby.

Leddy, S., & Pepper, J. (1985). *Conceptual bases of professional nursing.* Philadelphia: Lippincott.

Leslie, F. (1981). Nursing diagnosis: Use in long-term care. *American Journal of Nursing, 81,* 1012–1014.

Liston, E. H. (1982). Delirium in the aged. *Psychiatric Clinics of North America, 5,* 47–52.

Matteson, M. A., & McConnell, E. (1988). *Gerontological nursing.* Philadelphia: W. B. Saunders.

McCourt, A. (1987). Implementation of nursing diagnosis through integration with quality assurance. *Nursing Clinics of North America, 22*(4), 899–904.

McLane, A. (Ed.). (1987). *Classification of nursing diagnoses: Proceedings of the Seventh Conference.* St. Louis: C. V. Mosby.

Pinnell, N. L., & de Meneses, M. (1986). *The nursing process: Theory, application, and related processes.* Norwalk, CT: Appleton-Century-Crofts.

Rantz, M., & Miller, T. V. (1987). How diagnoses are changing in long-term care. *American Journal of Nursing, 87,* 360–361.

Roslaniec, A., & Fitzpatrick, J. (1979). Changes in mental status in adults with four days of hospitalization. *Research in Nursing and Health, 2,* 177–187.

Rowe, J., & Kahn, R. (1987). Human aging: Usual and successful. *Science, 237,* 143–149.

Specht, J., & Drey, K. (1987). The implementation of nursing diagnoses. *Nursing Clinics of North America, 22*(4), 917–929.

Thatcher, R. M. (1983). 98.6 F—What is normal? *Journal of Gerontological Nursing, 9*(1), 22–27.

Turkoski, B. (1988). Nursing diagnosis in print, 1950–1985. *Nursing Outlook, 36*(3), 142–144.

Williams, M., Campbell, E., Raynor, W., Musholt, M., Mlynarczyk, S., & Crane, L. (1985). Predictors of acute confusional states in hospitalized elderly patients. *Research in Nursing and Health, 8,* 31–40.

Yura, H., & Walsh, M. (1983). *The nursing process.* Norwalk, CT: Appleton-Century-Crofts.

Chapter 3

Nursing Assessment of the Elderly Person

Terry T. Fulmer and Eileen Quinlan

APPROACHES TO THE NURSING ASSESSMENT OF ELDERLY INDIVIDUALS

Parameters of the Assessment

Over the past decade, much has been done to emphasize the point that the health assessment of older individuals is specialized in nature. Just as children have special physiologic features which warrant particular interventions, members of the elderly population have specialized physiologic parameters as well. In the past, elderly persons were often assessed in the exact same manner as 30- or 40-year-old individuals. Today we know that this is inappropriate, and programs in nursing education have responded by developing curricular materials that teach students this information. Gerontological nursing as a specialty is now in its third decade and much progress is evident.

One of the most important changes in health assessment of the elderly is the improvement in attitudes toward older individuals. Gerontological nursing is a growing field in the nursing profession. Every year there is increased demand for the services of nurses who provide care to the elderly population. In a report by the National Institute on Aging (NIA) entitled, "Personnel for the Health Needs of the Elderly

Through Year 2020" (NIA, 1987), it is estimated that there will be a need for 12,000 to 20,000 gerontological nurse practitioners by the year 2010. In light of the fact that there are currently about 1,000 certified nurse practitioners certified in this field by the American Nurses' Association, and only about 6,000 adult and family nurse practitioners, there is clearly a need to attract individuals to this area.

The same NIA report documents that in 1984 a study of generic baccalaureate programs in nursing reported that 71% of the 197 schools responding had integrated gerontological content into their curriculum, and another 11% had specific courses on gerontological nursing. This is important information. It is only through a sound educational program that the parameters for assessing the elderly, as well as the attitudinal changes that enable positive approaches to assessing the elderly, will come about.

Eliopoulos (1983) described the necessity of what she calls "maintaining a therapeutic staff" in the creation of a therapeutic environment for the elderly. Her contention is that without a therapeutic staff there can be no therapeutic environment. The positive approaches that are necessary in assessing and caring for the elderly go hand-in-hand with the overall attitude of the nurses and nursing assistants who are delivering the care. It is important to look for the classic signals that indicate burnout, such as attendance problems, poor morale, withdrawal, rigidity, and poor performance. If nurses do not have a positive attitude about themselves, it is unlikely that they will be able to approach the care of elderly persons with the requisite enthusiasm and commitment.

Fitzsimons (1985) believes that attention to the developmental needs of older adults can bring about a more effective health care experience and reduce the risks of infantilization which occurs so frequently in care of the elderly. Table 3.1 outlines the potential developmental issues of older adults and describes nursing intervention options which address those issues.

Effective communication with elderly persons depends on several things: the attitudes of the interviewer; the environment; and the way the elderly person receives the communication. Stokes, Rauckhorst, and Mezey (1980) pointed out that it is important to be aware of any stereotypes that may come into play while communicating with the elderly and that interviewers should be mindful of the fact that the elderly may fear rejection in the same way that their younger counterparts do. A direct and mature approach that encompasses respect and a sense that each older person is in charge of his or her own health is important. It should not be assumed that the elderly person is hard of hearing or demented! These are examples of stereotypes which will damage the assessment process before it begins. It is important to take each individual and assess that person independently of the norms that have come to be expected with elderly clients.

TABLE 3.1 Attention to the Developmental Needs of the Older Adult Can Reduce the Risk of Infantilization

Potential development issues for the older adult	Behavioral signs	Possible client objectives	Nursing intervention options
		The client will	
Grief response over loss of health and displacement	Apathy	Seek contact with family	Meet basic client needs for comfort and safety. Meeting biologic needs may obliterate severe feelings of loneliness.
	Rigidity		
Social role devaluation	Boredom	Identify territory and boundaries	Reminiscing can be used as a therapeutic tool for the older adult.
Meaninglessness of daily routines	Ennui	Sense ability to control environment	Provide client with control over money in some way.
	Anger		
Lack of autonomy	Loneliness	Feel needed and useful	Arrange to have meaningful objects from home in the hospital environment.

Feelings of loneliness			Identify client's life contributions. Discuss these during nurse-client interactions.
Self-Absorption	Depression	Feel successful in coping with illness	Tactile needs can be met during backrub. Touch client's bed when speaking to him or her (it reduces distancing feelings between nurse and client).
Threat to independent role at home		Take opportunities to be assertive	Provide opportunities for socializing with other clients.
Fear of chronic illness (Older adults cite fear of chronic illness as greater than fear of death.)		Maintain adaptive flexibility	
		Establish appropriate relationships with staff and other clients	

Source: Fitzsimons, V. M. (1985). Maintaining a positive environment for the older adult. *Orthopaedic Nursing, 4*(3), 50. Reproduced with permission of the publisher, 1985, *Orthopaedic Nursing*, official publication of the National Association of Orthopaedic Nurses.

THE PERSON-CENTERED APPROACH:
A HOLISTIC VIEW OF THE ELDERLY

Just as there is no set formula for prescribing medications to the psychiatric client, there is no rigid formula for assessing older individuals. The person-centered approach, which allows for the individuality of each elder, is the most appropriate way to approach an assessment. Older people bring with them a life history full of events, people, and environments which shape the manner in which they react to interviews in the health-care setting. In the case of elders who have any degree of cognitive impairment, the complexity of the interview is compounded. However, even the presence of dementia does not preclude in all cases the elder's ability to give a health history. It may take longer, but it is important to try to get the elderly person to give the history whenever possible. This is a clear signal that the elder is valued as an autonomous, independent individual. This person-centered approach also minimizes the possibility of infantilizing and offending the older person. It is true, however, that certain interview techniques and pre-interview activities aid the process.

Whenever possible, and especially in the ambulatory setting, it is helpful to send a form to the client which lists in advance the questions that will be asked of the elder in order to let the person have some extra time to get his or her responses organized. Imagine trying to recall 85 years of information! A useful format is one which is straightforward with questions clearly stated. Such a form can be mailed to the elderly person's home a week in advance of the appointment and brought in the day of the appointment. In some cases, it may even be possible to have the elder mail the form in before the appointment so the nurse can review it and be better prepared. When the health assessment is being conducted under duress, as in the case of an emergency room visit, questions should be simple and straightforward, and elders should be reassured that they need only give it their best attempt. Opportunities for follow-up for greater detail can be arranged.

EFFECTIVE TECHNIQUES FOR
FOCUSING THE INTERVIEW

The interview will remain in focus if the nurse is clear from the outset about the information that is needed. However, there are times when an older person can digress from the required information. Usually, a gentle reminder, such as, "Can we come back to the topic of what is troubling your sleep?", will get the process back on track. Some elders (and, indeed, some young people) use the interview as a way of unloading all their problems; this makes it very difficult for the nurse to bring the assessment process into focus. If bizarre, erratic thought patterns seem present, note them, and discuss the behavior with other members of the health-care team involved with the case. It may also be helpful to ask older persons directly why they seem to need to digress. They may think they are being "good patients" by being more expansive. Alternatively, they may simply be nervous, or have a physical discomfort that is causing them to act in an unusual way. Input from friends and family regarding usual behavior is helpful, but the nurse should try to rely primarily on the elderly person and not solely on well-meaning friends and family who may dominate the interview in the name of "helpfulness."

It is useful to begin the interview with an explicit time frame. For example, the nurse might say: "We have a half-hour together, and I'd like to use the first 10 minutes to get your health background and the next 10 minutes talking about what brought you here today. We'll save the last part of the interview for you to fill in any gaps and ask any questions you may have." A clock in the room with large numbers for easy reading is helpful.

THE SETTING

As previously suggested, the setting has a great impact on the interview process. The nurse needs to take into account the environment as it affects the process of assessment and make any necessary adjustments. Physically, an interview should take place in an atmosphere of comfort where there is adequate lighting, comfortable furniture, and relative quiet. It is important for the nurse to sit at eye level while interviewing the older adult, and to utilize touch to convey a feeling of security and concern. In the community setting, it may be that the interview will take place in the elder's own home. As a "guest" in that setting, the nurse should be mindful of any family traditions and observe them when appropriate.

In the acute care setting, the nurse needs to anticipate that the elderly person's stress level may be very high and a second interview may be necessary to obtain additional details. It is also important to start the interview by assuring the elder and any family that you know how difficult it is for them to concentrate on questions which do not seem very important, but the interview will conclude as soon as possible.

The nursing home setting requires an altogether different approach, depending upon whether the interaction is an admission interview or an interview for an emerging health-care problem. For an admission interview, it will be helpful to schedule several appointments over the course of the first month in order to get information, but also to note the adjustment process of the elderly person. In the event of an emergent health problem, a brief interview will usually get the necessary information to treat appropriately.

THE DATA BASE

The Health History

The nursing process begins with the collection of data. An excellent health history is basic to the success of the plan of nursing care. This history can also be the most difficult information to obtain from any client, sometimes more so from the aged. The subjective data is the patient's history; the objective data is information gathered from the physical examination and laboratory tests. Table 3.2 summarizes some of the difficulties encountered in history-taking with elderly clients. An important aspect of the health history is the nurse's ability to ask the appropriate questions and listen to the client's answers. It is necessary to have a firm theoretical knowledge base of normal age-related changes which serves as the foundation for interpreting information gleaned during the interviews.

Elderly clients can be slow in response to questions; any attempt to hurry the response may lead to confusion and anxiety (Mezey, Rauckhorst, & Stokes, 1980). Many older persons attribute their aches and pains to old age. They believe, either as a result of popular myth or lack of information, that physical and psychological problems are part of the normal aging process and that nothing can be done about such problems. This is not true; any physical or psychological ailment warrants a careful medical examination and thorough nursing assessment, just as it does in a younger individual. Obviously, the reliability of a client must be determined. Any change in mental status will hinder the history-taking process, and it is important to supplement data from other sources of information such as, family or other caretakers.

Hearing and vision impairments may impose sensory deficits even with corrective devices. Techniques such as speaking slowly, in low tones, and toward the ear with better auditory acuity are often helpful. Sitting, being face to face, and maintaining eye contact may also assist with communication in that some lip reading may be possible.

At the same time, there are different physical and physiological responses to some disease processes with aging. For example, while most younger individuals present with chest pain during a myocardial infarction, elderly clients may report only fatigue or shortness of breath. The nurse must be knowledgeable about normal age-related changes and how they differ from disease-related symptoms.

The educational and cultural background of the elderly person will affect the responses elicited during the interviews. One-quarter of the current aged population in the United States is foreign born. (This

TABLE 3.2 Potential Difficulties in Taking Histories from the Elderly

Difficulty	Factors Involved	Suggestions
Communication	Diminished vision Diminished hearing	Use well-lit room Eliminate extraneous noise Speak slowly in a deep tone Face patient, allowing patient to see your lips If necessary, write questions in large print
	Slowed psychomotor performance	Leave enough time for the patient to answer
Underreporting of symptoms	Health beliefs Fear Depression Altered physical and physiological responses to disease process Cognitive impairment	Ask specific questions about potentially important symptoms Use other sources of information (relatives, friends, other caregivers) to complete the history
Vague or nonspecific symptoms	Altered physical and physiological responses to disease process Altered presentation of specific diseases Cognitive impairment	Rule out treatable diseases, even if the symptoms (or signs) are not typical or specific Use other sources of information to complete the history
Multiple complaints	Prevalence of multiple coexisting diseases Somatization of emotions —"masked depression"	Attend to all somatic symptoms, ruling out treatable conditions Get to know the patient and the patient's complaints; pay special attention to new or changing symptoms Interview the patient on several occasions to complete the history

Source: Kane, R. L., Ouslander, J. G., & Abrass, I. B. (1984). *Essentials of clinical geriatrics* (p. 38). New York: McGraw-Hill. Reprinted by permission.

percentage will drop to 10% in the year 2000.) Roughly, less than 50% of the current aged have not completed high school. Therefore, it is best if words chosen for the interview are clear and simple. Use of slang, while helpful with some age groups (e.g., adolescents), may not be understood by the elderly. Questions should be brief and to the point, requiring only one response at a time. For example, when asking a patient about peripheral neuropathy, secondary to diabetes mellitus, the question to ask is, "Do you have any change of feeling in your feet?" An incorrect question would be, "Do you have any numbness, loss of feeling, or tingling in your feet?" This second question requires three answers, which may be confusing to the client. It is also important to rephrase a question to get the essential information from the client. This is especially true in the elderly when symptoms are vague, non-specific, and often attributed to old age itself. For example, when questioning an elderly client about chest pain, the nurse must ask about chest tightness, heaviness, pain, throbbing, squeezing, but also about any new fatigue or change in usual activities in daily living.

There are many health history outlines available: Eliopoulos (1984); Mezey, Rauckhorst, and Stokes (1980); Carnevali and Patrick (1986); and Hogstel (1981). It is often useful to review and edit these outlines in order to fit the needs of a specific setting and the interviewer's personal style.

Each section of the history is equally important and the order in which information is elicited depends on the nurse's style and the elder's level of comfort. The social history is often perceived as a non-threatening way to begin a health history. However, sensitive topics such as finances may be explored more easily on the second interview when a nurse-client relationship has ben established. It is essential to assess the ability of the elder to perform activities of daily living (ADL). Kane, Ouslander, and Abrass (1984) identified tasks which are slightly more complex than ADL but necessary to function in our society. These tasks have been referred to as instrumental activities of daily living (IADL). Such tasks require a combination of physical and cognitive abilities. Examples of instrumental activities of daily living include: writing, reading, cooking, shopping, the ability to travel, manage money, and take medications. Again, there are a multitude of ADL scales varying according to setting (Duke University, 1978; Katz, et al., 1963). This information can come from the client and/ or caregiver. Often, it may prove helpful to have the client demonstrate the tasks during the interview. Obviously, the functional assessment of the patient in an acute care situation is of limited value. The area of functional assessment is one best handled by an interdisciplinary team over a period of time.

Another important area of assessment is that of medications. It is essential to ask about both prescribed and over-the-counter (OTC) drugs. Clients of all ages may not consider OTC drugs as "medications." Specific questions about laxatives, cold remedies, analgesics, vitamins, home remedies, and so on, need to be asked. Any history of previous allergies or reactions to medications should be noted. This is also a good time to review the current medication regime, checking for any beneficial or adverse side effects. Compliance, as well as the client's knowledge about the current medication regime, should be assessed and documented. This is often facilitated by having the client collect all current medications for review with the nurse, as well as discarding any that are outdated.

Physical Examination

The purpose of the physical examination is to verify, clarify, and amplify the health history. Often the physical examination will alert the nurse to new problems (e.g., newly-elevated blood pressure) or forgotten history (e.g., abdominal scars).

Knowledge of age-related changes is important to the interpretation of physical findings in the aged and can help determine the plan of nursing care. Table 3.3 outlines the effects of aging on various body systems (Adams, 1982). The first column lists the physical and physiologic changes associated with aging for the different body systems. The second column gives normal age-related changes. The third column lists examples of potential health problems. This outline is certainly not all-inclusive, but is meant to identify major changes and related health problems. For a more complete account, a detailed discussion of each bodily system should be reviewed.

The physical examination starts with the greeting of the client, when an overall impression of such obvious items as skin, hair, and mobility can be assessed. Although the physical assessment occurs during the entire history-taking process, actual disrobing should not be done until the time the nurse is ready to start to examine the entire body. Carnevali and Patrick (1986) warned that with the elderly, who are often cold and may be at risk for hypothermia, it is necessary to limit exposure of body parts to a minimum. This is accomplished by careful draping to expose only the area being examined. Appropriate techniques for the examination must be modified according to the client's difficulties with mobility, balance, or hearing, for example. In order to reduce client fatigue, it is essential that the physical examination entail a minimum amount of position changes. The examination should be done in a systematic way, which minimizes the client's movements and reduces missing data. Once the nurse has become comfortable with the process of physical examination, it also becomes an opportune time for health education. For example, when examining an ear, the nurse can inquire about how the client usually cleanses the external canal. The response given by the elderly client may lead to topics that require health education.

TABLE 3.3 Effects of Aging

Morphological age changes in various systems	Related 'normal' age changes	Clinical pathological trends
Skin		
Atrophy	Skin thinned, wrinkled, dry, fragile, and discolored	Abrasions and infections
epidermis		Pruritis; intertrigo
sweat glands	Greying and recession of hair	Ulcers
hair follicles	Nails thin, brittle, ridged, and slow-growing	Onychogryphosis and other nail changes; paronychia
Pigmentary changes	Senile lentigines and seborrheic warts	Solar keratoses
Epidermal hyperkeratosis		Carcinoma
		intraepidermal
		basal cell
		squamous cell
Degeneration	Loss of elasticity	
collagen	Senile purpura	
elastic fibers	Campbell de Morgan spots	
Sclerosis of arterioles	Less padding	Pressure sores
Reduced subcutaneous fat	Less insulation	Hypothermia
Central Nervous System: Special Senses		
Eye		
Loss of orbital fat	Sunken appearance of eye	Entropion
	Laxity of eyelids	Ectropion
	Senile ptosis	Trichiasis (ingrowing lashes)
		Basal-cell carcinoma of eyelid
Stenosis of lacrimal duct	Epiphora	Dacryocystitis
		Lacrimal abscess

Lipid deposits in cornea Conjunctivitis sicca	Arcus senilis Reduced tears; dry cornea	Necrotizing sclerokeratitis; corneal ulcers *Slow loss of vision*
Shallow anterior chamber	Reduced filtration angle Increased intraocular pressure	Glaucoma angle closure (acute) open angle (chronic)
Loss of elasticity and nuclear sclerosis in lens	Presbyopia	Cataract
Degenerative changes in muscles of accommodation, iris, vitreous, retina, and choroid	Contracted pupils, slowed reflex Impaired visual acuity and tolerance of glare Reduced fields of vision Defective color vision Slowing of dark-adaptation Muscae volentes (objects floating in field of vision)	Macular degeneration *Sudden loss of vision* Retinal detachment Occlusive vascular disease: 1 Central retinal artery or vein 2 Posterior cerebral artery—*cortical blindness* from bilateral occlusion; sometimes vision denied (Anton's syndrome); visual hallucinations common; pupils react normally. Macular or vitreous hemmorhage
Degeneration in cortical neurons relating to vision (occipital lobes) and of intrinsic or extrinsic ocular muscles	Visuo-spatial perception and discrimination less accurate Impaired accommodation Limitation of upward gaze	Confusional states caused by sensory deprivation
Ear Degeneration of organ of Corti (loss of hair cells) Loss of neurons in cochlea (ganglion cells) and temporal cortex	Presbycusis—impaired: 1 Sensitivity to tone (high frequency) 2 Perception (especially against background noise)	Psychological effects of deafness (isolation; suspicion; depression)

(continued)

TABLE 3.3 (continued)

Morphological age changes in various systems	Related 'normal' age changes	Clinical pathological trends
Impaired elasticity affecting vibration of basilar membrane	3 Sound localization 4 Cortical sound discrimination	
Otosclerosis of ossicular chain in middle ear		Conductive deafness
Excessive wax accumulation		
Atrophy of striae vascularis (impaired endolymph production)	Impaired reflex postural control	Ménière's syndrome
Degeneration of hair cells in semicircular canals	Uncertainty and unreliability in moving about in darkness	
Nose, throat, and tongue		
Atrophic changes in mucosae	Impaired sense of taste and of smell	Risks of gas or food posioning
Neuronal degeneration (taste buds reduced 64% by age 75)	Diminished responsiveness of reflex cough and swallowing	Anorexia Food fads
Atrophy and loss of elasticity in laryngeal muscles and cartilages	Vocal folds slack, voice tremulous and pitch raised; power and range reduced	Malnutrition Avitaminosis Sublingual varicosities and hemorrhages Carcinoma of larynx (men) Post-cricoid carcinoma (women)

Central Nervous System: Brain and Spinal Cord
Macroscopic changes
Meningeal thickening, cerebral atrophy (brain weight down 10% between ages 30 and 70)

Histological changes
Earliest is patchy loss of dendrite spines on neurons followed by swelling of dendrite shafts and cell bodies, progressing to fragmentation and cell deaths. (Loss of synaptic connections, impaired electrochemical reactions, and neural dysfunction are thought to follow from reduction in dendrite neuropil.) In all cells—deposits of lipofuscin ('wear-and-tear pigment' formed in degenerating cytoplasm probably from lysosomes or mitochondria)

In neurons:
1. Loss of RNA, mitochondria, and enzymes in cytoplasm
2. Hyaline and eosinophilic inclusions and Lewy bodies
3. Neurofibrillary tangles, senile plaques, and granulovacuolar degeneration.

Different degenerative changes occurring with increasing frequency in people over 60 years of age, but not directly related with each other
Corpora amylacea: occur anywhere in brain tissue

Diminished intellectual responsiveness, mental agility, and abstract reasoning capacity
Impaired perception, analysis, and integration of sensory input
Failing short-term memory and learning ability
Less resilient, more rigid in outlook, tending toward being more self-centered, withdrawn, and introverted

Impaired sensory awareness (of pain, touch, heat and cold, and joint-position sense)
Sensori-motor performance slower to achieve accuracy
Impaired mechanisms controlling posture, anti-gravity support, balance, and moving equipoise (nerve conduction velocity reduced 10% by age 75)

Reduced intellectual reserves predisposing to acute confusional states
Dementia—deficits in intellect and memory similar to those of normal senescence begin earlier and act with greater intensity progressing to the disorientation and sustained mental, behavioral, and motor changes of presenile and senile mental deterioration
Depression
Persecutory symptoms of paraphrenia

Defective appreciation and localization of pain
Predisposition to falls and injuries

(continued)

TABLE 3.3 (continued)

Morphological age changes in various systems	Related 'normal' age changes	Clinical pathological trends
Vascular changes Intimal and medial fibrosis: Siderosis, amyloid and hyaline degeneration Atheroma—increasing in extent with age, but pathogenesis is multifactorial		Multiple infarct dementia Transient ischemic cerebral episodes Impending, progressing, and completed strokes Postural instability
Autonomic Nervous System Neurotransmission depends on acetylcholine and on the catecholamines dopamine and noradrenalin. Autonomic reflex response is probably weakened in old age by age-dependent reduction in synthesis and hydrolysis of these neurotransmitters combined with receptor loss. Autonomic dysfunction accompanies the Shy-Drager syndrome, parkinsonism, cerebrovascular disease, and various causes of neuropathy, particularly diabetes and alcoholism.	Predisposition to postural hypotension (asymptomatic) Impaired response to Valsalva maneuver Diminished baroreflex sensitivity Impaired thermal regulation in response to heat and cold Loss of appreciation of visceral pain Impaired alimentary motility	Symptomatic postural hypotension Defective autoregulation in the cerebral circulation Liability to falls Predisposition to hypothermia or heat stroke Misleading presentations of illness
Locomotor System *Muscles* *Atrophy* affecting both number and size of fibres conditioned by metabolic disorder and 'functional denervation.'	Loss of muscle bulk Nocturnal cramp Herniae: extra- and intra-abdominal	Muscular wasting, especially distal extremities

Decline in physical strength—'physiological' weakness

Disability, and limitation of range and speed of movements—combined effects of muscular weakness, joint stiffness, and impaired central mechanisms for sensorimotor performance:

1. Less precision in fine movements and in rapid alternating movements
2. Irregular timing of action, loss of smooth flow of one form of action into another
3. Slowing down to avoid outcome of one action before planning the next.

Asymptomatic, or slight backache; kyphosis, stoop and loss of height

Bone loss
osteoporosis; thinning of trabeculae and enlarged cancellous spaces.

Pathological weakness:

1. Metabolism: deficiency in serum Ca, K, Vitamin D
2. Endocrine: thyrotoxicosis, Cushing's syndrome, cortisone myopathy
3. Cardio-respiratory disease, anemia (anoxia)
4. Carcinomatosis

Severe backache, kyphosis, and fractures (inadequate bone density)
Osteomalacia: deficient calcification of normal bone matrix. Bone pain; myopathy; fractures.
Paget's disease (osteitis deformans)
Bunions; subluxation of small joints in hands and feet
Painful feet (and other chiropody problems)

(continued)

TABLE 3.3 (continued)

Morphological age changes in various systems	Related 'normal' age changes	Clinical pathological trends
Joints Degenerative changes in ligaments, peri-articular tissues and cartilage Synovia are thickened with villous hypertrophy Cartilage becomes yellow and opaque; there may be superficial erosions; and biochemical changes lead to mucoid degeneration; cyst formation and calcification	Loss of elasticity and resilience in joints Stiffness and predisposition to aches and pains Confidence and reliability of activity reduced Difficulty with intricate tasks (especially if complicated by uncompensated visual defect) Stooped posture, loss of height, and other distortions owing to atrophy and effects of weakness in skeleton and major muscle groups responsible for posture and antigravity support.	*Arthritis:* leading to ankylosis and contractures: 1. Osteoarthritis: such a commonplace of old age as to be considered almost 'physiological' 2. Rheumatoid arthritis: a constitutional disorder with onset usually in earlier adult life but not uncommon over 60 in either sex 3. Gout and pseudo-gout 4. Neuropathic arthropathy
Gastrointestinal System Dental caries; gingival recession Atrophic changes in jaw	Problems of adaptation to dentures and altered alignment of bite	Retained carious stumps Cysts; dental sepsis Angular fissures Oral ulcers Risk of parotitis Temporo-mandibular arthritis
Atrophy of mucosa, intestinal glands, and muscularis	Capricious appetite Asymptomatic alterations in intestinal secretion, motility, and absorption occur in 'normal' aging	Anorexia Malnutrition Hiatus hernia Achlorhydria (incidence increases over age 60): related to defective absorption of iron and vitamins, and to pernicious anemia

No significant age changes described in liver, and there are as yet no tests of function sufficiently refined to detect the impairment sometimes suspected in older patients	Constipation (prolonged gastrointestinal transit time) Diverticulosis (anywhere in gastrointestinal tract, but in colon related to a lifetime of low-residue diet)	Dysphagia (pseudo-bulbar palsy: esophageal reflux, pouches, and carcinoma) Peptic ulcer Fecal impaction Diverticulitis

Respiratory System

Coalescence of alveoli (atrophy and loss of elasticity in septa) Sclerosis of bronchi and supporting tissues Degeneration of bronchial epithelium and mucous glands	Total lung volume unchanged but vital capacity is diminished, O_2 diffusion impaired and respiratory efficiency reduced; as are sensitivity and efficiency of self-cleansing mechanisms	Increased susceptibility to pneumonia
Osteoporosis thoracic vertebrae rib cage Reduced elasticity and calcification of costal cartilage Weakness of intercostal and accessory muscles of respiration	Kyphosis and increasing rigidity of chest wall Functional reserve respiratory capacity is therefore impaired in old age, but clinical evidence is minimal unless evoked by illness. Compliance changes little because the rise to be expected from diminished elastic recoil is offset by increased lung stiffness (fibrosis) and loss of flexibility in chest wall.	Chronic obstructive airways disease: owing to *emphysema* (which predominates in 'pink puffers') combined with *chronic bronchitis* (underlying 'blue boaters') Pulmonary tuberculosis (reactivation of 'healed' tuberculosis) Carcinoma of bronchus Pulmonary embolism Concurrent respiratory disease and cardiac failure

(continued)

TABLE 3.3 (continued)

Morphological age changes in various systems	Related 'normal' age changes	Clinical pathological trends
Cardiovascular System Aorta: loss of elasticity in media and intimal hyperplasia	Aorta dilated and unfolded (may obstruct venous return in left side of neck therefore assess jugular venous pressure on right)	Aneurysm Aortic stenosis Arrhythmias
Cusps of heart valves degenerate: less resilient with nodular sclerosis and sometimes calcification which may extend into interventricular septum	Apex beat difficult to locate if chest rigid or distorted by kyphoscoliosis Stiffened valves cause murmurs: aortic systolic, mitral regurgitant; not necessarily significant	Conduction defects: bundle branch block probably indicates significant heart disease Pulmonary heart disease (pulmonary embolism)
Myocardial changes: lipofuscin deposits, myocardial fibrosis, and amyloidosis Atrophy and fibrosis of media, and intimal hyperplasia in coronary arteries Brown atrophy only in association with debilitating states: malnutrition, cancer, pernicious anemia, etc. (heart weight correlates with body weight)	No specific age-determined changes or degeneration in the heart (i.e., no 'senile heart disease') can be correlated convincingly with impaired cardiac function in old age but it is accepted that: 1. cardiac output declines owing to reduced stroke volume; 2. therefore capacity for physical work is limited; 3. a given amount of exercise raises heart rate and blood pressure more in old age than in youth.	Blood-pressure changes: difficult to define hypertension over age 65. B.P. readings alone do not constitute a diagnosis (it requires evidence of adverse effects on eye, heart, brain, and kidney). Hypotension often more sinister in old age.

Atheroma—incidence increases with age, probably promoted by hypertension and cigarettes

Genito-urinary System
Thickening of basement membrane of Bowman's capsule and impaired permeability
Degenerative changes in tubules
Atrophy and reduced numbers of nephrons
Vascular changes affect vessels at all levels from intimal thickening of the smallest, to arteriolar hyalinization and intimal hyperplasia in large arteries
Prostatic atrophy—acini and muscle with local areas of hyperplasia
Benign nodular hyperplasia present in 75% of males over 80 years of age
Histological (latent) prostatic carcinoma demonstrable in most males aged over 90 years (clinical carcinoma very much less)

Mental confusion and *profound weariness* should raise suspicion of heart disease in old people. They are often more prominent than anginal pain or even breathlessness (because of restricted activity)

Renal efficiency in waste disposal impaired by reduced renal mass and functional decline:
1. The number of nephrons is halved in an average life span
2. Renal blood flow is also halved by age 75
3. Glomerular filtration rate and maximum excretory capacity reduced by same proportion. The aging kidney can still maintain normal homeostatic mechanisms and waste disposal within limits, but it is less efficient, needs more time, and its reserves may be minimal. Therefore relatively minor degrees of dehydration, infection, or impaired cardiac output may precipitate failure

Ischemic heart disease is the most common cause of heart failure in geriatric medical practice

Renal calculi
Renal infections: pyelonephritis, cystitis
Prostatic disease
Gynecological disorders
Retention
Incontinence

(continued)

TABLE 3.3 (continued)

Other Systems
Endocrine

Hormones are maintained at the serum levels required for various homeostatic mechanisms by the balance struck between the rate of synthesis, the rate of secretion, the concentration of specific carrier proteins (which determine the levels of free or active fractions of hormones in circulation), and the rate of metabolic disposal in the tissues. A change in one factor will be offset by a compensatory shift in another to ensure that the hormone blood level remains unchanged. These factors may be affected by aging (though differently in different systems) but compensation is so effective that serum levels give little indication of age-changes in endocrine function, and they are difficult both to demonstrate and to interpret. Responsiveness and the ability to adapt to changing conditions tend to alter so that, although endocrine failure is not a consequence of normal aging, it is difficult to distinguish physiological change and, as in other systems, it may be poverty of reserves that precipitates evidence of deficiency.

1. Age does not affect fasting lucose level, but there is an age-related decrease in glucose tolerance. Pancreatic cell secretion in response to hyperglycemia is diminished, and diabetic abnormality of glucose tolerance increases with age. It is not clear whether this should be attributed to the change in cell sensitivity, to reduced insulin sensitivity (owing to decreased gluco-receptor-response at the cell surface), or to the effects of changing body composition with age, especially obesity. Receptor loss, caused by complex changes in cellular enzyme activity, probably accounts for many age changes in endocrine regulation, but whatever the cause, aging is acknowledged to be the outstanding factor contributing to clinical diabetes.

2. Functional thyroid activity decreases with age; BMR and radioactive iodine uptake fall. The rate of metabolic disposal of thyroxine is probably decreased, and the gland compensates by reducing the secretion rate to keep the hormone blood level unchanged, but there is an age-related fall in plasma levels of triiodothyronine (T_3) converted from thyroxine (T_4). It is not known whether this indicates reduced thyroid production, impaired conversion, or altered disposal rate. The free thyroxine index (serum T_4 divided by T_3 uptake $\times$ 100) and serum TS level are probably the best indices of thyroid performance, but all tests of thyroid function are suspect in old people who are ill. *Myxedema* is three to four times more common than *thyrotoxicosis* in older people, and atypical presentation is common to both: non-specific debility, anemia, hypothermia and paranoid psychiatric illness in hypothyroidism; atrial fibrillation unresponsible to digitalis, heart failure, and osteoporosis in hyperthyroidism.

3. A post-menopausal fall in estrogen levels is associated with an increased rate of loss of bone in elderly women. Primary testicular failure in men over 50 leads to falling plasma testosterone levels and high levels of gonadotrophins. There is increased conversion of androgen to estrogen in peripheral tissues, declining sexual performance and fertility, and loss of muscle mass.
4. Changes in antidiuretic hormone secretion in the elderly affect responses to hemodynamic stimuli and to serum osmolality and so many induce postural hypotension or upset fluid balance.

Homeostasis

Particularly vulnerable in old age to plasma or blood loss, dehydration, potassium depletion, and metabolic acidosis. At rest the normal old person can maintain a constant internal environment, but capacity to react to stress, even the demands of daily living, is markedly lessened owing to two key characteristics of aging:

1. poverty of reserve which impairs the ability to restore systematic equilibrium quickly when it is upset;
2. breakdown in coordination because different organs age at different rates, and functions dependent on the performance of several systems are therefore impaired.

Age-related shortcomings in neuroendocrine control mechanisms underlying defective homeostatis have been discussed earlier.

Reprinted from: G. Adams (1982). *Essentials of geriatric medicine* (2nd ed.; pp. 11–19). Oxford: Oxford University Press.

Psychosocial Assessment

Psychological changes that are a normal part of the aging process (see Table 3.1) have implications for the evaluation of an elderly individual's personality, cognitive functioning, and affect. Oviously, there is also tremendous interplay among the elder's physical health, mental health, and social situation. An elderly person with cataracts may feel unable to continue to go out and grocery shop due to decreased visual acuity. This isolation can have profound effects on the phychological well being of the elderly person, as well as on physical health and social needs.

The major developmental tasks in old age include maintaining independence, relinquishing power, coping with losses, initiating a life review process, and developing a philosophical perspective on life (Mezey, Rauckhorst, & Stokes, 1980). Throughout the interview and assessment process, the nurse should keep in mind these tasks and note the degree to which the elder seems to be accomplishing them. Questions related to retirement adjustment, financial concerns, changes in family structure, and the death of dear friends can elicit much information that will help shape a successful plan of care.

SPECIAL CONSIDERATIONS

Elder Abuse

Currently, it is estimated that between 700,000 and 1.1 million incidents of elder abuse occur annually in the United States (Pillemer & Finkelhor, 1988). Most states now have mandatory reporting laws which require that nurses and a variety of other health-care professionals report any suspected cases of elder abuse, neglect, or mistreatment to appropriate state agencies (Thobaden & Anderson, 1985). Nursing has an important role to play in assessing the safety and well being of the elderly. In the past, when abuse or neglect was suspected, it was very difficult to know how to deal with such suspicions as these matters were often deemed to be private and beyond the purvue of a professional health assessment. Today, a more appropriate approach is one of advocacy and support.

Elders have a right to feel safe and secure from any physical or emotional battering. Within the context of the health assessment, the nurse should ask elderly persons if they have any safety problems at home. One way this might be asked is: "I know your daughter is responsible for most of your daily care. Is this a good arrangement? Are the two of you getting along as well as you always have?" This enables the elder to discuss any problems or at least to give clues if there is any trouble. When there is a complaint of elder abuse, the nurse should provide the elder with the appropriate agency telephone numbers in order to complain and request protective services. If the elderly person has a severe dementia and is documented to be incompetent, the nurse should proceed based on set agency policy. If no policy exists, discussion with a supervisor should ensue in order to use appropriate channels for action.

It should be noted that there are a number of age-related changes and disease-related signs and symptoms which may mask or exaggerate signs and symptoms of elder abuse. When in doubt, a consultation with other members of the interdisciplinary team or outside expert consultation should be sought.

At times, there may be suspicion of institutional abuse or neglect, as in the case of elders residing in nursing homes or recently discharged from hospitals. The same thoughtful review of the history, signs, and symptoms applies. Table 3.4 provides a list of possible manifestations of abuse or neglect.

Assessment of the Caregiver

Much has been written recently about the "old-old" and the burgeoning number of individuals who are living beyond 85 years of age. This group represents the fastest growing segment of America's aging population, and a new development which is evolving in tandem is the aging of the caregiver. Today, it is not unusual to have a 75-year-old woman bring her 95-year-old mother in for care, and it is important that the nurse be sensitive to the health and social support needs of such an elderly caregiver. It is not hard to understand how care provided can be minimal or inadequate when the person delivering that care may also be struggling with diminishing health.

Many families take enormous pride and derive great satisfaction from giving care to their elderly loved ones. It would be insensitive and unacceptable to suggest to these people that their parents need a nursing home. The nurse needs to work through, over a period of time, what the care needs are for the elder and the caregiver. As a result, the nurse can try to provide an assortment of services which will support the family unit. The assistance of social service departments can be invaluable in such cases. The most important nursing action is to continually reassess the stability of the situation on a regular basis in order to prevent its deterioration and subsequent consequences to the health of the elderly person and caregiver.

CASE STUDY

Mrs. T. is a 91-year-old caucasian widow of Irish descent who has lived with her daughter, Anne, and granddaughter, Annie, for the past 12 years. She is a tall woman, five feet nine inches, and weighs about 140

TABLE 3.4 Possible Manifestations of Elder Abuse and Neglect

Abrasions	Malnutrition
Lacerations	Inappropriate clothing
Contusions	Poor hygiene
Burns	Over sedation
Freezing	Over or under medication
Depression	Untreated medical problems
Fractures	Behavior that endangers
Sprains	Failure to meet legal obligations
Dislocations	
Decubiti	
Dehydration	

pounds. She has taken a "fluid pill" for the last several years along with her .125 mg (of digoxin). Mrs. T. appears to be in relatively good health, is able to fix her own meals with limited assistance, and can go up and down stairs alone. She has no difficulty going to the bathroom.

About two years ago, Mrs. T. was taking 2 mg of Coumadin qd for prophylactic anticoagulation due to a period of extended bedrest which was necessary to heal a pelvic fracture after a fall. She fell on an elevated step between two rooms and was immediately taken to the hospital where the diagnosis of a pelvic fracture was made. She recovered without complication and was fine until one year ago when, after Thanksgiving dinner, she vomited blood and was taken to the hospital. During that admission, her Coumadin was discontinued and she was transfused, stabilized, and discharged home.

This past summer, Mrs. T. was visiting one of her other daughters when she was noted to have memory loss. That is, she was uncertain as to whether she had taken her pills and unable to remember the names of her newest grandchildren. Her long-term memory was intact.

Mrs. T. is worried about these changes in her memory and her daughter is convinced it is the result of the discontinuation of the Coumadin. The physician can find no abnormal laboratory values and has said he believes that Mrs. T. is exhibiting changes consistent with aging.

A nurse practitioner has been assigned to Mrs. T. for her regular visits and knows that it is very important to include her daughter in the interview while ensuring that the daughter does not "do the talking" for Mrs. T.

Mrs. T. presents as a well groomed, pleasant woman who is somewhat distressed at her new memory lapses but says, "after all, I'm 91 years old." She states she has the most wonderful family in the world and that all her needs are attended to. The nurse notes that Mrs. T's vital signs are: T. 98.6°, P. 66 (regular), R. 18, B.P. 140/80. The only other physical complaint is that of arthritis in her knees, but she says it only flares "with bad weather." She is unable to recall what she ate for breakfast, but can recall that FDR was president during World War II and was married to Eleanor. "And they had a little dog," she adds. The nurse believes the best approach for Mrs. T. at this time is monthly coagulation studies along with regular mini-mental status examinations. The nurse offers to check on Mrs. T. and her daughter periodically and encourages them to call if they have any concerns.

CONCLUSION

Nursing assessment of elderly persons is a complex, multifaceted process which requires great skill and acumen. There is no substitute for experience, and the best way to become expert is to practice the process repeatedly under the guidance of someone who is adept in nursing assessment. In the following chapters of this book, specific physical and psychosocial needs of older adults will be addressed which will build upon the overview provided here.

REFERENCES

Adams, G. F. (1982). *Essentials of geriatric medicine* (2nd ed.). New York: Oxford University Press.

Carnevali, D., & Patrick, M. (Eds.) (1986). *Nursing management of the elderly.* Philadelphia: Lippincott.

Duke University Center for the Study of Aging and Human Development. (1978). *Multidimensional functional assessment: The OARS methodology.* Durham, NC: Author.

Eliopoulos, C. (Ed.) (1984). *Health assessment of the older adult.* Menlo Park, CA: Addison-Wesley.

Eliopoulos, C. (1983). *Nursing administration of long term care.* Rockville, MD: Aspen.

Fitzsimons, V. M. (1985). Maintaining a positive environment for the older adult. *Orthopaedic Nursing,* 4(3), 48–51.

Hogstel, M. (Ed.) (1981). *Nursing care of the older adult.* New York: John Wiley & Sons.

Kane, R. L., Ouslander, J. G., & Abrass, I. B. (1984). *Essentials of clinical geriatrics.* New York: McGraw-Hill.

Katz, S., Ford, A. B., Moscowitz, R. S., Jackson, B. A., & Jaffe, M. W. (1963). Studies of illness in the aged. The index of ADL: A standard measure of biological and psychosocial function. *Journal of the American Medical Association,* 185, 94–98.

Mezey, D. M., Rauckhorst, L. H., & Stokes, S. A. (1980). *Health assessment of the older individual.* New York: Springer Publishing Co.

National Institute on Aging. (1987). *Personnel for health needs of the elderly through year 2020.* September 1987 Report to Congress, United States Department of Health and Human Services.

Pillemer, K., & Finkelhor, D. (1988). The prevalence of elder abuse: A random sample survey. *The Gerontologist, 28,* 51–57.

Stokes, S. A., Rauckhorst, L. H., & Mezey, M. D. (1980). Health assessment: Considerations for the older individual. *Journal of Gerontological Nursing, 6*(6), 328–337.

Thobaden, M., & Anderson, L. (1985). Reporting elder abuse: "It's the law." *American Journal of Nursing, 85,* 371–374.

Part II

Physical Needs In
The Elderly

The central chapters in this book address specific areas of need or concern with respect to nursing care for elderly persons. These areas of concern have to do with functional well being, whether that relates to the promotion of wellness, the maintenance of present quality in living, or the correction of some disorder. The point is to identify areas in which elderly persons might stand in need of or benefit from nursing intervention in relationship to an actual or potential health problem.

In each case, these chapters take their primary structuring principles from the nursing process and specified nursing diagnoses. The *nursing process* is the single, common method whereby nurses organize their professional activities, approach clients in a systematic and scientific problem-solving manner, and establish accountability for what they do. *Nursing diagnoses* already are, and will increasingly become, the language of nursing care and the professional responsibility of each individual nurse. For these reasons, after a brief introduction to its particular topical area, each of the 10 central chapters that follows is organized around the structure of the nursing process and model nursing diagnoses.

Within each chapter, the section on *assessment* identifies important factors to consider when entering into a nursing relationship with an elderly person. In assessment, it is essential to distinguish normal age-related changes from those which may represent or serve as clues to some sort of alteration in health status. Assessment leads naturally to the formal statement of a *nursing diagnosis*, which specifies both a category of nursing concern and specific etiologies from which the concern has arisen or might arise in particular cases.

On the basis of one or more nursing diagnoses, *planning* sets forth an overall strategy of general goals and measureable objectives to guide client behaviors designed to redress or ameliorate problems or to enhance wellness. From this flow nursing *interventions* and an ongoing process of *evaluation* to determine whether or not appropriate outcomes have been achieved. When that is not the case, evaluation becomes the basis for reassessment and renewed initiation of the entire nursing process.

In the chapters that follow, contributors have been asked to organize what is known about nursing care of the elderly in light of their own clinical expertise, the best available research, and current literature in the field. Their shared aim has been to combine these elements in ways that serve the needs of nursing practice and nursing education. Concrete examples appear throughout the text and longer case studies are introduced as appropriate.

Because psychosocial and spiritual issues that are distinctive in human life can rarely be addressed fully or satisfactorily in the presence of underlying physical distress, chapters in this Part begin with analyses of a broad range of physical needs: Betty Ferrell and Bruce Ferrell take up comfort in terms of pain, hygiene, skin, mouth care, and sleep; Pamela Duchene and Joan LeSage examine hydration and nutrition, which have broad ramifications for obesity, failure to meet bodily requirements, bowel elimination, skin integrity, and deficits in self-care or knowledge; Mary Jirovec explores problems of urinary and fecal incontinence; Jean Wyman considers issues of mobility and safety, including falls; Barbara Brandt addresses issues in sensory functioning; and Stephanie Nagley discusses issues in cognitive functioning in the form of acute ard chronic brain syndromes.

Chapter 4

Comfort

Betty R. Ferrell and Bruce A. Ferrell

INTRODUCTION

The challenge to "comfort always" in the old adage, "To cure some-times, to relieve often, to comfort always," has become a familiar one in the areas of palliative care and hospice nursing in recent years. This same challenge is appropriate to the emerging field of gerontological nursing care. For the elderly person, comfort is a very appropriate goal for health promotion, as well as in times of acute or chronic illness.

The concept of comfort is frequently cited in the literature and is accepted as a universal goal for nursing. The concept, however, has not been thoroughly defined. Many words have been used to describe comfort, including such terms as to soothe, to aid, to ease, to offer consolation or solace, or to palliate.

Comfort can be thought of as closely associated with the "art" of nursing. Nursing as a caring profession has as an essential activity the goal of comfort. Comfort is also a distinguishing characteristic of the nursing profession. The goals of geriatric medicine are focused on prevention, diagnosis, and treatment of disease. Gerontological nursing focuses on well being, the nursing diagnosis of actual or potential health problems, and the elderly person's experience of illness. It is evident that interventions of comfort are consistent with the basic aims of gerontological nursing.

Although central to gerontological nursing, comfort in the elderly offers particular challenges. Older adults often have multiple chronic illnesses with many threats to comfort. These chronic illnesses, as well as normal physiologic processes of aging, are often not amenable to cure or even relief. Often, comfort is all that is available to elders. With an ever-aging population, many ethicists and policy makers would contend that aggressive curative treatments will no longer be available in an environment of cost containment and limited resources. Thus, palliative treatment and goals of comfort may increasingly be the choice of care for the elderly, but this does not exclude approaches to gerontological nursing which involve aggressive treatment of problems that pose threats to the comfort of elderly persons. Goals of maintaining mobility and avoiding social isolation are applicable to all comfort interventions, whether for healthy elders or for those with acute or chronic illness.

Comfort is not an isolated concept in gerontological nursing; rather, it is closely related to other critical concepts in care of the elderly. For example, there are strong correlations between comfort and patient satisfaction with care (Merskey, 1976; Sternbach & Timmermans, 1975). Comfort is also associated with overall quality of life (Ferrell, Wisdom, & Wenzl, 1989). Interventions aimed at the elderly person's comfort have the ability to influence the total quality of care for the individual.

Gerontological nursing is family-centered nursing. Care of the elderly involves sensitivity to the larger family unit and active family involvement in the plan of care. Nurses in various settings, including acute care hospitals, long-term care facilities, and home health, are well aware that patient comfort is a major priority of nursing care as perceived by family members (Kristjanson, 1986).

Comfort is most often equated with assessment and intervention for physiological needs. In fact, however, comfort is a multidimensional concept involving physical, psychological, and emotional needs. This chapter addresses five major areas of comfort for the elderly: pain, hygiene, skin care, mouth care, and sleep. Each of these is a major area of threat to comfort in the elderly, as well as an opportunity for improving functional well being and quality in living.

Comfort implies successful intervention for an actual or potential problem, but also involves a personal and individual experience. Use of the nursing process provides assessment of the problem area, diagnosis of the problem amenable to nursing intervention, collaborative planning with the elderly person and family, implementation of comfort interventions, and evaluation of these interventions in terms of goals and objectives based on client perceptions of comfort. The nursing process thus provides a cycle of dynamic activity with a central goal of comfort.

ASSESSMENT

Pain

Although pain is considered a universal sensation, perception of pain is an individual experience involving both nociceptive and affective components. Nociception refers to the sensory reception of pain. The affective component includes modification of pain reception by higher cortical functions, such as attention, memory of past experiences, and other emotional or behavioral expressions of the perceived pain.

In clinical practice, pain should be assessed from the perspective of the person experiencing it. In the words of McCaffery (1979, p. 8), "Pain is what the patient says it is and exists when he says it does." The person who is hurting is the chief source of information for nursing assessment of pain.

The demography and epidemiology of pain in the elderly has not been well studied. Elderly persons do suffer disproportionately from chronic illnesses and, therefore, also disproportionately suffer chronic pain. Recent research (Bayer, et al., 1986; Yoshikawa & Norman, 1987) has suggested that the elderly frequently exhibit atypical presentations of pain. Silent myocardial infarctions and silent abdominal emergencies suggest that the elderly may have decreased pain perception. Other research (Harkins, Kwentus, & Price, 1984) is contradictory as to whether elderly persons have increased or decreased pain perception when compared to younger people.

Assessment of chronic pain in the elderly is essential as pain is the most common symptom of disease. Assessment is also important for evaluation of intervention effectiveness. Frail elderly are vulnerable to both undertreatment and overtreatment of pain. Further, assessment differentiates acute endangering pain from longstanding chronic pain. For example, a patient hospitalized with chronic arthritis and a long history of pain may develop an acute pain warning of myocardial infarction. Accurate nursing assessment of pain is critical to early diagnosis and treatment of potentially life-threatening health problems.

Because pain is such an individual experience, a multidimensional approach to assessment is required. Assessment should include physical, psychosocial, and functional dimensions. Table 4.1 lists some important features of a pain assessment. This assessment should be preceded by an accurate medical history and medication history. Assessment of any trauma should be thoroughly evaluated because of concerns about elder abuse. Pain from traumatic causes would include falls, a common problem in the elderly (see Chapter 7).

The elderly may present special problems in obtaining an accurate pain history due to memory impairment, depression, and cognitive

TABLE 4.1 The Clinical Assessment of Pain

History	Physical exam	Pain assessment tools	Assessment of other constructs
Medical history	Routine exam	Visual analog Scale	Physical symptoms Fatigue
Pain history	Signs of trauma		Sleep
Location		Pain graphs	Appetite
Frequency	Musculoskeletal		
Duration	examination	Pain diaries	Depression
Severity	Trigger points		
Interventions	Swellings		Anxiety
Exacerbations	Masses		
Alleviations	Tender spots		Activities of
	Inflammation		daily living
History of trauma			
	Range of motion		Quality of life
Medications	Joints		
Drug	Muscles		Cognitive function
Dose			
Route	Functional		
Frequency	impairment		
Efficacy			
Reactions			
Previous pain experiences			

impairment. Underreporting of symptoms may result because elderly persons expect pain associated with aging and disease. Elders may not report their pain because they fear the meaning of the pain. They may fear taking medications or they may feel that the pain cannot be relieved (Ferrell & Schneider, 1988). The importance of family and caregivers as a source of information for the pain assessment cannot be overemphasized (Ferrell & Ferrell, 1989).

Psychological assessment related to pain should include evaluation of mental status and evaluation for depression. These concepts are discussed more fully elsewhere in this book (see Chapters 9 and 12), but it is important to recognize the close relationship between these concepts and pain.

Many instruments have been developed to assist clinicians and researchers to measure, document, and communicate accurately pain in elderly persons. Figure 4.1 illustrates examples of tools for use in pain assessment. The pain graph can be used to help individuals identify their daily pain experience in relation to medication use and activity. The visual analog scale helps to quantify pain intensity for better communication between caregivers and elders. It is more effective to

A

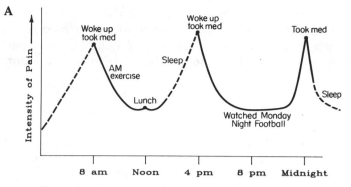

Example of a pain graph showing irregular pain
medication administration resulting in wide swings
in pain intensity and decreased night time sleep

B

Date/ Time	Activity	Medication	Pain Intensity*	Other Symptoms+

* Pain Intensity: A number of scales may be used
   Example: 0 = no pain; 1 = mild; 2 = discomforting;
                     3 = distressing; 4 = horrible; 5 = excruciating

+ Other Symptoms: Possibilities exist for other measures
   such as functional status, side effects or other symptoms
   of greatest concern.

C

Visual Analog Scale

No Pain   The Worst Pain
                                                               I have ever had

Directions: Please make a mark on the line
indicating the amount of pain you are
experiencing now.

FIGURE 4.1 Examples of three tools useful in the clinical assessment of pain: a)
Pain Graph; b) Pain Diary; c) Visual Analog Scale.

report that the person "had a pain intensity of 88 which decreased to 29 thirty minutes after receiving pain medication," than to simply chart "patient complains of moderate pain." A pain diary is also a useful tool to assist elderly persons in recording their pain experience more objectively.

Hygiene

An individual's ability to perform self-care activities, such as feeding, grooming, bathing, and toileting, is basic to the goal of comfort. These essential activities satisfy fundamental needs and, in so doing, make a major contribution to the comfort of the elderly.

Determination of functional status and the ability to accomplish activities of daily living is a primary component of the assessment of hygiene needs. Specifically, nurses should assess the elderly person's self-care abilities and personal care routines. Nurses should also assess the elder's own perceptions of hygiene needs, as well as determining who, if anyone, assists with the person's hygiene.

Observation can be an important skill in assessment of hygiene needs. Nurses should observe the individual's dress, general appearance, personal habits, body odor, and condition of hair and skin. Assessment of cognitive ability can also provide useful information in the assessment of hygiene needs. Neglect of self-care needs is often an early sign of cognitive impairment, such as dementia. Awareness of previous hygiene patterns may facilitate detection of behavior changes indicative of possible pathology. Incontinence assessment is also an important prerequisite to planning for hygiene needs. Both cognitive assessment and incontinence are discussed elsewhere in this book (see Chapters 6 and 9) but should be considered in planning comfort needs of the patient (Moseley, 1985).

Skin

The skin serves as the body's chief protection and is, therefore, critical to the comfort of elderly persons. The skin protects from bodily injury and also assists in the regulation of temperature. Skin problems can result in potential threat to comfort, ranging from mild irritation to severe discomfort. Wrinkled skin, "old age spots," and grey hair are the stereotypical signs of age in our society. Appearance of the skin is important to psychological comfort of the older adult.

Nurses should be aware that there are many normal physiological changes in the skin associated with aging. Table 4.2 outlines some of these changes. The skin has a decreased thickness of the epidermis, delayed healing time, and decreased cutaneous cellular immunity. Decrease in ground substance and subcutaneous fat results in increased

TABLE 4.2 Normal Skin Changes with Aging

Element	Change	Clinical consequences
Epidermis	Thinning	Fine wrinkles, scaling
	Reduced melanocyte	Ultraviolet sun sensitivity
Dermal junction	Reduced corrugation	Increased shearing, tearing, blister formation
Dermis	Altered collagen	Increased fragility, reduced elasticity, decreased turgor
	Altered elastin	
	Thinning	
Sebaceous glands	Reduced activity	Increased dryness
Sweat glands	Reduced number	Increased dryness
	Reduced activity	Altered thermal regulation
Hair	Altered regional growth	Baldness in males, increased facial hair in females
Nails	Reduced growth	Irregular thickness, susceptibility to trauma

risk for trauma and decubitus ulcer formation. Also, there is altered elastin and collagen resulting in common wrinkling of skin and decreased turgor in the elderly. The capillaries become fragile resulting in the bruises under the skin surface known as senile purpura. Also, the number and function of sebaceous and sweat glands decrease, resulting in dryness of the skin (Gilchrest, 1986). Proliferative and repair mechanisms of skin cells are altered with age. Hair, nails, and skin may show a 50% reduction in cell myotic activity and growth. Finally, altered central nervous system thermal regulation operating through vascular control of the skin contributes greatly to morbidity and mortality from heat strokes, as well as hypothermia in the elderly (Berlinger, 1986).

In addition to physiologic changes associated with the passage of time, many elderly persons suffer skin abnormalities due to years of environmental influences. Environmental exposure to solar radiation, chemical substances, or medications early in life may result in altered skin repair mechanisms and increased risk of cancer (Shelley & Shelley, 1982).

Because of the changes outlined above, elderly persons are at great risk for trauma and pressure sores. Because of decreased sensitivity to pain and the fragile nature of skin, serious injury, disruption of skin, and infection may go unrecognized from what seemed to be minor trauma. Cognitive impairment, agitated behavior, gait instability, falls, and physical restraints represent significant risks for skin injuries in the elderly.

Changes in other body systems greatly influence the skin. Alterations in circulation, pigmentation, and nutritional state influence the vulnerability of the skin. Wound excretions and urinary or bowel incontinence create major skin irritation. Elders often present with complaints of skin irritation as an initial sign of undiagnosed incontinence. Nurses should also be aware that the patient who simply presents with poor skin hygiene and self neglect may be showing early subtle signs of significant cognitive impairment and dementia.

The prevention and treatment of *pressure sores* (decubitus ulcers or bed sores) is one of the most frustrating problems in gerontological nursing. Pressure sores are a major cause of discomfort and morbidity in elderly persons, as well as being responsible for tremendous resource expenditure. The term, "decubitus," from the Latin root meaning "lying down," is really a misnomer in that these sores may develop in any position. The term, "pressure sore," is more desirable because it is more accurate and describes the pathophysiology (Reuler & Cooney, 1984).

The incidence of pressure sores is difficult to estimate. Reports range from an incidence of 10 to 25% for elderly patients in acute care hospitals (Allman, et al., 1986) to an estimate that 20% of all nursing home patients will develop a pressure sore at some time (Reuler & Cooney, 1984).

Factors implicated in the development of pressure sores can be divided into primary and secondary categories based on their direct role in causality. Primary causes of pressure sores include pressure, friction, and shear; secondary causes include moisture, immobility, malnutrition, anemia, vascular insufficiency, cognitive impairment, and denervation.

Pressure on the skin surface resulting in capillary insufficiency and tissue ischemia is the most important cause of pressure sores. The maximum pressure at which no ischemia will occur has not been defined. Several animal studies have demonstrated a definite pressure-time relationship for the development of necrosis, as well as the effect of alternating pressure (Kosiak, 1961). Clinical evidence suggests that two-hour turning does prevent ischemia and necrosis for most patients. Although no controlled clinical trials exist, it has been accepted that reduced skin surface pressure below capillary filling pressure (25–35 mm Hg) will also prevent ischemia and necrosis (Seiler & Stahelin, 1985a).

Friction is the force created when two surfaces in contact move across each other, as when a patient is slid across the bed sheets. Friction causes skin shear, skin ischemia, and necrosis. Friction also results in abrasion, enhancing the risk for infection. Shear forces result from traction of the skin and lead to interruption of the blood supply to the skin and subcutaneous tissue. For example, when the head of the bed is raised, this causes the torso to slide down and traction occurs on the skin. The blood supply to the skin is then interrupted over the sacrum, deep fascia, and buttocks. The result is sacral ischemia, skin necrosis, and pressure sore formation (Bennett, et al., 1984).

Moisture macerates the skin and enhances infection. This occurs clinically where patients constantly perspire or are incontinent. Maceration softens the skin and results in edema. Macerated skin is more susceptible to abrasion and infection.

Contributing factors, such as immobility, malnutrition, anemia, vascular insufficiency, fecal incontinence, cognitive impairment, and a host of others, may be considered risk factors for the development of pressure sores (Allman, et al., 1986). Assessment of these factors has been valuable in trying to assess and prevent risk of pressure sore development in individual patients. The Norton Risk Assessment Scale (Norton, McLaren, & Exton-Smith, 1975) is one such scale that uses these factors to identify patients at risk for pressure sores, although it has been criticized for poor clinical accuracy in predicting sores (Lincoln, et al., 1968). Recently, the Braden Scale has been considered more promising (Bergstrum, et al., 1987), but it is still undergoing clinical trials for predictive accuracy.

Finally, staging of existing sores is important in documenting their severity, choosing initial therapy, and assessing prognosis. The Shea Scale is the most widely used scheme for staging pressure sores (Shea, 1975). Stage I is indicated by erythema, edema, and induration, but skin remains intact. This lesion will heal spontaneously in a few hours or days if pressure and shear are removed. Stage II is indicated by those changes described in Stage I, but the skin is broken. The skin has abrasion or blister formation. In addition to the removal of pressure and shear, this lesion requires a dressing and careful attention to prevent wound contamination and infection. Stage III is indicated by ulcer formation and is usually accompanied by purulent drainage and some eschar formation. Stage III ulcers are limited to the dermis and subcutaneous fat. These ulcers usually require debridement, extensive nursing care, and protracted lengths of time to heal; sometimes surgical excision and reconstruction is needed. Stage IV is indicated by infection extending into underlying muscle, bone, and deep tissue planes. These ulcers are frequently associated with sepsis and high mortality. Treatment is similar to Stage III ulcers but frequently requires surgery and prolonged systemic antibiotics.

Assessment of healing of pressure sores remains difficult. Although the Shea Scale is widely used, it is not very sensitive to small changes. Pressure sores do not frequently heal in the predictable, progressive, systematic fashion that the Shea classification would suggest. Our experience suggests that surface area measurement is more sensitive and useful for the measurement of pressure sore healing (Ferrell & Osterweil, 1989). Surface area may be estimated by the cross product of the largest diameter of the sore, by comparison to a circular or elliptical template of known area, or by integrating the area of a wound tracing (Braden, 1988). Table 4.3 summarizes the scales frequently cited in the assessment of pressure sores.

The incidence of skin malignancies is higher in the elderly. Premalignant skin changes, known as keratoses or leukoplakia, are early signs for the development of skin cancers. An important nursing intervention in these premalignant conditions is to instruct the patient to avoid sun exposure and to use sun screens. Common malignant conditions in the elderly include basal cell carcinoma, squamous cell carcinoma, and melanoma.

Nurses should also assess for skin allergies, including acute and delayed hypersensitivity. A common example is that of acute dermatitis resulting from exposure to detergents used in laundering of bed linens.

Skin reactions to medications are frequently seen in the elderly as in the case of skin reaction to tetracycline with sun exposure. Many other medications have side effects involving skin reactions and, therefore, a careful medical history is important during skin assessment.

Finally, nurses should be aware that skin problems may relate to some cardinal signs of elder abuse and neglect. The dependent patient who exhibits poor hygiene, chronic rashes from incontinence, and bruises in locations not associated with falls or extensor surfaces, may be manifesting the first signs of family fatigue, neglect, or abuse.

An outline of sample criteria for skin assessment is included in Table 4.4. As with all nursing assessment, an important issue is the communication of assessment data to other nurses and to the patient's physician. Precision of language is important in such communication,

TABLE 4.3 Instruments for Pressure Sore Assessment

Instrument	Purpose	Ease of administration	Reliability/ validity	Reference
Shea Scale	Severity	Easy	Fair	Shea, 1975
	Healing	Easy	Poor	Ferrell & Osterweil, 1988
Surface Area	Healing	Fair-Hard	Fair-Good	Ferrell & Osterweil, 1988 Braden, 1988
Norton	Risk	Easy	Poor-Fair	Norton, McLaren, & Exton-Smith, 1975 Lincoln, et al., 1968
Braden	Risk	Easy-Fair	Fair-Good	Bergstrum, et al., 1987 Braden, 1988

TABLE 4.4 Skin Assessment in the Elderly

History	Physical exam	Assessment of age-related problems
Rashes	Inspection of entire	Specific neoplastic lesions
Eruptions	skin surface	Squamous cell
Irritations	Overall pigment	Basal cell
Itching	Color	Melanoma
	Trauma	
Trauma		Trauma
Blisters	Inspection of moist	
Abrasions	epithelial borders	Nutritional assessment
Bruises		
	Inspection of specific	Medication evaluation
Abnormal growths	skin lesions	
Moles	Distribution	Cardiovascular assessment
Warts	Pattern	
"Age Spots"	Margins	Pressure sore risk
	Centers	
Sun exposure	Size	Incontinence evaluation
Exposure to allergens	Palpation of skin	
Plant	Turgor	
Animal	Moisture	
Mineral (nickel)	Thickness	
Food	Subcutaneous fat	
Pollens		
Medications	Palpation of skin	
	lesions	
Exposure to toxins	Texture	
Chemicals	Elevation	
Cleaning Fluids	Density	
	Vascularity	
Skin care products	Tenderness	

since observations of skin features depend upon detailed characteristics of interest.

Mouth Care

Mouth care is a key component of patient comfort and also an example of an area of health promotion activity which can enhance comfort. Contrary to common belief, natural teeth do last a lifetime with appropriate hygiene. Many health care providers, as well as elderly people, mistakenly feel that the loss of teeth is an unavoidable phenomenon. The ability to retain one's own teeth is a great asset to comfort by avoiding painful conditions of dentures and assisting in normal nutrition.

The cause of tooth decay in the elderly is poor dental hygiene. Proper cleansing of the teeth using a fluoride toothpaste remains essential through the later years. Nurses should be particularly attuned to the needs of elderly persons who are unable to provide their own mouth care. This may include individuals with limited motor skills, cognitive impairment, or functional impairments.

There are normal physiological changes associated with aging that have implications for dental health. A decrease in saliva production results in decreased ability to cleanse the mouth and remove food particles. Decreased saliva may also result in a feeling of mouth dryness. There are also changes associated with the oral mucosa. Oral tissue becomes less vascular and more fibrous, resulting in greater risk of injury and infections. Oral infections in the elderly can be fatal and are associated with other disease, such as endocarditis (Baum, 1985).

Commonly, older people will have partial or complete loss of teeth, making the need for dentures inevitable in many individuals. Forty-two percent of all people over the age of 65 are edentulous (DHHS, 1987). Sixty to 90% of individuals with their own teeth have dental caries and periodontitis. Maxillary and mandibular ridges shrink after teeth are lost, so eventually all dentures inevitably create oral problems. It is no wonder, then, that many persons become disenchanted with the frustration of denture use, even to the point of malnutrition.

Nursing assessment should also include appraisal of the oral cavity for cancer. Persons with history of tobacco use are at greatest risk. Leukoplakia, or white patches in the mouth, are an early sign of oral cancer. Leukoplakia may appear on any surface of the oral cavity, including the tongue and lips. Early diagnosis of oral cancer is critical, as advanced oral cancers are a major illness and create significant discomfort for elders.

Dental health can greatly influence social comfort for the individual. The mouth is important to self-esteem and the person's ability to express feelings, such as with a smile or frown. The ability to communicate verbally is also impacted by the state of the mouth. Table 4.5 includes criteria for mouth assessment in the elderly.

Sleep

It has been accepted that increasing age is associated with increasing sleep disturbances. Complaints of sleep disturbances are common in the elderly population; thus, the use of sleeping pills increases with age. Individuals commonly make subjective complaints of poor sleep, even while caregivers paradoxically report increased total sleep time and more frequent daytime naps. Studies revealing a variety of sleep changes with advancing age can generally be summarized as indicating that age is associated with a decrease in both quality and quantity of

TABLE 4.5 Oral Assessment in the Elderly

Oral history	Oral examination
Oral hygiene habits	Inspection
Routine dental exams	Facial symmetry
Prior dental problems	Moist membrane borders
	Gingiva
Previous oral surgery	Teeth
Chewing problems	Tongue
	Palate
Dentures	Pharynx
Partial	Observe movements
Complete	Salivary volume
Fit and security	Tongue
Taste	Palate
Oral skin lesions	Gag reflex
Dry mouth	Swallow
Swallowing problems	Palpation
Change in voice	Lips
	Floor of mouth
Tobacco history	Palate
	Tongue
	Specific lesions
	Submandibular nodes
	Cervical nodes

sleep (Clark, 1985; Lerner, 1982). Table 4.6 lists some of the changes in sleep associated with age.

Sleep disorders can be classified into four general categories: disorders of initiating and maintaining sleep (e.g., those caused by discomfort, depression or anxiety, sleep apnea, or "restless legs"); disorders of excessive sleep (e.g., those caused by overmedication, narcolepsy, or sleep apnea); disorders of the sleep-wake cycle (e.g., those related to dementia, delerium, or jet lag); and dysfunctions associated with sleep, sleep stages, or partial arousals (e.g., sleepwalking or sleep-related seizures). Probably the most common causes of sleep disturbances are situational, or related to symptoms of specific diseases. Some of the more common serious sleep disorders in the elderly include psychologic disturbances, such as anxiety or depression, drugs or alcohol, and physiologic abnormalities such as sleep apnea or restless legs.

It is ironic that medications for sleep may be one of the most common causes of sleep disturbance. Indeed, it is common for sleeping pills to simply perpetuate sleep disturbances. Sleeping pills, though usually effective in initiating sleep, frequently reduce the quality of sleep. Most hypnotic drugs reduce REM (rapid eye moment) sleep and alter the amount of other stages of sleep resulting in overall decreases in quality

TABLE 4.6 Changes in Sleep with Aging

Measurement	Change with aging
Subjective	
Insomnia	Increased
Total sleep time	Increased
Night time awakenings	Increased
Daytime naps	Increased
Wake time after sleep onset	Increased
Objective	
Rapid eye movement (REM)	Unchanged
Non-REM sleep	Decreased
Stage 1–3	Unchanged
Stage 4	Decreased
Total sleep time	Decreased
Sleep latency	Increased
Awakenings during sleep	Increased

of sleep. Moreover, hypnotic drugs in the elderly have high potential for oversedation, confusional states, agitation, restlessness, hypotension, and falls. In the final analysis, the risks frequently outweigh the indications for these medications. Many hypnotics have other systemic effects, such as exacerbating sleep apnea, resulting in addiction and interactions with other medications. Finally, most elders develop tolerance to hypnotic medications, resulting in loss of effectiveness and potential for abuse.

Depression is a very common cause of sleep disturbance in the elderly. Depression usually manifests difficulties in initiating and maintaining sleep, but some depressed persons may actually have increased sleep. Other neurovegetative signs may also be present, such as anorexia and nervousness, although pure anxiety disorders are less frequent in the elderly. In the more severe forms of depression, psychotic features such as delusions and hallucinations may be directly exacerbated by sleep deprivation. Thus, a vicious cycle of psychopathology may exist.

It is important to differentiate depression from other causes of sleep disturbances because treatment with conventional sleeping pills will usually exacerbate the depression. By contrast, management with sedating antidepressant medications is usually quite effective for correction of the sleep impairment as well as the overall mood disorder. It is also interesting that Electro-Convulsive Therapy (ECT or shock treatments), which may be the treatment of choice for many elderly patients with significant depression, usually results in an immediate and dramatic return to normal sleep habits.

Sleep apnea can be a life-threatening cause of sleep disturbance. This disease is usually associated with chronic lung disease or a history of midbrain damage. It may also be associated with profound hypothyroidism and micro agnathia or deficient development of the lower jaw. The sleep apnea syndrome is usually classified as a disorder of excessive sleep since the etiology seems to lie in the midbrain control of respiration during sleep. In general, sleep apnea can further be divided into three categories: obstructive, central, or mixed. Obstructive sleep apnea involves the relaxation of the hypopharynx during sleep and partial or complete obstruction of air flow at the glottis. Although this syndrome has been associated with loud snoring, snoring *per se* is a result of nasopharyngeal relaxation, rarely resulting in airway obstruction. During obstructive sleep apnea, chest wall respiratory movements continue in spite of upper airway obstruction. During central sleep apnea, complete respiratory movement will cease. Mixed varieties do occur, but in any event, when systemic oxygen saturation falls low enough, individuals wake with a startle response, resume regular respiration, and eventually doze back off to sleep. This pattern will continue as often as every three or four minutes throughout the night, resulting in very poor quality sleep. These persons wake in the morning, being very tired and drowsy all day, but having little insight into their sleep behavior.

It is important to recognize the syndrome of sleep apnea because left untreated, many individuals will develop congestive heart failure and arrhythmias associated with chronic intermittent hypoxemia, and nocturnal sudden death is not an uncommon outcome. Moreover, sleep apnea is frequently a curable (or at least treatable) disorder. Obstructive apnea is prevented by a nocturnal tracheostomy button, whereas central apnea may be greatly ameliorated by nighttime low-flow oxygen and/or medications that may stimulate the central respiratory center.

Another common cause of sleep disorder in the elderly has become known as "restless legs." The term has become a catchall description for a variety of musculoskeletal causes of sleep-related complaints, including muscle cramps, aches, fatigue, and restlessness. This syndrome has been associated with nocturnal myoclonus and peripheral neuropathies. Nocturnal myoclonus is a neuromuscular disorder of myoclonal jerks, usually occurring during sleep latency and REM periods. Nocturnal myoclonus may be caused by certain physiologic states including chronic uremia, hyperthyroidism, and medications including beta blockers. In some persons, however, symptoms are purely subjective and no true myoclonus is observable. In these persons a higher incidence of peripheral neuropathies is found, resulting from diabetes, although many may be idiopathic (Guilleminault, 1984).

A thorough sleep history is important to assessment. Nurses should determine prior sleep habits, use of sleep medications, and other aids to sleep (Johnson, 1986). There are signs to observe for sleep disturbances, such as yawning, difficulty in concentrating, dozing, and dark eyes.

NURSING DIAGNOSIS

After thorough assessment of areas of comfort, the nurse proceeds through the nursing process by formulating a nursing diagnosis. A nursing diagnosis is a conclusion or judgment about a client which derives from assessment data and which is amenable to nursing intervention. In the case of comfort, the diagnosis will judge deficiencies or threats to the client's comfort for which nursing actions can offer increased comfort (Rantz & Miller, 1987).

Table 4.7 lists the North American Nursing Diagnosis Association (NANDA) diagnosis and etiologies related to comfort in each of the five subject areas addressed in this chapter. In addition, sample nursing diagnoses follow within the framework of the subsequent steps of the nursing process.

PLANNING

Planning is the process in which nurses consider the nursing diagnosis, establish goals, define measurable objectives, and select interventions consistent with those goals and objectives. This step is essential to insuring the comfort of the elderly person. Although true in all areas of planning, because comfort is such an individual experience, this area critically demands involvement by elderly clients in order to establish desirable and realistic goals. Table 4.8 lists comfort goals and objectives in each of the five areas discussed in this chapter.

INTERVENTION

Intervention is the implementation of nursing actions to meet established goals and objectives. In the case of comfort, interventions are selected nursing actions directed at specific problems to meet established goals of comfort (Strauss & Corbin, 1984). Because of the broad scope of this chapter, nursing interventions related to comfort are illustrated in two ways. First, Table 4.8 includes a list of possible interventions associated with nursing diagnoses, goals, and objectives taken from each of the five areas addressed in this chapter. Second, because

TABLE 4.7 Nursing Diagnoses Related to Comfort in the Elderly

Diagnostic category	Etiologies—related to:
COMFORT, ALTERATION IN: Pain, Acute Pain, Chronic	Biologic injuring agents Chemical injuring agents Physical injuring agents Psychologic injuring agents
SELF-CARE DEFICIT: Feeding, Bathing/Hygiene, Dressing/Grooming, Toileting	Intolerance to activity, decreased strength & endurance Pain, discomfort Perceptual or cognitive impairment Neuromuscular impairment Musculoskeletal impairment Depression, severe anxiety Impaired transfer ability Impaired mobility status
SKIN INTEGRITY, IMPAIRMENT OF: Actual Potential	External (environmental) Internal (somatic)
ORAL MUCOUS MEMBRANE, ALTERATION IN	Pathologic condition—oral cavity Dehydration Trauma Nothing by mouth (NPO) instructions for more than 24 hours Ineffective oral hygiene Mouth breathing Malnutrition Infection Lack of or decreased salivation Medication
SLEEP PATTERN DISTURBANCE	Internal factors External factors

Source: T. A. Duespohl (1986). *Nursing diagnosis manual for the well and ill client.* Philadelphia: W. B. Saunders.

TABLE 4.8 Examples of Planning and Intervention

NURSING DIAGNOSIS: Comfort, Alteration in: Pain, Acute

GOAL: The client will experience a decrease in pain intensity as measured by a visual analog scale.

OBJECTIVES:

1. Client will be able to move about and walk without pain within 48 hours.
2. Client will be able to write a pain diary and make use of a visual analog scale to identify severity of pain within 48 hours.
3. Client will be able to select activities and alternatives to promote relaxation and pain relief within one week.

NURSING INTERVENTIONS:

1. Assess current medication use and instruct client regarding principles of analgesia.
2. Instruct client on the use of a pain diary and a visual analog scale to identify pain patterns.
3. Assist client in identifying possible non-drug pain relief measures, such as relaxation, distraction, heat/cold, massage, etc.

NURSING DIAGNOSIS: Self-Care Deficit: Hygiene

GOAL: The client will be able to meet basic needs for bathing and grooming as evidenced by personal appearance and reports of self esteem.

OBJECTIVES:

1. Client will be able to state goals for oral care and body hygiene within 48 hours.
2. Client will be able to bathe self with assistive devices, such as a shower chair, within 24 hours.
3. Client will plan a schedule of daily activities within 48 hours to help lessen fatigue.

NURSING INTERVENTIONS:

1. Assess client's current abilities and environment.
2. Identify with client desired bathing and grooming goals.
3. Provide assistive devices to enhance mobility and function for grooming.
4. Assess client for incontinence and skin care needs.

NURSING DIAGNOSIS: Skin Integrity, Impairment of: Potential

GOAL: Client will demonstrate behaviors to prevent skin breakdown associated with incontinence.

OBJECTIVES:

1. Within one week, the client will be able to explain the need for skin hygiene after each toileting.
2. Client will be able to demonstrate self-care within 48 hours.
3. Client will be able to select proper incontinence aids at own discretion within one week.

INTERVENTIONS:

1. Assess functional and pharmacologic causes of incontinence.

(continued)

TABLE 4.8 (continued)

2. Instruct client regarding incontinence, moisture, chemical irritation, and skin integrity.
3. Instruct client regarding control of moisture, chemical and infectious contamination.
4. Assess client for incontinence, skin care hygiene, and such needs as incontinence pads or pants.

NURSING DIAGNOSIS: Oral Mucous Membrane, Alteration in:

GOAL: To minimize breakdown of integrity of oral mucosa as determined by oral inspection and client's reports.

OBJECTIVES:

1. Client will be able to report beginning signs of oral mucosa breakdown as they occur.
2. Client will be able to establish a mouth care routine four times a day.
3. Client will be aware of comfort measures to be used as prescribed by the physician.
4. Client will be able to select aids to stimulate salivation within 24 hours.
5. Client will be able to perform a daily oral self-assessment of condition of oral mucosa during hospitalization.

NURSING INTERVENTIONS:

1. Instruct client regarding danger of infection with breakdown of integrity of oral mucosa.
2. Establish routine mouth care QID, including brushing and normal saline rinse.
3. Provide comfort measures, such as cool drinks, rinses, and prescribed medications, e.g., anesthetic lozenges, viscous lidocaine, or analgesics.
4. Assist client in selection of aids that stimulate or replace saliva, and choice of foods (e.g., lemonade, lemon drops).
5. Perform oral assessment daily/p.r.n. for signs of infection or ulceration. Instruct client on self oral assessment post hospital care.

NURSING DIAGNOSIS: Sleep Pattern Disturbance

GOAL: The client will report feelings of increased rest and decreased fatigue.

OBJECTIVES:

1. Client will be able to resume normal sleep patterns as supportive measures become effective.

NURSING INTERVENTIONS:

1. Instruct client on appropriate use of analgesic or hypnotic medications.
2. Discuss, with family, sleeping aids, such as massage, quiet or soothing music, warm food or beverages, appropriate temperature and lighting control.
3. Assist client and family with a sleep diary to determine patterns and cycles.
4. Formulate a schedule for exercise and rest.
5. Explore possible psychological causes, such as grief, anxiety, and depression.

of the high incidence of morbidity in the elderly related to pressure sores, possible interventions in that area are explored in greater depth.

Nursing interventions related to pressure sores include relief of pressure, debridement, control of infection, use of dressings, and nutrition. Relief of pressure is the single most important aspect of prevention and treatment of pressure sores. Pressure relief can be accomplished in a variety of ways, including frequent turning, the use of local padding, and various pressure reducing beds.

Frequent turning of immobilized patients has been the mainstay of pressure relief since Kosiak (1961) identified the two-hour critical time interval at which constant local pressure resulted in irreversible ischemic injury. In addition to diligent turning, patients should be placed in 30 degree oblique positions to relieve pressure over bony prominences and the most common ulcer location (Seiler & Stahelin, 1985a). Various local skin padding devices, such as "donuts," are poor interventions because they actually impede local circulation. Nevertheless, heel protectors may be quite useful in preventing friction, but require careful monitoring to avoid strap pressure and tourniquet effect.

Many types of beds and mattresses are available to reduce pressure, including foam mattresses, water beds, various air mattresses, and air fluidized beds. Of the bedding choices, foam mattresses are probably the least expensive and most convenient. These advantages are offset by the fact that foam mattresses offer the least pressure reduction (Redfern, et al., 1973). Foam mattresses can also be criticized for their frequent contamination by urine, feces, and wound drainage. Water beds are available, but their pressure reduction is modest and their inflation pressure is critical. Overinflation or underinflation results in less than optimal pressure reduction (Lilla, Friedrichs, & Vistnes, 1975). These beds are usually rubber or plastic; thus, perspiration and moisture may be a problem. Weight may require special facilities and has limited use of water beds. Various types of air mattresses have also been introduced, but even with alternating air mattresses, pressure reduction is modest. Air mattresses also require specific inflation, and alternating air mattresses can be criticized for their expenses and noise of operation.

"Air fluidized" beds involve a levitation medium (either glass beads or air) that has been altered by turbulent air flow in order to enhance pressure dispersion. These beds offer the greatest potential for pressure reduction and labor conservation by not having to turn patients as often. Other potential benefits include a dry environment that may decrease the effects of perspiration and incontinence, and a freely movable surface that may reduce friction and shear forces. Although initially criticized for the limited posture they afforded patients, newer models now allow patients a variety of positions, including semi-fowelers. Air fluidized beds have not been widely used because of their cost and weight, although one randomized trial argues their effectiveness over conventional beds (Allman, et al., 1987).

Debridement can be accomplished in the operating room, or, more commonly, it is carried out over several days at the bedside with gauze abrasion or biologically using proteolytic enzymes to help liquify the necrotic tissue. Available enzymes include trypsin, papain, collagenase, and sutilains. Of these, only collagenase is capable of digesting undenatured collagen as is found in most eschar. Unfortunately, we lack clinical trials comparing the results of various enzymes available. Some studies do support the use of these products over dry gauze dressings alone (Yucel & Basmajian, 1974).

Most pressure sores become infected at some time during this course. Infection is a major cause of delayed healing, long-term morbidity, and mortality in patients with pressure sores (Daltry, Rhodes, & Chattwood, 1981). Complications related to infection include sepsis, sinuous tract formation, and osteomyelitis. Debridement, drainage, and removal of necrotic material alone will control most infections. Systemic antibiotics are of no proven benefit in most ulcers probably because of reduced vascularity in the region. Their use should be reserved for patients who appear septic, have cellulitis, or have osteomyelitis. Topical antiseptics may decrease bacterial counts, but may also be harmful. Iodine and hexachlorophene are toxic to granulation and young epithelial tissue (Rodeheaver, et al., 1982). Topical antibiotics may temporarily reduce bacterial counts, but typically result in emergence of resistant organisms.

Dressings are essential for the maintenance of a microenvironment conducive to healing by secondary intention. Both granulation and epithelialization are impeded by dessication and lack of oxygen (Seiler & Stahelin, 1985b). Therefore, maintenance of a moist environment and exposure to oxygen are important. Occlusive dressings should not be used if they are impermeable to oxygen and water, since they may enhance infection. Several semi-permeable dressings are available, but none have been shown clearly superior to saline soaked gauze dressings for advanced ulcers. Semi-occlusive dressings are helpful in reducing contamination. Urine and feces may continuously contaminate pressure sores and prolong healing. However, in many cases there is no substitute for diligent nursing care in keeping patients clean and dry.

It has been accepted that malnutrition is common in frail elderly and a major impairment to wound healing (Morley, 1986). Many patients in nursing homes with pressure sores are malnourished. Once nutritional status has been assessed, intervention should consist of supplying sufficient calories to cover needs due to fever, infection, and other stresses that may be present. The use of enteral or parenteral hyperalimentation may be required in patients whose appetite or disability impairs adequate intake. Nutritional assessment must continue throughout the treatment course to insure adequate replenishment of deficits and to prevent complications, such as hyperglycemia and fluid volume and electrolyte disturbances. Besides protein and calories, vitamins and minerals may also affect wound healing. There are suggestions that zinc and Vitamin C accelerate wound healing (Morley, 1986).

EVALUATION

The nursing process is incomplete without the final step of evaluation. Evaluation occurs as the nurse assesses the effectiveness of the interventions in achieving the established goals. Evaluation is a dynamic process frequently involving alteration and reformulation of goals, objectives, and interventions to meet the client's changing needs.

Comfort, as a multidimensional construct, is also dynamic. The client is the best authority in evaluating his or her own comfort. The exception is with the cognitively-impaired elderly for whom the nurse will have a challenging task of evaluating comfort through observations.

HEALTH PROMOTION AND WELLNESS

Comfort is often considered to be a concept appropriate during times of injury or illness. To comfort implies that a discomfort exists. Nursing care is also focused on the well individual for health promotion and disease prevention. The elderly person should be encouraged to seek health behaviors which promote continued comfort and limit discomforts associated with normal physiologic changes accompanying aging or with illness.

Elderly persons must understand that health promotion can reduce the negative consequences of aging and that one's level of comfort is amenable to influence. For example, adequate dental care, routine dental examinations, and oral hygiene can greatly influence painful oral problems and nutrition with life-long consequences.

A major problem in our aging society has been the misconceptions surrounding normal aging versus disease. Many people assume that aging must be characterized by discomfort, and that pain and other symptoms are unavoidable in old age. An important intervention for the well elderly is education regarding the pathology of disease versus normal aging.

Nurses also need to be involved in education of the public regarding principles of preventive care and early diagnosis of illness. Breast cancer, for example, is a major concern for the older woman and yet is curable if diagnosed early. Breast self-examinations and routine health assessments including mammography are life-saving activities for many women.

As an example of health teaching, nurses should encourage elderly women to seek health activities which minimize the effects of disease. Such women should be counseled regarding calcium supplements to avoid bone loss. Elderly persons with arthritis should assume an adequate program of exercise and rest to avoid bone injury and complications of illness. A healthy lifestyle can make a difference between a person effectively coping with a chronic illness and experiencing minor discomforts versus the individual with major complications from a chronic illness experiencing major discomforts.

CONCLUSION

Comfort is an important concept on which all nursing care should be based. Comfort is the individual's perception of well being and should serve as an evaluation criteria for all nursing interventions. Advances in the field of gerontological nursing will develop new instruments and technologies for improvement in nursing care. The evolution of this field should also be concerned with improved interventions for comforting elderly persons.

Nurses should be reminded that comfort as an outcome does not result from a passive approach. Comfort is the result of skilled assessment, accurate diagnosis and planning, and skilled intervention and evaluation in areas of threats to comfort. This philosophy is inherent in the Latin origin of the word comfort, *comfortis*, meaning intensive (*com*) and strong (*fortis*). An intensive and strong approach to comfort for the elderly will greatly contribute to quality of life and health.

REFERENCES

Allman, R. M., Laprade, C. A., Noel, L. B., Walker, J. M., Moorer, C. A., Dear, M. R., & Smith, C. R. (1986). Pressure sores among hospitalized patients. *Annals of Internal Medicine, 105,* 337–342.

Allman, R. M., Walker, J. M., Hart, M. K., Laprade, C. A., Noel, L. B., & Smith, C. R. (1987). Air fluidized beds or conventional therapy for pressure sores—a randomized trial. *Annals of Internal Medicine, 107,* 641–648.

Baum, B. J. (1985). Alterations in oral function. In R. Andres, E. L. Bierman, & W. L. Hazzard (Eds.), *Principles of geriatric medicine* (pp. 288–296). New York: McGraw-Hill.

Bayer, A. J., Chadha, J. S., Farag, R. R., & Pathy, M. S. (1986). Changing presentation of myocardial infarction with increased age. *Journal of the American Geriatrics Society, 34,* 263–266.

Bennett, L., Kavner, D., Lee, B. Y., Trainor, F. S., & Lewis, J. M. (1984). Skin stress and blood flow in sitting paraplegic patients. *Archives of Physical Medicine and Rehabilitation, 65*, 186–190.

Bergstrum, N., Braden, B. J., Laguzza, A., & Holman, V. (1987). The Braden Scale for predicting pressure sores. *Nursing Research, 36*, 205–210.

Berlinger, H. (1986). Aging skin, Parts I & II. *American Journal of Nursing, 86*, 1138–1141, 1259–1261.

Braden, B. J. (1988). Measuring skin integrity. In M. Frank-Stromborg (Ed.), *Instruments for clinical research* (pp. 379–390). East Norwalk, CT: Appleton & Lange.

Clark, H. (1985). Sleep and aging. *Occupational Health Nursing, 33*, 140–145.

Daltry, C. W., Rhodes, B., & Chattwood, J. G. (1981). Investigation into the microbial flora of healing and non-healing decubitus ulcers. *Journal of Clinical Pathology, 34*, 701–705.

Department of Health and Human Service [DHHS]. (1987). *Oral health of the United States adults: The national survey of oral health in U.S. employed adults and seniors, 1985–86.* Washington, DC: U.S. DHHS, Public Health Service, National Institutes of Health, NIH Publication #87–2868.

Ferrell, B. A., & Ferrell, B. R. (1989). Assessment of chronic pain in the elderly. *Geriatric Medicine Today, 8*(5), 128–134.

Ferrell, B. A., & Osterweil, D. (1989). Measuring the volume of pressure sores [Letter to the editor]. *Journal of the American Geriatrics Society, 37*, 288.

Ferrell, B. R., & Schneider, C. (1988). Experience and management of cancer pain at home. *Cancer Nursing, 11*, 84–90.

Ferrell, B. R., Wisdom, C., & Wenzl, C. (1989). Quality of life as an outcome variable in management of cancer pain. *Cancer, 63*, Supp. Issue, 2321–2327.

Gilchrest, B. A. (Ed.) (1986). The aging skin. *Dermatologic Clinics, 4*(3).

Guilleminault, C. (1984). Sleep and sleep disorders. In C. K. Cassel & J. R. Walsh (Eds.), *Geriatric medicine* (Vol. II, pp. 192–210). New York: Springer-Verlag.

Harkins, S. W., Kwentus, J., & Price, D. D. (1984). Pain and the elderly. In C. Benedetti, C. R. Chapman, & G. Moricca (Eds.), *Advances in pain research and therapy*, Vol. 7 (pp. 103–121). New York: Raven Press.

Johnson, J. E. (1986). Sleep and bedtime routines of non-institutionalized aged women. *Journal of Community Health Nursing, 3*, 117–125.

Kosiak, M. (1961). Etiology of decubitus ulcers. *Archives of Physical Medicine and Rehabilitation, 42*, 19–29.

Kristjanson, L. (1986). Indicators of quality of palliative care from a family perspective. *Journal of Palliative Care, 1*(2), 8–17.

Lerner, R. (1982). Sleep loss in the aged: Implications for nursing practice. *Journal of Gerontological Nursing, 8*(6), 323–326.

Lilla, J. A., Friedrichs, R. R., & Vistnes, L. M. (1975). Flotation mattresses for preventing and treating tissue breakdown. *Geriatrics, 30*(9), 71–75.

Lincoln, R., Roberts, R., Maddox, A., Levine, S., & Patterson, C. (1986). Use of the Norton Pressure Sore Risk Assessment Scoring System with elderly patients in acute care. *Journal of Enterostomal Therapy, 13*, 132–138.

McCaffery, M. (1979). *Nursing care of the patient in pain.* Philadelphia: Lippincott.

Merskey, H. (1976). Psychiatric aspects of the control of pain. In J. J. Bonica & D. Albe-Fessard (Eds.), *Advances in Pain Research and Therapy*, Vol. 1 (pp. 711–716). New York: Raven Press.

Morley, J. E. (1986). Nutritional status of the elderly. *American Journal of Medicine, 81,* 679–695.

Moseley, J. R. (1985). Alterations in comfort. *Nursing Clinics of North America, 20,* 424–438.

Norton, D., McLaren, F., & Exton-Smith, A. (1975). *An investigation of geriatric nursing problems in hospital.* Edinburgh: Churchill Livingston.

Rantz, M., & Miller, T. (1987). How diagnoses are changing in long-term care. *American Journal of Nursing, 87,* 360–361.

Redfern, S. J., Jeneid, P. A., Gillingham, M. E., & Lunn, H. F. (1973). Local pressures with ten types of patient-support systems. *Lancet, 2,* 277–280.

Reuler, J. B., & Cooney, T. C. (1984). Pressure sores. In C. K. Cassel & J. R. Walsh (Eds.), *Geriatric medicine* (Vol. I, pp. 508–516). New York: Springer-Verlag.

Rodeheaver, G., Bellamy, W., Kody, M., Spatafora, G., Fitton, L., Leyden, K., & Edlich, R. (1982). Bactericidal activity and toxicity of iodine-containing solutions in wounds. *Archives of Surgery, 117,* 181–185.

Seiler, W. O. & Stahelin, H. B. (1985a). Decubitus ulcers: Preventive techniques for the elderly patient. *Geriatrics, 40*(7), 53 60.

Seiler, W. O., & Stahelin, H. B. (1985b). Decubitus ulcers: Treatment through five therapeutic principles. *Geriatrics, 40*(9), 30–44.

Shea, J. D. (1975). Pressure sores: Classification and management. *Clinical Orthopedics and Related Research, 112,* 89–100.

Shelley, W. B., & Shelley, E. D. (1982). The ten major problems of aging skin. *Geriatrics, 37*(9), 107–113.

Sternbach, R. A., & Timmermans, G. (1975). Personality changes associated with the reduction of pain. *Pain, 1,* 177–181.

Straus, A., & Corbin, J. (1984). Comfort work in the hospital. In *Chronic illness and the quality of life* (pp. 152–169). St. Louis: C. V. Mosby.

Yoshikawa, T., & Norman, D. (1987). *Aging and clinical practice: Infectious diseases.* New York: Igaka-Shoin.

Yucel, V. E., & Basmajian, J. V. (1974). Decubitus ulcers: Healing effect of an enzymatic spray. *Archives of Physical Medicine and Rehabilitation, 55,* 517–519

Chapter 5

Hydration and Nutrition

Pamela Muhm Duchene and Joan LeSage

INTRODUCTION

The accomplishments of Eubie Blake (1883–1983) as an American jazz pianist and composer are well recognized. Almost as famous is Mr. Blake's comment reported in the *London Observer* (February 13, 1983): "If I'd known I was going to live this long, I'd have taken better care of myself." Concerns with regard to aging and nutrition appear to be twofold: enhancing quantity and quality of life. Many have concerns centering around the issue of longevity and whether or not a particular diet will result in a long existence. They wonder whether a "fountain of youth" is linked with specific foods and eating styles. Animal research involving dietary restrictions, which cannot be ethically replicated in humans, confirms that nutrition can influence aging (Masoro, 1984). Study of centenarians suggests an association of longevity with agrarian culture, diet, and work patterns (Mazen & Forman, 1979).

The second focus of concerns about aging and nutrition relates to quality rather than quantity of life. This is the concern of the present chapter, whose purpose is to discuss factors affecting hydration and nutritional status in older persons, and to present possibilities for promotion of optimum hydration and nutritional status of the aged through the nursing process.

ASSESSMENT

Relationships among aging, nutrition, and disease are not well understood. Nutritional adequacy, however, is of fundamental importance to health and well being. To assess the nutritional and health status of the elderly, one must consider: criteria for nutritional adequacy; psychological, physical, and socioeconomic factors affecting dietary intake; components of nutritional history; clinical observations; and age-related factors affecting nutritional status. A single assessment method is usually inadequate on its own, so several techniques are needed to determine nutritional status.

Criteria for Nutritional Adequacy

Anthropometric measurements provide information about body proportions, size, and weight, including information about body stores of fat and muscle. Serial assessments can help monitor nutritional interventions. When height and weight are difficult to obtain for non-ambulatory persons, wheelchair scales are useful. Formulas to estimate stature (knee-height measurement and weight), as well as norms for those aged 75 years and older, are available (Chumlea, Roche, & Mukherjee, 1987). Interpretation of data may be affected by individual differences in age-related changes, such as reduction in height, variation in the amount and distribution of body fat, and change in tissue compressibility and elasticity. The individual's current weight, usual weight, and ideal body weight should be determined. Edema can mask weight loss. Anthropometric measurements require little other than a tape measure and skinfold calipers (Shuran & Nelson, 1986).

Laboratory tests which may be beneficial in determining nutritional status include: total count lymphocytes, serum albumin, total iron binding capacity, transferrin, urinary creatinine, hematocrit, and hemoglobin (Bistrian, et al., 1975). A significant difficulty exists with regard to interpretation of biochemical measurements in the elderly, as norms for most measurements in older individuals have not been clearly established. Thus, in addition to laboratory measures, nutritional assessment of older people should encompass other methods, i.e., history taking and physical assessment (Foley, Libow, & Sherman, 1981). Assessments should include determination of protein-calorie nutrition, as protein-calorie malnutrition leads to impaired immunologic defense and increased susceptibility to infection.

Recommended Dietary Allowances (RDAs; Whitney & Cataldo, 1983) do not give recommendations for higher nutrient requirements for the elderly. Older adults are included in RDAs for groups of males and females over age 50. The only special recommendation for age 65 and over is the reduction in total caloric intake for people over 75 years old. RDAs are set above average requirements and reflect current knowledge, but they will not always meet the need of any one individual, especially one with illness. Nutrient dense foods are necessary to keep the required reduction in caloric intake from causing deficiencies of essential nutrients.

Selection and analysis of a diet, using food groupings which supply the Basic Four nutrients, is convenient. While this method does not regulate intake of cholesterol, saturated fats, and sodium, it can guide older adults to improve their nutritional state.

Factors Affecting Dietary Intake

Psychological

The psychological status of an individual affects food intake and preferences. Nutritional deficiencies may be associated with psychological problems, such as anxiety, apathy, depression, and confusion. For example, anxiety frequently provokes self-selected therapeutic measures, such as reduction or increase of food or alcohol intake. Apathy and depression can be contributors to anorexia. Confusion may result in altered food intake. Individuals who are disoriented may fail to recall when they last ate; therefore, they may eat meals too frequently, or fail to eat at all. Disorientation may result in a failure to prepare food safely, leading to risks of food poisoning, contamination, or fire. In some cases, confusion may be the result of nutritional deficiency. Low blood pressure, low blood sugar, congestive heart failure, and vitamin deficiencies can cause cerebral anoxia or reduce essential nutrients to the cerebrum. The aged brain, which is particularly vulnerable to anoxia, may display signs of organic brain syndrome.

Physical

Physical factors, such as smoking, excretion, dentition, weakness, and chronic disease, have a tremendous impact on nutritional status. Cigarette and cigar smoking affect taste and smell, with damage occurring over time to these senses. Impairment of the senses of taste and smell may lead to improper nutritional intake. That is, individuals fail to eat adequate amounts because foods have little taste, or alternatively, they may use extra seasoning or eat excessively. Constipation, an excretory problem, can cause or be caused by improper dietary habits. Inadequate physical activity, emotional stress, and medications are other predisposing factors. Usually, constipation is correctable through increasing the levels of bulk and water in the diet. Exercise is also beneficial. Poor dentition is a common problem of older adults, with more than 50% of those 65 years or more completely edentulous (Hickler & Wayne, 1984).

Dentition problems, including ill-fitting dentures, may lead to rejection of food or insufficient processing of eaten foods. One means of preventing nutritional deficiencies due to poor dentition is to consume liquids with high nutritional value. Physical weakness due to arthritis, bursitis, and joint immobility may make eating painful and handling utensils difficult. Chronic diseases such as diabetes, atherosclerosis, and renal failure, may contribute additional stress to an individual's system and impair the system's ability to use ingested nutrients properly.

Socioeconomic

One must also consider social and economic factors that affect nutritional intake. While these are somewhat self explanatory, they merit discussion. The living situation of elderly persons may affect their nutritional status. An elder whose spouse provided all shopping and cooking, may be compromised nutritionally following the spouse's hospitalization or death. Facilities for food preparation must be assessed. Older adults may find it impossible to prepare low-cost, nutritious meals if they have no cooking facilities or are limited to just a hot plate in a hotel room. The cost of food high in nutritional value is often prohibitive to the elderly. Requirements of special, modified diets can be costly. For example, salt-free foods, although accessible in many grocery stores, are more expensive than foods with salt. Prices of fresh fruits and vegetables consistently exceed those of canned or processed foods and carbohydrates. Transportation is frequently a factor affecting the accessibility of food. Individuals may not have resources or physical stamina to get to shopping facilities or to congregational dining locations. Accessible food may not be the food of choice. Community food agencies, such as "Meals on Wheels" and senior center meals, provide a much-needed service to the elderly. However, the frequency of meals may be inadequate, and foods served may not routinely appeal to ethnic and personal preferences.

Nutritional History

Methods of nutritional assessment are diverse, but a nutritional history is essential for evaluation of nutritional adequacy of the elderly. Has the elder had a loss of appetite? Are taste and smell senses intact? Does the elder have difficulty swallowing or chewing? Are indigestion or elimination disturbances present? What medications, including laxatives, is the elder taking? Does the elder drink alcoholic beverages? Has the elder experienced a recent weight loss, prolonged illness, or hospitalization? Such questions give a general indication of the nutritional status of the older adult. Weight loss, in particular, needs to be given careful consideration, and is a critical symptom related to its link with cancer, thyrotoxicosis, and other diseases (Morley, et al., 1986). Weight gain is equally serious, as it may be indicative of water retention associated with congestive heart failure.

A socioeconomic history should be taken, and should include an assessment of marital status, social support systems, home circumstances, financial status, and mental state. Methods of food storage and preparation, cooking facilities, accessibility of food sources, and shopping habits should be investigated. In addition, a dietary history should be taken. The individual should be asked to recall his or her food intake for the past 24 hours. This 24-hour nutritional recall enables nurses to assess an aspect of short-term memory and provides a snapshot of an elder's nutritional patterns. In addition, a three-day diary of food and fluid intake can provide a means of assessing typical meal and snacking patterns. For example, there is risk in low-calorie diets because of limited nutrients per 1000 Kcal unless nutrient-dense foods have been selected. Also, fluid intake may have been restricted voluntarily to avoid incontinence. Thus, food patterns and habits over the past year—food preferences, allergies, and aversions—and dietary restrictions or prescriptions, plus the use of nutritional supplements, should also be ascertained. Another method of assessment of nutritional patterns is a food frequency questionnaire to determine dietary diversity. Lack of variety in the diet directly affects its quality. From the three-day diary and the 24-hour dietary recall, the nurse should determine typical calorie, fluid, and Basic Four intake.

A significant component of the nutritional assessment is the medication record. Not infrequently, drugs interfere with nutrients. Common drugs, such as barbiturates and salicylates, interact with ascorbic acid and folic acid metabolism. Individuals taking corticosteroids need to be assessed for deficiency of vitamin A, pyridoxine, vitamin D, and potassium. If an elder reports a high to moderate alcohol intake, he or she should be examined for clinical signs of deficiency of folic acid, iron, and zinc. Anticonvulsants may interfere with metabolism of pyridoxine, vitamin B12, vitamin D, vitamin K, and calcium. Individuals should be assessed for use of over-the-counter drugs, in addition to prescribed medications. In particular, the use of salicylates, laxatives, and antacids should be assessed—it is not uncommon to find a pattern of abuse of over-the-counter medications. When self-report is not possible or reliable, interviews with significant others or direct observation of those in health care facilities should be done.

Clinical Observations

The clinical examination should include a dental assessment and observation for signs of vitamin and mineral deficiency. Signs and symptoms may be due to disease states other than malnutrition, so alternatives must be considered. Lowered serum levels of vitamins and minerals are not always compatible with clinical observations; they may precede clinical signs of deficiency. Validation of a clinical or medical diagnosis may depend on resolution of the condition following specific nutritional intervention. Observations of chewing, swallowing, and feeding skills can be helpful. Information regarding the individual's activity level should be obtained.

Age-Related Factors Affecting Nutritional Status

Physical activity often declines with age. Furthermore, there is a gradual loss of functioning cells from many organs and tissues in the body. This loss of functioning cells results in a decrease in the basal oxygen uptake. Concurrently, with age there is a decline in the basal metabolic rate. The age-related reduction in energy requirement increases the risk of obesity unless calorie intake is reduced with aging. Another age-related change affecting nutritional status occurs with body composition. With age, fat deposition is increased, and body water is lost. Water, although the most critical nutrient for life, is typically given too little consideration in nutritional assessments. Even with enteral or parenteral feedings, there remains danger of insufficient water or fluid intake. A loss of only 20 to 22% of body water is fatal. Therefore, the elderly, with less body water, are at a greater risk for dehydration and water deficit (Morley, 1986). Intake and output fluid measurements are complicated by incontinence. Skin coloring is altered through aging, with a decrease in skin capillaries, skin, and subcutaneous tissue thickness, resulting in pallor. Body contour also changes with age, with a reduction in muscle mass and redistribution of fat, especially to the trunk.

NURSING DIAGNOSES

Older adults are at risk for multiple nutritional and hydration problems, most of which are related to specific disease states with nutritional components, such as hypertension, diabetes, and osteoporosis. The following discussion presents nursing diagnoses and associated medical conditions with descriptions of the problems and characteristics of elders who are predisposed to them.

Alteration in Nutrition:
More than Body Requirements; Obesity

Obesity during adulthood is associated with a decrease in life expectancy (Rossman, 1986). This risk of a reduction in life expectancy with obesity may be attributed to the health problems in which overweight serves as a predisposing factor, including diabetes, hypertension, and cardiovascular, liver, and gallbladder disease. A positive correlation has been found between weight and systolic and diastolic pressures. The link betwen diabetes and obesity may be attributed to the positive correlation between fasting serum glucose and weight. In contrast, there is not a clear association with weight, anthropometric measures, and serum cholesterol (Yearick, 1978). Obesity is recognized as a complication for the treatment and therapy for arthritis, Parkinson's disease, and surgery. Predisposing factors for obesity include sedentary lifestyle, immobility, failure to reduce caloric intake with aging, appetite stimulating drugs, and stress. Obesity does not exclude a state of undernutrition for essential nutrients.

Obesity is an impediment to physical care for those with problems of immobility, as nurses and caregivers may not be able to complete effectively positioning and range of motion. When an elder is both obese and immobile, activity may be impaired, as caregivers may be unable to transfer the individual safely to the chair or commode. Not only is the obese, immobile individual at risk for less than optimal rehabilitation, but the caregiver is at risk for physical strain and back injury. Obesity has negative effects on quality of life. The obese individual may have difficulty making trips outside the home and will fatigue easily with activity.

A difficulty with studies of obesity in older adults is the problem with norms and measurements. Obesity in adult men (25% over desirable weight) and women (20% over desirable weight) is well defined. However, these standards are not applicable to individuals over 65 years of age, as the studies did not include older adults (Damon, 1988). In assessing the prevalence of obesity, Albanese (1980) reported a lower incidence in black males and white women aged 20 to 74 years.

Obesity over the age of 65 years is associated with few drawbacks and may have some benefits. Overweight older individuals on prolonged bedrest are at less risk for pressure sores than those who are underweight.

Alteration in Nutrition: Less than Body Requirements

Anemia

Although anemia is not a routine consequence of aging, it is a frequent problem of older individuals, with iron deficiency anemia as the most common type. The physical signs of anemia in the elderly are: tachycardia, cardiac murmurs, headaches, angina, mucal pallor, and congestive heart failure. Anemia may be caused by gastrointestinal tract disorders resulting in poor vitamin B12 absorption, or by nutrient deficiency. Frequently, elders are susceptible to anemia related to dietary inadequacies (Harrell, 1988).

Anorexia

Older adults are susceptible to anorexia related to social, psychological, and physical factors. On a social basis, many elderly reside alone and therefore are not able to socialize during mealtimes. Food has strong social meaning, and there may be less enjoyment associated with mealtimes if all meals are eaten in solitude. The economic status of older adults is a factor if cost prohibits a diet high in nutritional quality or variety. When economic and isolation factors are compounded by impaired mobility, older adults may not have the energy or desire to eat sufficiently.

With regard to psychological factors, older adults struggling with grief or depression may lose their desire to eat. Food is often associated with pleasure, and older individuals who are having difficulty finding enjoyment in living may neglect to eat appropriately. Confusion may lead to anorexia, as individuals may forget when or if they have eaten.

There are numerous physical factors that impede the ability to receive adequate nutrition. These include decreased feeding drive, reduced demand for food, poor dentition, medications, and chronic illness. The anorexia of aging is a phenomena attributed to decreased activity and metabolic rate, compounded by increased satiety, and exacerbated by impaired olfaction, vision, and gustation (Morley, et al., 1986).

Undernutrition

Although it is difficult to define normal aging and concomitant nutritional changes, elderly persons frequently experience varying degrees of malnutrition. Such problems with undernutrition, related to a variety of nutrients, are difficult to detect, as their presentation often is insidious and may be attributed to old age (Gupta, Dworkin, & Gambert, 1988). An additional problem in the detection of malnutrition in the aged is that classic clinical indicators of nutritional status may not be adequate assessors of nutritional status for the age group of older adults. Rather, several clinical and biochemical markers (norms may lack agreement) should be checked to determine nutritional status (Kergoat, et al., 1987).

Low food intake may be an important cause of malnutrition in the elderly (Suter & Russell, 1987). Problems of poor nutritional habits are intensified by frequent gastrointestinal changes with aging. Secretion of hydrochloric acid, required for bacterial destruction and food break-

down, is reduced with age. Decreases in enzymes and bile salts may lead
to further impaired digestion and absorption of nutrients. Changes in
blood supply to the gut may result in abdominal cramping following
meals. Pain from intestinal angina may be sufficient to cause a fear of
eating (Matteson, 1988).

Protein Caloric Malnutrition

Protein caloric malnutrition may be a result of anorexia or of food
refusal. Older individuals may refuse to eat in order to receive attention
from distant caregivers. The result of protein caloric malnutrition in
the aged is poor wound healing, apathy, depression, irritability, weakness, lethargy, weight loss, cachexia, and skin breakdown (Weinsier &
Butterworth, 1981).

Dehydration

The most common fluid disorder of older adults is dehydration (Lavizzo-Mourey, Johnson, & Stolley, 1988). Residents of nursing homes
are at high risk for development of dehydration which may occur when
daily fluid intake is inadequate, that is, less than 1200 to 1500 cc per
day. When fluid is lost due to vomiting or diarrhea, the actual fluid loss
may be small, with dehydration sometimes associated with losses of
only 2%. Clinical symptoms of dehydration include less than 500 cc
daily urine output with increased specific gravity, dry skin and parched
tongue, altered mental status, low blood pressure, and drowsiness
(Albanese, 1980).

Specific risk factors for dehydration in the elderly have not been
definitively identified. However, in a study of 339 nursing home residents developing acute illness, the primary risk factor was that of
inability to self-feed (Lavizzo-Mourey, Johnson, & Stolley, 1988).

Alteration in Bowel Elimination

Constipation

At one time, it was believed that constipation resulted in an accumulation of body poisons. Inaccurate but widespread beliefs such as this and
the impression given by laxative commercials that grandpa is "not
himself" due to irregularity have resulted in the commonly held notion
that daily bowel movements are necessary for a happy existence. Constipation is prevalent among the elderly and, in some cases, may be
attributed to excessive use of laxatives and enemas taken to ensure that
a daily stool occurs. Laxatives have been found to be used twice as often

by individuals over 70 in comparison with those 40 to 50 years of age. Even if laxative abuse is not a factor, the elderly are at high risk for constipation related to inadequate fiber and fluid intake, reduced activity, decreased bowel tone, and medications such as antacids and sedatives (Natow & Heslin, 1983).

Diarrhea

One cause of diarrhea in the aged is lactose intolerance. This intolerance is of particular concern when enteral feedings are required for nutritional maintenance. Administration of tube feedings containing lactose to individuals with lactose intolerance will result in high osmotic pressure due to intact lactose in the intestine. Osmotic pressure will draw fluid from the body into the intestine resulting in gut distension, rapid peristalsis, diarrhea, and a loss of fluid and electrolytes (Albanese, 1980). Another cause of diarrhea is laxative abuse, evident in a pattern of alternating constipation and diarrhea. Additional causes of diarrhea are antibiotics, drugs, and bacterial infections. With diarrhea there is the risk of involuntary stools, resulting in embarrassment and decreased social contacts.

Impairment of Skin Integrity

Surgery

Elderly, chronically ill, and inactive individuals are at high risk following surgery. A study of elderly females who required surgery found that the most effective nutritional support, which facilitated wound healing, was prevention of starvation, and supplemented but not excessive caloric administration (Clark, et al., 1988). Of particular concern with elders are complications of surgery. Infection results in increased energy expenditure and a need for increased fluids and calories (Whitney & Cataldo, 1983).

Pressure Ulcers

Problems to which older individuals are susceptible increase the risk of development of pressure ulcers. Obesity, underweight, anemia, hyperglycemia, and dehydration are considered predisposing factors for pressure sore development. Risk factors, including immobility, bedrest, hypotension, and low serum albumin, when combined with persistent pressure, may lead to development of pressure sores (see Chapter 4). An inadequate nutritional status will predispose one to pressure ulcer development and will impair healing of the ulcer (Agate, 1986).

Self-Care Deficit: Feeding

Musculoskeletal Impairment

Musculoskeletal impairment, especially in the form of arthritis, is common in older adults. Nutritional therapy is not usually the mainstay of treatment for these conditions, but may serve as an adjunct. For example, the primary nutritional concern of older adults with arthritis is that of weight. Excessive weight causes care to be difficult for the caregiver. The result of impaired mobility and pain with the disease may be weight loss, as movement associated with self-feeding may impede adequate intake. Hand deformities may lead to difficulty in grasping utensils and holding cups (Hennig, 1981).

Neuromuscular Impairment

Neuromuscular impairment, such as Parkinson's disease, results in slow, rigid movements with tremors. Such effects impair self-feeding abilities. Individuals may have difficulty holding eating utensils, and tremors may cause a lack of coordination with the hand-to-mouth movements required for self-feeding. Muscles of the mouth and throat are often affected by neuromuscular impairment, and individuals with such conditions may not be able to close their lips or suck on a straw. They may not have the strength or coordination to bite, chew, or swallow. Self-feeding often becomes a long, slow, tedious process. The individual becomes frustrated at the time and energy required for eating, and may eat less than necessary (Carter, 1986).

Enteral Nutrition

Enteral nutrition may provide a viable alternative for individuals who are unable to ingest sufficient nutrients orally. In nursing homes, enteral feeding may be suggested if staff are required to devote excessive amounts of time to mealtime assistance. In a study of indications for tube feedings, the two primary reasons for the decision to feed through enteral nutrition were refusal to swallow and dysphagia (Ciocon, et al., 1988). In order for enteral nutrition to be a viable alternative route, the gastrointestinal tract must be intact and functioning adequately. Tubes may be a mechanical irritant or resented by individuals who believe their lives are being prolonged when they wish to die.

Total Parenteral Nutrition

Total parenteral nutrition (TPN) is the delivery of a concentrated, high-caloric solution for individuals unable to take sufficient nutrition orally or enterally. The solution may deliver as much as 5000 calories daily and is administered through a catheter inserted in the superior vena cava. If an elderly person requires enteral nutrition for more than 10 days, TPN should be considered. TPN may be used for extended periods of time to provide nourishment. In individuals over 65 years of age hyperosmolar, nonketotic hyperglycemia may result from TPN. The solution is hypertonic, and if administered quickly, can cause osmotic diuresis, weakness, dehydration, and convulsions. Careful monitoring of blood and urine glucose levels can alert caregivers to the problem of TPN-related hyperglycemia (Whitney & Cataldo, 1983).

Alteration in Thought Processes

There is an increased incidence of alteration in thought processes with the aging of the population. Thus, older adults with such conditions as Alzheimer's disease are at high risk for nutritional deficiencies. Such risks may be attributed to mental changes, including decreased attention span. During the middle stage of the disease, elders may forget to eat or may overeat. In the latter stages, individuals may not be able to self-feed, and may resist feeding by caregivers (Sandman, et al., 1987). Continuous wandering and movement may increase caloric requirements. Polyphagia can lead to ingestion of plants and other objects.

Knowledge Deficit: Nutrition

Hyperglycemia

Since 60% of those newly diagnosed each year with diabetes are over 54 years of age, diabetes is of concern in any discussion of geriatric nutrition. Abnormal blood glucose tests are found in 50% of elders over the age of 60 years; however, the standards for such tests are based on studies of young, healthy individuals and may not be applicable to those over that age range (Albin, Ross, & Rifkin, 1986). It is believed that glucose tolerance levels increase 10 to 13 mg/100 ml for every 10 years of age. Even with this increase taken into account, there is a high percentage of individuals over age 65 with hyperglycemia. A normogram is available to interpret oral glucose tolerance tests at various ages (Andres, 1971). Some investigators have attributed the prevalence of hyperglycemia among the aged as a normal consequence of aging, while others have related it to insulin inhibitors, reduced insulin response, functional declines in glandular secretory activity, and glucose metabolism. A primary concern regarding nutrition and diabetes in older individuals is that of nutritional education which is addressed in the following intervention section.

Cardiovascular Impairment

The risk for cardiovascular impairment is positively correlated with age. Elders with hypertension who smoke are susceptible to cardiovascular problems. Inactivity, diabetes, obesity, and stress are associated with atherosclerosis and cardiovascular impairment. Many of the risk factors and aspects in management of cardiovascular impairment are amenable to dietary control. Circulatory problems with the lower extremities may lead to the development of stasis ulcers; arterial insufficiency may lead to a need for amputation. Cardiovascular impairment influences quality of life through increased fatigue with activity, shortness of breath upon exertion, and difficulty resting (Fleg & Lakatta, 1986).

Hypertension

Hypertension may occur at any age, with one in four Americans affected (Heinz, 1984). With aging, arteriosclerosis and vascular stiffening occur resulting in a disproportional increase in systolic pressure. Aging is associated with hypertension, particularly in industrialized societies. Aged blacks have a higher incidence of hypertension than whites of the same age group. Geriatric hypertension frequently stems from salt sensitivity, which may be attributed to an age-related renal function decline resulting in inappropriate salt load excretion (Zemel & Cowers, 1988). Diuretic treatment for hypertension may result in hyperglycemia, dehydration, and electrolyte problems. Hypertension drug therapy may lead to incontinence and adverse effects on functional status.

PLANNING

Regardless of the underlying nutritional problem or nursing diagnosis, a critical element in treatment is planning *with* individuals and their caregivers rather than *for* them. Since nutritional habits are established over a period of six or seven decades of life, it is unlikely that even the best-intentioned clinician can alter such patterns without integrally involving individuals and their caregivers in planning. Nurses should address individual life styles, ethnic backgrounds, food preferences, desires, economic status, functional status, and living situations when formulating patient goals and measurable objectives for older adults.

Nurses need to define measurable objectives in care plans or other health records. Older adults or caregivers must share in identifying both short- and long-term goals, although they may not always agree with nurses on the desirable outcomes. When writing patient objectives, nurses should consider how much; how long; how many consecutive successful repeats; display of knowledge through verbal, written, or actual performance; level of functional independence; number of social contacts per defined time period; and acceptable level of drug use. Nurses should document successful interventions and progress, or lack of success, of the nutritional care plan.

Nurses need to be cognizant of the meaning of food to each individual. In institutional settings, changes in food preferences may reflect anxiety, stress, or depression. Decreases in food intake may reflect depression or stress. Through careful on-going assessment of nutritional intake patterns, nurses may be able to anticipate and intervene early in mental health problems. Nurses may be able to optimize nutritional plans through observing individual appetite patterns. Typically, older adults receive the first meal of the day with the greatest degree of enthusiasm, and may eat a greater percentage of breakfast than other meals. Through observing patterns such as this, nurses may make the most of such habits by structuring dietary plans around existing habits and trends.

In formulating goals and objectives for older adults, nurses should assess the social support situation. Those who are living alone by choice may lack the desire to participate in shopping, meal preparation, and even eating. Additionally, grief may lead others living alone without choice to have no desire to prepare and eat meals. Homemaker services are available for meal preparation and shopping.

Nurses should consider the following services when planning a nutritional program with an older adult. Congregate dining provides a hot prepared meal in a group setting. Although congregate dining programs vary with regard to the number of meals and days of the week served, most programs provide for the noon meal at least five days a week. Home delivered meals or "Meals on Wheels" uses volunteers to deliver a prepared meal to homebound elders. Geriatric day care is available in many communities at an economical cost. Day care programs provide social activities with supervision and one to two meals per day (Natow & Heslin, 1983). Services such as geriatric day care, Meals on Wheels, and congregate dining enable older adults to receive nutritious meals while in a community setting. Such services maximize the potential for individuals to remain in a home situation.

INTERVENTION

Alteration in Nutrition: More than Body Requirements; Obesity

Interventions with persons who are obese should center around changing patterns of eating and weight reduction. Such interventions include presenting examples of pattern changes and the dangers of fad diets, and giving positive reinforcement for changes made. The use of life-size food models to teach portions and working with a dietician may facilitate educational programs. Interventions directed toward physical care should include the observation of body folds for moisture and maceration. If osteoarthritis is also a problem, obesity may exacerbate the disease process and pain, which may cease with weight loss. However, although weight loss may be essential for management of arthritis and diabetes, reduction plans for older adults should be moderate and not aggressive. A 500 Kcal per day decrease in intake should result in a loss of one pound per week, enough to minimize the risks of poor nutritional intake and optimize benefits of the reduction.

Alteration in Nutrition: Less than Body Requirements

Just as aggressive weight reduction plans are apt to be inappropriate for older adults, aggressive weight gain programs are equally inadvisable. A well-balanced diet providing 500 calories over the daily requirement should result in a gain of one pound per week weight. Providing large amounts of food during meals may cause individuals to become discouraged and decrease their appetites. Giving snacks between meals may be beneficial, but should be carefully timed, as snacks that are too close to meals may reduce the appetite further. Finger foods that can be kept at the bedside may provide a significant difference in caloric intake. Preferred foods should be presented attractively and incorporated in the diet, and mealtimes should be unrushed with socialization.

Correction of the underlying disease state linked to anemia is necessary for prevention and remediation of inadequate nutrition associated with anemia. A diet containing adequate protein and calories, and a daily multivitamin with iron or provision of the specific mission nutrient such as B12, should be of assistance. A side effect of the use of iron supplements is the masking of gastrointestinal bleeding. Anemia may be due to a drug and food interaction; correction of the problem may require a change in prescribed medications.

Inadequate nutrition due to dehydration should be corrected gradually. Medication changes, including reducing or discontinuing tranquilizers, hypnotics, diuretics, and laxatives, may be necessary for correction of dehydration. Frequently, correction of the fluid deficit occurs when the individual's thirst is satisfied, and urinary output and blood pressure return to normal. The fluid needs of older individuals at risk for dehydration are often overlooked. Nurses need to monitor closely the intake and output, and the fluid status of individuals with diarrhea, fever, polyuria, and vomiting. Older adults residing in tropical climates or exposed to high environmental temperatures are at high risk for dehydration and should be carefully assessed for the presence of fluid deficit. One means of preventing dehydration is through the use of a fluid prescription. Such an intervention should not be limited to intravenous fluids, but should apply to all fluid intake.

Alteration in Bowel Elimination

Depending on the cause of constipation, stool softeners and dietary fiber may be beneficial. Inadequate fluid intake is a frequent cause of constipation, and should be correctable with an intake of 36 to 48 ounces of fluid daily, if not contraindicated. Bowel habits should be identified and complied with to the extent possible. Individuals who have for 90 years had a bowel movement at 8:00 A.M. following a hearty breakfast and two cups of strong black coffee, should not have to reschedule their bowel functions to accommodate a therapy or treatment schedule. Exercise and a diet high in fiber content with prune juice, warm water, or fruit may result in correcting constipation. Providing privacy, use of a bedside commode, and eliminating bedpan use may facilitate healthier bowel habits. Interventions may need to be directed toward weaning from enemas and regular laxative use, if possible.

Impairment of Skin Integrity

Optimal nutrition status is necessary for effective wound healing, whether the wound is due to pressure or surgery. Nutrients involved in wound healing include protein, vitamins, and minerals. Although increasing specific nutrients may not speed wound healing, retardation of the healing process will occur if the diet is lacking. If the disease state is associated with nutritional deficiency, it must be treated for effective wound healing to occur.

Self-Care Deficit: Feeding

For individuals with mobility and feeding difficulties, nurses need to be aware of self-help eating devices. Aids that enable elders to eat independently will minimize embarrassment and maximize the enjoyment of mealtime. Table 5.1 identifies feeding difficulties and self-help aids. In addition to using such aids where appropriate, energy saving techniques may be of benefit. Cutting meats, buttering breads, and opening milk cartons prior to serving meals, along with the use of finger foods, may reduce the frustration experienced during mealtime by individuals with mobility and energy problems. Clothing protectors, not referred to as "bibs," may prevent soiling of clothes.

Knowledge Deficit: Nutrition

Problems with inadequate nutritional knowledge should be corrected through educational programs involving the individual. Such programs are discussed in detail in the following teaching section; however, a few comments will be made here about specific nutritional programs.

TABLE 5.1 Self-help Aids for Feeding

Feeding difficulty	Self-help aid
Weak hand grasp	Built-up handles, such as plastic molded handles or foam curlers placed over utensils Cloth covers over drinking glasses
Tremors, reduced coordination	Plate guard or dishes with curved sides Suction cups under dishes, rubber mats, or sponge cloths under plates to prevent sliding Two-handled cups
Weak oral muscles	Spouted cup Extended and bent straws for liquids
Limited use of one arm	"Spork" to replace the need for multiple utensils Clip to maintain the placement of a straw in a glass

Diet treatment for diabetes may be one of three basic types: free, weighed, or measured. Free diets are best suited to younger diabetics as they match caloric intake to expenditure. Weighed diets are rigid and often meet with noncompliance. Measured diets, which make use of food exchanges and caloric allowances, are most frequently prescribed for older diabetics.

The American Heart Association has made recommendations for healthy cardiac diets. Basically, the recommendations include optimal caloric intake for attainment of a desirable weight, reduction of fat and cholesterol intake, elimination of simple sugars, and limited use of salt (Weinsier & Butterworth, 1981).

For older individuals with hypertension, "limited use of salt" may be ineffective in correcting elevated blood pressure. Based on assessment of the older hypertensive person, a salt-restricted diet may be prescribed. A mild salt restriction (two to three gm of sodium daily) involves not using the salt shaker at the meal table. A moderate salt restriction (1000 mg of sodium daily) reduces the intake of high salt vegetables (beets, kale, celery, and carrots). A strict salt restriction (300–250 mg of sodium daily) is difficult and costly to implement. Salt substitutes may be of benefit in assisting individuals to reduce salt intake. Excessive use of salt substitutes may present a risk for electrolyte imbalance, as many contain potassium.

EVALUATION

In evaluating the effectiveness of nutritional planning and intervention for older adults, nurses should consider the degree to which nutritional problems are corrected. Measurable outcomes defined in the planning process facilitate objective evaluation of plans and interventions. Elders should be questioned to determine if they found the plans and interventions effective and efficient. Were plans appropriate? Did plans and interventions meet needs and preferences? Does the individual plan to continue with the interventions? If the plans were ineffective, can the rationale for failure be identified? When outcomes have not been achieved, appropriate steps of the nursing process need to be repeated. Positive reinforcement should be provided to enable an individual to move from short-range to long-range goal achievement.

HEALTH PROMOTION AND WELLNESS

The best teaching plans are those that are practical, effective, and based upon input from the older adult. Nutrition education programs should be respectful of individual preferences, likes, and dislikes. Programs should be formed with consideration of the participant's learning style and specific communication needs, such as hearing and visual considerations. Adequate lighting without glare should be provided. Such programs should be directed at promoting health, wellness, and maintenance of independence. Nutrition education may be provided on a one-to-one basis or in groups. The use of groups for educational programs is cost effective and encourages socialization and group problem resolution. There is a wealth of practical knowledge among the elderly that is not apt to be located in any text. Therefore, nurses facilitating group nutritional classes should expect to learn from participants.

Although a variety of subjects may be appropriate for nutrition education programs, topical interest will vary considerably. Programs that address the cost of meals, meal preparation, shopping for one or two persons, and the safe use of leftovers may be popular with older adults. Classes on cooking, brand names, and label reading may be beneficial. An additional topic that nutrition education programs should address is that of nutritional folklore, since it is essential that nurses investigate which, if any, beliefs of nutritional folklore are held by individuals. Safety and food preparation tips are good subjects for inclusion, as is information about use of microwave ovens to facilitate preparation of "leftovers" and smaller portions.

Food is often the highest expense in the budget of a retired elder. In spite of this, many older adults have not learned how to shop successfully. Many who shop when hungry and tired buy foods on impulse. Purchase and preparation of small amounts of food may be difficult. Nonfat dry milk may be a better purchase than liquid milk due to its long shelf life. Loaves of bread may be frozen following purchase to prolong storage potential. Older adults should be advised against storing large quantities of food, due to the risk of spoilage. However, storage of foods in preparation for emergencies, such as snow storms, should be encouraged. Individuals should be instructed to keep a supply of liquid and soft foods that are prepared easily for sick days.

CASE STUDY

Mrs. S was admitted to a medical unit of an acute care hospital with a diagnosis of dehydration and fever. Mrs. S's sister and niece accompanied her to the hospital, and commented that Mrs. S had recently moved to the area. She and her sister were living alone in an apartment in a small village near the hospital. Their income consisted of the sister's social security checks and the scant funds Mrs. S had brought with her from her previous residence.

Nutritional Assessment

Mrs. S's diet consisted of under 800 Kcal daily. Recently, she had been eating only small quantities of bread, gelatin, and milk. At the time of admission, Mrs. S was lethargic and responded minimally to verbal and environmental stimuli. Her fever was 103.2. Physical examination revealed that she was a thin, white, elderly female, aged 80. Her skin turgor was poor, and she moaned softly when touched or repositioned. There was a 5 cm epidermal break noted in the skin integrity over her coccyx. Mrs. S's weight was 80 pounds, and she was 64 inches tall. Her skinfold thickness of the triceps was 8 mm, which is smaller than 95% of women over 80 years of age (Chumlea, Roche, & Mukherjee, 1987).

Nursing Diagnoses

Two nursing diagnoses were identified: 1) alteration in nutrition: less than body requirements related to dehydration and protein-calorie malnutrition; and 2) impairment of skin integrity related to a pressure ulcer over her coccyx.

Planning

Immediate goals for Mrs. S revolved around: (1) correction of the dehydration; (2) facilitation of wound healing; and (3) determination of cause of fever (e.g., infectious process or dehydration). Examples of measurable objectives for this client would be: (1) after cessation of IV tube feedings, Mrs. S will drink at least 1500 cc each day; and (2) Mrs. S will identify foods high in vitamins, minerals, and protein before discharge. Following correction of the crisis situation, long-term goals involved assessment of the home and a social support situation.

Nursing Interventions

Rehydration was accomplished within 48 hours through intravenous feeding. Mrs. S was monitored for intake and output, and her blood pressure was checked every 8 hours. The social worker assigned to the unit was contacted to investigate the home and financial situation, and to determine possible socioeconomic alternatives for Mrs. S and her sister. An occupational therapist examined the home environment to assess cooking facilities and the need for environmental modification. Interventions for the pressure ulcer included placing Mrs. S on a "q 1 hour" turn schedule related to her size and poor nutritional status. The ulcer was cleansed every 8 hours and covered with a light dressing to prevent contamination of the wound during incontinence.

Evaluation

At the end of a week of hospitalization, Mrs. S was alert and responsive to verbal and environmental stimuli. Her skin turgor had improved and the pressure ulcer showed signs of healing. The social worker was able to arrange Meals on Wheels and an application for food stamps to support Mrs. S and her sister's food supply. Discharge plans included involvement of a home health nurse for weekly visits to continue the nutritional education initiated during hospitalization. Mrs. S's niece agreed to call or visit Mrs. S daily. Volunteers from Mrs. S's church agreed to visit semi-weekly to assist with cleaning and shopping.

Teaching

The teaching plan for Mrs. S included instruction on a balanced diet and the need to seek medical attention early during episodes of illness. Instruction on the effects of pressure and need for frequent position changes was given, in addition to teaching care of the small pressure ulcer. At the time of discharge, Mrs. S was weak, but ambulatory with minimal assistance, and was eating 1200 calories daily. At six weeks after discharge, the home health nurse reported that plans had been successful, that Mrs. S had gained four pounds, and that the ulcer had healed. Mrs. S and her sister no longer required Meals on Wheels, but were participating in congregate meals.

CONCLUSION

A careful and varied approach to nutritional assessment should result in the identification of actual and potential nutritional problems through specified nursing diagnoses. To increase the possibility of success, established plans and interventions should include the involvement of the older adult and caregivers, with determination of measurable outcomes. The satisfaction of the older adult with the plans should be considered in addition to the attainment of outcome goals in evaluation of the plans and interventions. In summary, good nutrition can be a significant factor in promoting a high quality of life for elderly persons.

REFERENCES

Agate, J. (1986). Special hazards of illness in later life. In I. Rossman (Ed.), *Clinical geriatrics* (3rd ed.; pp. 125–137). Philadelphia: Lippincott.

Albin, J., Ross, H., & Rifkin, H. (1986). Diabetes in the elderly. In I. Rossman (Ed.), *Clinical geriatrics* (3rd ed.; pp. 629–640). Philadelphia: Lippincott.

Albanese, A. (1980). *Nutrition for the elderly*. New York: Alan R. Liss.

Andres, R. (1971). Aging and diabetes. *Medical Clinics of North America, 55*, 841.

Bistrian, B., Blackburn, G., Sherman, M., & Scrimshaw, N. (1975). Therapeutic index of nutritional depletion in hospitalized patients. *Surgical Gynecology and Obstetrics, 141*, 512–516.

Carter, A. (1986). The neurologic aspects of aging. In I. Rossman (Ed.), *Clinical geriatrics* (3rd ed.; pp. 326–351). Philadelphia: Lippincott.

Clark, N., Rappaport, J., DiScala, C., Lamothe, P., & Blackburn, G. (1988). Nutritional support of the chronically ill elderly female at risk for elective or urgent surgery. *Journal of the American College of Nutrition, 7*, 17–26.

Chumlea, W., Roche, A., & Mukherjee, D. (1987). *Nutritional assessment of the elderly through anthropometry*. Columbus, OH: Ross Laboratories.

Ciocon, J., Silverstone, F., Graver, L., & Foley, C. (1988). Tube feedings in elderly patients. Indications, benefits, and complications. *Archives of Internal Medicine, 148*, 429–422.

Damon, J. (1988). Nutritional considerations. In M. Matteson & E. McConnell (Eds.), *Gerontological nursing: Concepts and practice* (pp. 623–647). Philadelphia: W. B. Saunders.

Fleg, J., & Lakatta, E. (1986). Cardiovascular disease in old age. In I. Rossman (Ed.), *Clinical geriatrics* (3rd ed.; pp. 169–193). Philadelphia: Lippincott.

Foley, C., Libow, L., & Sherman, F. (1981). Clinical aspects of nutrition. In L. Libow & F. Sherman (Eds.), *The core of geriatric medicine: A guide for students and practitioners* (pp. 280–299). St. Louis: C. V. Mosby.

Gupta, K., Dworkin, B., & Gambert, S. (1988). Common nutritional disorders in the elderly: Atypical manifestations. *Geriatrics, 43*(2), 87–89, 95–97.

Harrell, J. (1988). Age-related changes in the cardiovascular system. In M. Matteson & E. McConnell (Eds.), *Gerontological nursing: Concepts and practice* (pp. 193–217). Philadelphia: W. B. Saunders.

Heinz, J. (Ed.) (1984). *Aging America: Trends and projections*. Washington, DC: United States Senate Special Committee on Aging.

Hennig, L. (1981). Rheumatic disease. In N. Martin, N. Holt, & D. Hicks (Eds.), *Comprehensive rehabilitation nursing* (pp. 605–643). New York: McGraw-Hill.

Hickler, R., & Wayne, K. (1984). Nutrition and the elderly. *American Family Physician, 29*(3), 137–145.

Kergoat, M. D., Leclerc, B. S., PetitClerc, C., & Imbach, A. (1987). Discriminant biochemical markers for evaluating nutritional status of elderly patients in long-term care. *American Journal of Clinical Nutrition, 46*, 849–861.

Lavizzo-Mourey, R., Johnson, J., & Stolley, P. (1988). Risk factors for dehydration among elderly nursing home residents. *Journal of the American Geriatrics Society, 36*, 213–218.

Masoro, E. (1984). Nutrition as a modulator of the aging process. *The Physiologist, 27*, 98–101.

Matteson, M. (1988). Age-related changes in the gastrointestinal system. In M. Matteson & E. McConnell (Eds.), *Gerontological nursing: Concepts and practice* (pp. 265–277). Philadelphia: W. B. Saunders.

Mazen, R., & Forman, S. (1979). Longevity and age exaggeration in Vilcamba, Ecuador. *Journal of Gerontology, 34*, 94–98.

Morley, J. (1986). Nutritional status of the elderly. *The American Journal of Medicine, 81*, 679–695.

Morley, J., Silver, A., Fiatarone, M., & Mooradian, A. (1986). Geriatric grand rounds: Nutrition and the elderly. *Journal of the American Geriatrics Society, 34*, 823–832.

Natow, A., & Heslin, J. (1983). *Nutrition for the prime of your life*. New York: McGraw-Hill.

Rossman, I. (1986). The anatomy of aging. In I. Rossman (Ed.), *The anatomy of aging* (3rd ed.; pp. 1–11). Philadelphia: Lippincott.

Sandman, P., Adolfsson, R., Nygren, O., Hallmans, G., & Winblad, B. (1987). Nutritional status and dietary intake in institutionalized patients with Alzheimer's disease and multiinfarct dementia. *Journal of the American Geriatrics Society, 35*, 31–38.

Shuran, M., & Nelson, R. (1986). Updated nutritional assessment and support of the elderly. *Geriatrics, 41*(7), 48–70.

Suter, P., & Russell, R. (1987). Vitamin requirements of the elderly. *American Journal of Clinical Nutrition, 45*, 501–512.

Weinsier, R., & Butterworth, C. (1981). *Handbook of clinical nutrition*. St. Louis: C. V. Mosby.

Whitney, E., & Cataldo, C. (1983). *Understanding normal and clinical nutrition*. St. Paul, MN: West Publishing Co.

Yearick, E. (1978). Nutritional status of the elderly: Anthropometric and clinical findings. *Journal of Gerontology, 33*, 657–662.

Zemel, M., & Sowers, J. (1988). Salt sensitivity and systematic hypertension in the elderly. *American Journal of Cardiology, 61*, 7H–12H.

Chapter 6

Continence

Mary Marmoll Jirovec

INTRODUCTION

Maintaining continence or the ability to control bodily wastes is a goal for all who have passed beyond the stage of toilet training. In Western cultures, in particular, people are expected to relieve themselves of bodily wastes at designated toileting facilities and, depending on the facility, in some degree of privacy. Incontinence is expected and readily accepted in infants, but adults are devalued if they are unable to control elimination.

Incontinence can be devastating for elderly persons and their caregivers. Incontinent individuals are shunned by society which is repulsed by the incontinence. Frequently, what happens is that incontinence is hidden by the elderly person. Rather than seeking help for the problem, the person is embarrassed by the soiling and often learns to handle the soiling rather than to seek help for the incontinence. Elderly women who do seek assistance from their physicians are often told that the incontinence is a normal part of aging for women and that they need to learn to live with the problem.

Incontinence, both urinary and fecal, is *not* a normal part of aging. It is a problem caused by some type of medical or functional disorder that may be ameliorated with medical treatment and/or nursing intervention. The nursing approach must be to promote continence and, if necessary, to address the incontinence problem first, along with its possible causes, rather than focusing care on management of the soiling. This chapter will examine problems of urinary and fecal incontinence. Greater emphasis will be placed on problems in urine control because of the widespread incidence of urinary incontinence in elderly persons.

URINARY INCONTINENCE

Urine control is an extremely complex phenomenon. It requires a variety of factors functioning appropriately in order to maintain control. These include an adequate stimulus to initiate the micturition reflex, neuromuscular and structural integrity of the genitourinary system, the cognitive ability to interpret adequately the sensation of a full bladder and to know how to respond appropriately, and the motivational basis to want to inhibit the passage of urine. At the same time, the individual must be mobile enough to be able to react to a full bladder before the urge to urinate overwhelms inhibiting ability. Finally, the person must attend to body sensations and environmental cues in order to know when and how the flow of urine should be controlled. Each of these factors is multifaceted and can impinge on urine control if altered.

Elderly persons are more likely than younger people to encounter problems with urine control. Estimates indicate that from 10 to 20% of older adults living at home have urine control problems. For those elderly living in some type of institution, incidence studies have shown more than 50% can be incontinent of urine (Ouslander, et al., 1985). The extent and severity of the incontinence problem in the elderly make assessing and planning care to promote continence a nursing priority. Promoting high level wellness in elderly persons through continence care makes urinary incontinence an exciting challenge to nurses.

Types of Urinary Incontinence

Urinary incontinence can generally be classified as acute or chronic.

Acute Incontinence

Most frequently occurring in acute care settings, acute incontinence is generally sudden in onset and limited in duration to the acute conditions with which it is associated (Ouslander, et al., 1985). Examples of these are illnesses that limit mobility or impair cognitive functioning, acute urinary tract infections, fecal impactions, or drug therapies. A common cause of acute incontinence in elderly is urinary tract infection. Often the initial episode of incontinence is related to a bladder infection. The infection inflames the bladder and urethral walls, making the bladder itself more irritable. The frequency and strength of bladder contractions result in frequent urination and feelings of urgency. Often elders will complain of burning or pain; however, some persons experience less discomfort than others.

An often-overlooked cause of acute urinary incontinence is fecal impaction or severe constipation. The fecal mass compresses the urinary outlet causing urinary retention. As the bladder fills to capacity, small amounts of urine are forced through the urethra to keep the bladder from bursting. Consequently, the person loses small amounts of urine throughout the day until the obstruction is relieved and the bladder can empty.

Medications also can contribute to acute incontinence. Tranquilizers, hypnotics, and sedatives can reduce the elderly person's sensitivity to body sensations. The individual may be less aware of the need to urinate. This may especially be the case if the elderly person is heavily sedated. Diuretics may be given at a time when their optimal effect makes it difficult to maintain continence. If the diuretic medication is not being given so that maximal output occurs during the morning and afternoon when the person has the most energy, incontinence is likely to develop.

Chronic Incontinence

This is a more persistent form of incontinence involving repeated, involuntary instances of urine loss. Chronic incontinence includes four sub-types: stress incontinence, urge incontinence, overflow incontinence, and functional incontinence.

Stress incontinence is associated with the leakage of small amounts of urine at times when intraabdominal pressure increases. Most evident is urine loss during sneezing, laughing, coughing, straining, exercise, and/ or upon rising. Circumstances that increase pressure on the bladder will cause the leakage. Stress incontinence is found most frequently in women and is related to a weakening of the urethral sphincter musculature and surrounding tissues. Surveys of women living at home have found stress incontinence to be the most common type of incontinence reported (Campbell, Reinken, & McCosh, 1985). Common causes are previous physical trauma associated with childbirth or pelvic surgery, and postmenopausal tissue atrophy and/or vaginitis associated with decreased estrogen.

Urge incontinence involves the loss of varying amounts of urine because of an inability to inhibit bladder contractions until the toilet is reached. It is accompanied by a feeling of urgency, that is, a felt need to get to the bathroom almost immediately. This can result from a variety of central nervous system changes anywhere along the nerve pathways to and from the bladder. The loss of the brain's ability to inhibit bladder contractions can result in this type of incontinence in the late stages of Alzheimer's disease.

Overflow incontinence is associated with loss of small amounts of urine when the bladder is excessively full. Elderly persons often have difficulty starting their stream. Overflow incontinence can occur when the detrusor muscle fails to contract or contracts weakly so that it is unable to overcome the normal intraurethral pressure. This can happen in spinal cord injury, as a complication of diabetes, or because of drugs, such as anticholinergic medications, that inhibit bladder contractions. More frequently, it occurs in combination with a mechanical obstruction that constricts the urethra. The most common cause of this is enlargement of the prostate gland in men.

Functional incontinence involves the inability to reach the toilet before urine is lost (Ouslander, et al. 1985). Functional incontinence is a broad classification that encompasses individuals with any number of impairments related to mobility, cognitive functioning, self-care abilities, motivation, or environmental factors. The origin of this type of incontinence lies outside the genitourinary system.

Normal Age-Related Changes

In addition to pathological conditions that can cause incontinence, there are also changes in the lower urinary tract associated with normal aging that can make maintaining urine control more difficult. Researchers found that almost all of one sample of incontinent elderly women had abnormal bladders (Brocklehurst & Dillane, 1966). Forty-three percent had bladder capacities of 250 ml or less. Normal bladder capacity is about 500 ml. Half of the elderly subjects had residual urine of 50 ml or more after voiding and almost three-quarters did not empty their bladders completely. A normal bladder empties completely with each voiding sequence. The majority did not evidence a desire to void until their bladders were at capacity and many evidenced uninhibited detrusor contractions.

These changes are so prevalent with the elderly that they are considered normal age-related changes. Their impact on elderly persons often results in urinary frequency because of decreases in bladder capacity and residual urine, as well as feelings of urgency due to uninhibited bladder contractions. In addition to normal age-related changes, several studies have established an abrupt increase in the incidence of urinary tract infections with age (e.g., Boscia, et al., 1986a & 1986b; Goldman, 1977; Kaye, 1980). A study of 557 elderly persons (Brocklehurst, et al.,

1968) found that 17% had infected urine. In addition, the female urethra is hormone dependent and susceptible to menopausal changes.
The prevalence of postmenopausal tissue atrophy, previous trauma
during childbirth, and gravitational forces over time make these
changes in women almost a normal age-related occurrence. These
changes make maintaining urine control more of an issue for all elderly.

Assessment

The nursing assessment should begin with a health history. In addition
to standard information obtained during a health history, questions
should be asked specifically related to any problems with urine control.
If problems exist, the elderly person should be asked to describe the
incontinence. When the incontinence occurs, the amounts of urine lost,
the circumstances surrounding the episodes, the presence of burning or
pain when passing urine, and the individual's perceptions of his or her
ability to control urine should be elicited. In addition, the person should
be questioned about any nocturnal enuresis, nighttime awakening to
void, and feelings of urgency and/or frequency. For elders with some
type of dementia, the caregiver should be questioned for information
that the person is unable to provide.

A standard physical examination should be provided with special
attention given to the genitourinary system. This includes attention
particularly to the abdomen and genitalia. Any scars which may indicate previous urological surgery should be noted. In addition, the
bladder should be percussed and palpated for distension. For women,
the perineal skin should be inspected for evidence of growths, color
changes, or other abnormalities. The condition of the urethra should be
evaluated for tightness, gaping, and the like, or the presence of a
urethrocele and/or carbuncle. The elderly person should be asked to
cough or bear down, and any stress urine leakage should be noted.

The introitus should be inspected for discharge, stenosis, or evidence
of prolapse such as cystocele, rectocele, or uterine prolapse. Manual
examination should be done with a well-lubricated, gloved finger. Persons with severe vaginal stenosis may be unable to tolerate even a
single-finger manual examination. Palpation of the vagina may reveal
the presence of any structural alteration, such as a prolapse, which
might contribute to urinary incontinence. In addition, the presence of a
pessary can be ruled out. These are soft rubber devices inserted into the
vagina to support tissue and reduce structural prolapses. Inserted correctly, pessaries can improve stress urinary incontinence. If inserted
incorrectly, they can obstruct urine outflow and may contribute to
infection, painful urination, or discomfort. Long-time, unattended pessaries can become incarcerated and lead to infection or fistula development (Poma, 1981). The rectal examination should also be completed,

with attention given to the presence of impaction or constipation which may influence urine control.

For males, the perineal area should be inspected for skin color, rash, growths, or discharge. The retractability and cleanliness of foreskin, if present, and the size, symmetry, and tenderness of the scrotum should be noted. The rectal examination is done to determine the presence of impaction or constipation, as well as to assess the lower one-third of the prostate gland for size, symmetry, consistency, and tenderness.

The physical examination part of the nursing assessment may identify treatable causes of urinary incontinence that require medical attention. A physician or urologic nurse practitioner may seek further testing to identify appropriate treatments. This usually involves obtaining a clean, voided urine specimen for culture and sensitivity testing, catheterizing the person for the presence of residual urine after voiding, and, if indicated, urodynamic studies to identify bladder activity more specifically. In addition to medical referral, the nursing assessment must include a careful functional assessment of the elderly person and the individual's environment in order to identify factors contributing to the urine control problem.

Functional Assessment

Functional assessment includes evaluation of the elderly person's cognitive abilities, mobility, and self-care abilities (see Table 6.1). Memory problems may contribute to incontinence if the person cannot find the toilet or is unable to remember what the sensation of a full bladder means. Evidence of restlessness or increased confusion before the incontinence may indicate the person's uncertainty regarding how to respond to the sensation of a full bladder.

Cognitive ability is always impaired in dementia. As the urinary bladder fills, impulses reach the cerebral cortex from the bladder with information on urine volume. This causes the person to become aware of the need to urinate. For urine control to be maintained, the individual must be able to interpret the meaning of the impulses from the bladder appropriately in order to consciously inhibit urination. Elders with dementia often have difficulty understanding the meaning of the sensations they are experiencing or remembering the proper response to the sensations, where to go in response to a full bladder, or how to remove clothing and assume the position needed to maintain urine control. These have been learned by the older adult previously and are, therefore, subject to the memory losses associated with dementia. Functional incontinence in dementia is very likely to be caused at least in part by memory defects.

Information that provides estimates of the individual's potential ability to control urine if toileted will also be useful. Further, it is useful to

TABLE 6.1 Functional Assessment of Urine Control Problems

Assessment area	Indications
Does the elder take a long time to find the toilet? Does the elder know where the bathroom is located? Does the elder evidence restlessness before an incontinent episode? Is confusion increased before an incontinent episode?	Provides information regarding *memory* problems that may contribute to incontinence.
Does the elder ask to go to the bathroom? If placed on a toilet, does the elder urinate? Is the elder concerned after incontinent episodes?	Provides information regarding potential *ability to control* urine if toileted.
What amounts of urine does the elder lose? What are the usual times the elder urinates? Does the elder drink adequate amounts of fluid? Is fluid intake regular?	Provides information about *voiding patterns* useful for planning care to promote continence.
Is the elder able to get to the bathroom alone? How quickly is the elder able to get to the bathroom? Can the elder balance alone while standing? Is the elder generally mobile? Is the elder free to move around at will?	Provides information regarding *mobility* problems that may contribute to incontinence.
Is the elder able to manipulate clothing? Is the elder able to button and zipper clothing? Can the elder dress self alone? With help? Does the elder perform hygiene activities for self?	Provides information regarding *self-care* abilities used to self-toilet.

establish the elderly person's usual voiding pattern as much as possible. Assessment of cognitive deficits related to urinary incontinence will prove invaluable in planning care to improve urine control.

Mobility difficulties may also contribute to or cause the urine control problem. In order to maintain urine control, individuals must be physically able to get to the bathroom. Mobility deficits were found to be closely related to urinary incontinence (Jirovec & Wells, 1985). Elderly persons who are able to ambulate alone are most likely to be continent; individuals who need help with ambulation are most likely to be incontinent. Disturbances in gait can often accompany dementia. If the elderly person resides in some type of institutional setting, restraints are frequently used to insure safety by not allowing the individual to walk alone. Unfortunately, restraining elderly persons often results in serious impairments to mobility (Warshaw, et al., 1982), and may lead to a variety of other harmful short- and long-term consequences (see Chapter 7). Many of the urological changes that occur with increased frequency as a person ages result in some type of urgency. Impaired mobility decreases the likelihood that elderly persons will be able to maintain continence. The functional assessment should address any mobility problems that may contribute to incontinence.

In addition to cognitive abilities and mobility, the functional assessment should include an evaluation of the elderly person's self-care abilities. Inability to perform self-care may impair the person's ability to maintain urine control. Concomitant with cognitive impairment are difficulties with manipulating clothing and performing basic hygiene activities. The person may be having difficulty reaching the toilet quickly because he or she is unable to unfasten clothing. Self-care ability needs to be evaluated. Difficulties managing basic self-care may be reflected in urinary incontinence, while information about the individual's ability and interest in toileting will provide information on that person's potential to respond to a structured toileting program. In addition, information about fluid intake will aid in planning nursing care.

Environmental Assessment

An area that can have substantial impact on behavior is the elderly person's environment. The environment should be analyzed for factors that foster or impair urine control. Much of the incontinence found in dementia patients occurs in nursing homes. This is partly because incontinence is often a reason to seek nursing home placement. Similarly, the nursing home is more likely to care for dementia patients late in the course of their illness. Nevertheless, the incontinence may be in part a function of what individuals learn from the environment.

A number of environmental characteristics have been identified within nursing home settings that influence motor activity, verbal behavior, and self-care ability (McClannahan, 1973). A review of several studies demonstrated the impact of environmental factors on residents' behavior (Hoyer, 1973). Lester and Baltes (1978) studied nurses' verbal responses to patient behaviors and found that when patients evidenced dependent behavior, they were most often reinforced with a positive verbal response by the nurse. In contrast, independent behavior by the patient was generally followed by no response. Other studies have demonstrated that changing environmental contingencies can alter the behavior of elderly nursing home residents in areas related to self-care (Gottfried & Verdicchio, 1974), eating behavior (Geiger & Johnson, 1974), activity level (McClannahan & Risley, 1975), socialization (MacDonald, 1978), and memory (Langer, et al., 1979).

Factors associated with institutionalization that may impact on urine control include staff shortages, crowded conditions, inadequate or insufficient equipment and/or facilities, inadequate lighting, low visibility of toileting facilities, impediments to mobility, and the overall nursing care approach. Caregivers often approach the problem of incontinence with resignation. After incontinent episodes, methods are quickly instituted to handle the consequences of the incontinence. Seldom does the solution include some mechanism to compensate for a cognitive deficit in order to maintain continence. If disposable briefs are worn by the elderly resident, removing the brief is often difficult. As a result, the brief makes it more difficult for the resident to use the bathroom. The resident may learn that further attempts to control urine are futile. The environment is structured in such a way that the focus of care is to manage the incontinence rather than to maximize continence.

Other skills necessary in maintaining urine control may also be impeded by the environment. Residents with dementia often wander. When gait disturbances begin to develop or the environmental structure is unable to accommodate unlimited wandering, the resident is often restrained to insure safety (Evans & Strumpf, 1989). Other residents may be restrained in the interest of safety in order to prevent them from walking alone. Unless the restraints are accompanied by frequent, regular opportunities to exercise, mobility skills will soon atrophy. Similarly, it is often quicker for caregivers to dress residents rather than allowing the time and assistance needed for residents to dress themselves. These skills also will diminish. Research has demonstrated that persons can erroneously infer their own incompetence from situational factors (Langer & Benevento, 1978).

The impact of the environment, particularly in nursing homes, is highlighted by social breakdown theory. This theory suggests that a person's sense of self, ability to interact with the social environment, and feelings of self-efficacy are related to the social labeling processes that the individual experiences (Kuypers & Bengston, 1973). Labeling processes are especially influential when people are deprived of important roles, normative information, and reference groups. This is the situation upon entering a nursing home. Previous roles are relinquished and the new role of the resident is assumed. The person's reference groups are gone and the norms used to guide behavior have been altered. The new reference group includes other residents, many of whom spend the day doing nothing. Some are restrained and/or incontinent. According to social breakdown theory, the new resident begins to believe he or she is like the other residents. Because of this belief, many behaviors are not attempted and skills atrophy. Passivity and helplessness are reinforced by the environment. This results in the resident demonstrating the incompetence he or she has come to accept and internalize (Kuypers & Bengston, 1973).

The environment needs to be carefully examined for factors that tend to impede urine control. The toileting facilities themselves should be evaluated. Are the facilities adequate for the number of persons using them? Is the room well lit and cheerful, making it a more inviting place? Bathrooms at home are usually bright and cheerful. Most residents will be accustomed to using a similar bathroom. Is the bathroom readily visible? Visibility may be a factor in maintaining or losing urine control. Are the toilet facilities comfortable? Is the toilet seat at a comfortable height? Residents with arthritic hips may find using the toilet adversive if they have to sit on a toilet that is too low and causes pain. If the facilities are used by more than one person, is privacy provided?

The environment also needs to be examined for other messages that impede maintaining continence. Are residents dressed appropriately for daytime? Similarly, are incontinence pads or disposable briefs used as if incontinence is expected? Are other residents incontinent, resulting in a dominant urine smell? How do caregivers respond to an incontinent episode? Is it accepted or are residents encouraged to use the bathroom in the future? Are the furnishings homey and attractive so that residents feel like they are in their own living rooms? Especially important, are residents free to move about? If restrained, residents will be unable to go to the bathroom unless a caregiver removes the restraint. Since some urgency in urination is fairly common in the elderly, restraints may make it impossible for residents to maintain continence unless caregivers are extremely vigilant and readily available.

Nursing Diagnosis

A person with urine control problems will have a primary nursing diagnosis of *altered urinary elimination pattern*. According to North American Nursing Diagnosis Association (NANDA) (Duespohl, 1986), this diagnosis will be related to one or more of the following etiologies: sensory motor impairment, neuromuscular impairment, or mechanical trauma. In this chapter, these etiologies have been described as related to urological pathology or functional difficulties. That is, persons with stress incontinence will evidence urine leakage especially noted during times when intraabdominal pressure is increased. Individuals with urge incontinence will evidence feelings of urgency and an inability to inhibit urination until a toilet is reached. With overflow incontinence, dribbling will occur throughout the day and will be accompanied by bladder distension. Some elderly persons will have an altered urinary elimination pattern with evidence of more than one type of incontinence, as when an elderly woman might experience leakage when rising, in combination with feelings of urgency.

For elderly persons with functional incontinence, an *altered urinary elimination pattern* may be related to *impaired physical mobility* caused by conditions such as gait disturbances and arthritis, or by environmental barriers to mobility such as restraints. The altered pattern may be related to *impaired thought processes* causing confusion and impairing the individual's ability to maintain continence. *Total self-care deficit* may make it difficult for an elderly person to perform activities needed to maintain urine control. A person with *impaired verbal communication* may be unable to communicate to caregivers needs related to urine control. Thus, functional incontinence provides a good example of the need to identify specific etiologies in addressing a urine control problem.

The incontinence, itself, can lead to a separate nursing diagnosis of *social isolation* as people around the incontinent person are repulsed by the incontinence and tend to withdraw. In a nursing home, residents may no longer be encouraged to participate in group activities. Family and friends may no longer feel comfortable taking the elder out of the home on day trips.

Planning

Urinary incontinence should be approached as other problems are approached. Medical approaches seek to identify the presence of urological problems that can be treated by pharmacological or surgical approaches. Some of the medical treatments and nursing implications considered for urge and stress incontinence are summarized in Table 6.2. Nursing assessment and diagnosis leads to planning that states specific goals and objectives for elders to accomplish in order to promote urine control and resolve problems of urinary incontinence.

For persons with stress incontinence, the goal may be to decrease urine leakage by strengthening perineal musculature. For elders with urge incontinence, the goals may be to increase bladder capacity and to decrease circumstances that lead to loss of urine. For instance, the plan may be to increase the interval between micturition and to provide greater regularity in fluid intake.

The goal of decreasing susceptibility to altered urinary elimination is often established regardless of the cause of the incontinence. When the urinary incontinence is secondary to impaired physical mobility, a goal of increasing mobility skills may be established. This may include daily ambulation the length of the hallway every two hours during waking hours with assistance, assistance every two hours in getting to a toilet, and fluid intake of 2600 cc. fluid including cranberry juice distributed systematically over a 24-hour period.

For persons with urinary incontinence related to impaired thought processes or impaired verbal communication, the goal may be to increase congruence between the individual and the environment. For incontinent elders with a total self-care deficit, the goal may be to compensate for activities the elderly person is unable to perform independently.

TABLE 6.2 Medical Treatments for Urinary Incontinence and Nursing Implications

Type of incontinence	Medical treatment	Nursing implications
Stress	Artificial sphincters	Post surgical care
		Patient teaching regarding use
	Surgical procedures (Bladder-neck suspension)	Post surgical care
	Medications (Ephedrine, Phenyl-propronolamine, Estrogen)	Patient teaching regarding use and side effects
	Pelvic floor exercises	Patient teaching and monitoring of exercises
Urge	Surgical procedures (Bladder-neck transsection, cystolysis, therapeutic bladder distension, etc.)	Post surgical care
	Medications (Propantheline, Imipramine, Flavoxate, Oxybutrin)	Patient teaching regarding use and side effects
	Biofeedback	

Intervention

Nursing interventions focus on the appropriateness of continence (McCormick, Scheve, & Leahy, 1988). Urine containment strategies should be minimized and any necessary approaches should be implemented in a way that does not impair urine control. Disposable briefs should be readily removable or removed for the patient at regular intervals. Similarly, restraints should be regularly and religiously removed. The overall attitude of caregivers should include an expectation that continence can be maintained. Accidents can be expected to happen. However, if caregivers give patients the impression that accidents are normal, patients will come to believe they cannot control urine. Rather, accidents should be cleaned courteously without reinforcing incontinence. Successful toileting should be praised so that patients obtain more positive feedback for continence as opposed to incontinence.

The impact of environmental manipulations on the toileting behavior of patients has been demonstrated by several researchers (Carpenter & Simon, 1960; Grosicki, 1968; Pollack, & Liberman, 1974; Sanavio, 1981;

Schnelle, et al., 1983). Thus, the environment needs to be structured to compensate for memory deficits. Specific strategies will evolve from the nursing assessment. For instance, making the toilet more visible with color contrast around the door or a sign on or near the door may help a dementia patient who is having difficulty finding the toilet. Providing a raised toilet seat may remove discomfort associated with using the toilet. Repeated discomfort during toileting will discourage toilet use. Velcro closures on clothing may help the elderly person who is having difficulty manipulating buttons and zippers. Table 6.3 summarizes some intervention strategies to be considered when planning nursing care for individuals who are functionally incontinent.

Interventions need to be individualized in order to promote continence. Often they include some type of environmental supports to establish a toileting routine. Habit training involves encouraging elderly persons to toilet according to their bladder patterns. As accidents occur, individuals are encouraged to toilet sooner until they are able to maintain continence. Elders without cognitive deficits may benefit from such a program. Similarly, behavior modification techniques may be helpful if individuals have learned to be incontinent from their environment. This generally involves a system of positive and negative reinforcement in order to promote continence and extinguish incontinence. These assume that incontinence is not due to cognitive impairment or mobility difficulties.

A bladder retraining program in which a routine of fluid intake and toileting is established with progressive lengthening of toileting intervals may aid in increasing bladder capacity for elderly persons without dementia who have urge incontinence. For individuals with cognitive impairment, some type of scheduled toileting that can be feasibly implemented should be considered. At home the schedule may be individualized to the person's bladder patterns. In an institution it may be more feasible to establish one schedule to which all caregivers adhere.

Interventions should also address mobility in the elderly person. If the individual does not ambulate independently, he or she should be helped to walk about regularly. As noted above, the use of restraints should be avoided in all but the most serious, short-term emergency (Evans & Strumpf, 1989). If their use is thought to be necessary, help should be provided so that individuals can ambulate on a regular basis. Mobility skills should not be allowed to atrophy. Even the person who needs help with ambulation will be more easily toileted if he or she is able to walk about with assistance.

The environment must also provide adequate fluid intake. Inadequate hydration causes the kidney to conserve fluids, producing only small amounts of highly concentrated urine which irritate the bladder wall. The bladder is seldom stretched and the stimulus of a full bladder can be so weak that the person no longer has the signal learned pre-

TABLE 6.3 Nursing Interventions Related to Functional Urinary Incontinence

Causes	Impact	Interventions
Impaired mobility	Inability to rise from chair Inability to walk to toilet Inability to reach toilet fast enough Inability to manipulate clothing Inability to maintain balance Inability to perform self-care without assistance	Assistive devices Assistance readily available Accessible call light Accessible facilities Commode available if needed Easily manipulated clothing Velcro closures, etc. Railings Raised toilet seats
Cognitive Impairment	Inability to find toilet Slowness in finding toilet Inability to identify proper response to a full bladder Inability to identify meaning of a full bladder	Environmental supports to compensate for cognitive difficulties
Inaccessibility of facilities	Toilet too far away Toilet seat too low or too high Toilet area too small for assistive devices Bedpan too small Facilities poorly lit	Readily accessible facilities (may include commode) Assistive devices Proper equipment
Psychological	Decreased attention to bladder cues; isolation/depression Loss of bladder control as attention-seeking device "Learned" incontinence through negative reinforcement of toileting attempts and no response or positive reinforcement of incontinence	Psychological care Offer positive reinforcement when dry Reinforce dryness and discourage incontinence

viously for urine control. The nursing literature repeatedly addresses the importance of sufficient fluid intake in controlling urine (Maney, 1976; Spiro, 1978; Wells & Brink, 1981). Patients should be offered adequate amounts of fluid at regular times in order to insure a regular pattern of urination. The practice of restricting fluids in order to decrease urination should be avoided. If elderly persons have been offered unusually large amounts of fluids as a result of a change in routine such as a party, caregivers can expect to toilet such persons more frequently during those times. Consideration of the regularity and amount of fluid intake will greatly aid in planning a successful continence plan.

Flexibility needs to be maintained throughout intervention. Much will be learned from the individual's response to the care provided. It may become evident that the incontinence is due to more than was originally identified from the initial assessment. Urine control is extremely complicated and can be impacted by a myriad of factors both internal and external to the person. Reassessment to discover previously unidentified factors that are contributing to the incontinence will increase the likelihood that care will be effective.

Evaluation

The success of the nursing care plan will vary with the elderly person's ability to cooperate, the caregiver's ability to implement the plan consistently, and the severity of the causes of the incontinence. Incontinence of urine is not a normal part of aging. Effective medical care and professional nursing care can be expected to significantly decrease, if not reverse, the incontinence. Individuals with functional incontinence or some type of urge or stress incontinence in combination with functional incontinence can be expected to respond dramatically to appropriate nursing interventions. Only in the late stages of Alzheimer's disease is incontinence to be expected; in earlier stages, environmental manipulations effectively and consistently implemented will decrease the incidence of incontinence.

FECAL INCONTINENCE

Fecal incontinence distresses elders who experience it, is especially unpleasant for caregivers, and repulses family members and friends. Repeated episodes of fecal incontinence will most often result in institutionalization as families find the incontinence intolerable. Nursing home studies have shown the prevalence of fecal incontinence to be between 10 to 14% (Tobin & Brocklehurst, 1986). Fecal incontinence, however, is often curable and preventable.

Assessment

Fecal stasis is the most common cause of fecal incontinence in the elderly (Brocklehurst, 1972). This is associated with an increase in the transit time through the colon. In almost all cases, as stasis progresses a large fecal mass is formed in the rectum causing fecal impaction. As the rectum becomes overdistended and too full, the sphincters lose their tone, the anus begins to open, and fecal incontinence results. Often there is a continuous leakage of fluid or semiformed feces. Unlike a normal bowel, the gastrocolic reflex does not produce bowel movements in association with meals.

Neurologic disorders can also cause fecal incontinence. The most common of these in the elderly is associated with the loss of central nervous system inhibition of the defecation reflex. Most frequently, this is associated with severe mental impairment. As a fecal mass stimulates rectal contractions, the elderly person is unable to inhibit the contractions resulting in evacuation of the fecal mass. The defecation pattern often follows the gastrocolic reflex occurring after meals.

As with urinary incontinence, elderly persons should be assessed for treatable medical problems contributing to the fecal incontinence. Medical evaluation should be followed by a nursing assessment that assesses the individual's cognitive abilities and mobility similar to that done for urinary incontinence. Much of the discussion in the section on urinary incontinence will be relevant when planning care related to fecal incontinence. In addition, in cases of fecal incontinence nurses must also assess for diarrhea, constipation, or other problems (see Chapter 5), the person's history of stool pattern, laxative use, physical findings (e.g., fecal impaction, bowel sounds), activity status, medications, fluid intake, and present diet.

Nursing Diagnosis

The principle nursing diagnosis in this area is *alteration in bowel elimination: incontinence*, for which the defining characteristic is involuntary passage of stool. This diagnosis may be based on any of the following NANDA-identified etiologies: neuromuscular involvement, musculoskeletal involvement, depression, perception or cognitive impairment (Duespohl, 1986).

Planning

The goal for all elderly, particularly those with altered bowel elimination, incontinence, is an established bowel pattern that maximizes fecal control. In order to achieve this, an objective should be to toilet elderly persons for fecal evacuation on a regular basis. Usually, this is most effectively done 30 minutes after eating. The time should be individualized depending on the elderly person's bowel habits. Besides regular toileting, other objectives, such as a high fiber diet, fluid intake of approximately 2000 ml., and regular exercise, should be established (see Chapter 5). What promoted bowel regularity in earlier days is also likely to be effective as the person ages. For this reason, elderly persons or family members should be questioned about the person's previous bowel habits. Something as simple as a second cup of coffee after breakfast may be the one added intervention in combination with intake and exercise that the elderly person needs to maintain bowel habits.

Intervention

Establishing a regular evacuation pattern will aid in maintaining fecal continence. Once the rectum has been cleared of any impaction, a high fiber diet (e.g., bran, fruits, vegetables) should be insured in order to stimulate intestinal peristalsis. In addition, fluid intake should be maintained at approximately two liters per day. Exercise is important as an aid to stimulating large bowel functioning. The gastrocolic and duodenocolic reflexes should be used to establish a fecal evacuation pattern. These reflexes cause mass movements in the large intestine after eating, most often after breakfast. Another important intervention is to offer encouragement and praise for efforts on the part of the elderly person.

Irregular bowel habits developed through a lifetime of inhibition of the normal defecation reflex are a frequent cause of constipation. If defecation reflexes are inhibited repeatedly or laxatives overused, clinical experience shows that the reflexes themselves will weaken over time. Eventually, the colon will become atonic. Noncognitively impaired individuals generally monitor their bowel habits and seek help if constipation becomes severe. Dementia patients will require assistance to insure that constipation does not develop into fecal impaction.

Fecal incontinence should not be passively accepted in patients with dementia. Even severely demented patients can have incontinence minimized with proper diet, fluid intake, exercise if feasible, and toileting. Little research has been done related to fecal incontinence in dementia patients. Tobin and Brocklehurst (1986) used two management protocols depending on the cause of the fecal incontinence. Patients with fecal impactions were given daily enemas until clear, followed by lactalose daily and weekly enemas. Patients diagnosed with neurogenic incontinence were constipated using codeine phosphate and given an enema every third day. The researchers reported improvement in the degree of fecal incontinence. While more research is needed, our understanding of the functioning of the normal bowel provides guidelines that can aid in reducing fecal incontinence.

Evaluation

The success of maintaining regular bowel habits will depend on achievement of objectives related to diet, fluid intake, exercise if possible, and regular toileting routine. The large intestine and rectum are organs amenable to regular evacuation. Careful attention to bowel habits will allow elderly persons to adjust the routine when needed to maintain proper evacuation. Fecal impaction should be suspected when small amounts of liquid stool are lost. Digital examination may identify the development of fecal impaction which, after clearing with digital manipulation and/or some type of enema, will allow for the reestablishment of regular bowel habits.

REFERENCES

Boscia, J. A., Kobasa, W. D., Abrutyn, E., Levison, M. E., Kaplan A. M., & Kaye, D. (1986a). Lack of association between bacteriuria and symptoms in the elderly. *The American Journal of Medicine, 81*, 979–982.

Boscia, J. A., Kobasa, W. D., Knight, R. A., Abrutyn, E., Levison, M. E., & Kaye, D. (1986b). Epidemiology of bacteriuria in an elderly ambulatory population. *The American Journal of Medicine, 80*, 208–214.

Brocklehurst, J. C. (1972). Bowel management in the neurologically disabled. The problems in old age. *Proceedings of the Royal Society of Medicine, 65*, 66–69.

Brocklehurst, J. C., & Dillane, J. B. (1966). Studies of the female bladder in old age. I. Cystometrograms in non-incontinent women. *Gerontologia Clinica, 8*, 285–305.

Brocklehurst, J. C., Dillane, J. B., Griffiths, L., & Fry, J. (1968). The prevalence and symptomatology of urinary infection in an aged population. *Gerontologia Clinica, 10*, 242–253.

Campbell, A. J., Reinken, J., & McCosh, L. (1985). Incontinence in the elderly: Prevalence and prognosis. *Age and Ageing, 14*, 65–70.

Carpenter, H. A., & Simon, R. (1960). The effect of several methods of training on long-term, incontinent, behaviorally regressed hospitalized psychiatric patients. *Nursing Research, 9*, 17–22.

Duespohl, T. A. (1986). *Nursing diagnosis manual for the well and ill client.* Philadelphia: W. B. Saunders.

Evans, L. K., & Strumpf, N. E. (1989). Tying down the elderly: A review of the literature on physical restraint. *Journal of the American Geriatrics Society, 37*, 65–74.

Geiger, O. G., & Johnson, L. A. (1974). Positive education of elderly persons: Correct eating through reinforcement. *The Gerontologist, 14*, 432–436.

Goldman, R. (1977). Aging of the excretory system: Kidneys and bladder. In

C. E. Finch & L. Hayflick (Eds.), *Handbook of the biology of aging* (pp. 409–431). New York: Van Nostrand Reinholdt.

Gottfried, A. W., & Verdicchio, R. G. (1974). Modifications of hygienic behaviors using reinforcement therapy. *American Journal of Psychotherapy, 28*, 122–128.

Grosicki, J. P. (1968). Effect of operant conditioning on modification of incontinence in neuropsychiatric geriatric patients. *Nursing Research, 17*, 304–311.

Hoyer, W. J. (1973). Application of operant techniques to the modification of elderly behavior. *The Gerontologist, 13*, 18–22.

Jirovec, M. M., & Wells, T. J. (1985). Factors associated with urine control in elderly nursing home residents with chronic degenerative brain disease. Paper presented at the meeting of the Gerontological Society of America, New Orleans, LA.

Kaye, D. (1980). Urinary tract infections in the elderly. *Bulletin of the New York Academy of Medicine, 56*, 209–220.

Kuypers, J. A., & Bengston, V. L. (1973). Social breakdown and competence: A model of normal aging. *Human Development, 16*, 181–201.

Langer, E. M., & Benevento, A. (1978). Self-induced dependence. *Journal of Personality and Social Psychology, 36*, 886–893.

Langer, E. J., Rodin, J., Beck, P., Weinman, C., & Spitzer, L. (1979). Environmental determinants of memory improvement in late adulthood. *Journal of Personality and Social Psychology, 37*, 2003–2013.

Lester, P. B., & Baltes, M. M. (1978). Functional interdependence of the social environment and the behavior of the institutionalized aged. *Journal of Gerontological Nursing, 4*(2), 23–27.

MacDonald, M. L. (1978). Environmental programming for the socially isolated aging. *The Gerontologist, 8*, 350–354.

Maney, J. Y. (1976). A behavioral therapy approach to bladder retraining. *Nursing Clinics of North America, 11*, 179–188.

McClannahan, L. E. (1973). Therapeutic and prosthetic living environments for nursing home residents. *The Gerontologist, 13*, 424–429.

McClannahan, L. E., & Risley, T. R. (1975). Design of living environments for nursing-home residents: Increasing participation in recreation activities. *Journal of Applied Behavior Analysis, 8*, 261–268.

McCormick, K. A., Scheve, A. A. S., & Leahy, E. (1988). Nursing management of urinary incontinence in geriatric inpatients. *Nursing Clinics of North America, 23*, 231–264.

Ouslander, J., Kane, R., Vollmer, S., & Menezes, J. (1985). *Technologies for managing urinary incontinence* (Health Technology Case Study 33), OTA-HCS-33. Washington, DC: U.S. Congress, Office of Technology Assessment.

Pollack, D. D., & Liberman, R. P. (1974). Behavior therapy of incontinence in demented inpatients. *The Gerontologist, 14*, 488–491.

Poma, P. A. (1981). Management of incarcerated vaginal pessaries. *Journal of the American Geriatrics Society, 29*, 325–327.

Sanavio, E. (1981). Toilet retraining psychogeriatric residents. *Behavior Modification, 5*, 417–427.

Schnelle, J. F., Traughber, B., Morgan, D. B., Embry, J. E., Binion, A. F., & Coleman, A. (1983). Management of geriatric incontinence in nursing homes. *Journal of Applied Behavior Analysis, 16*, 235–241.

Spiro, L. R. (1978). Bladder training for the incontinent patient. *Journal of Gerontological Nursing*, 4(3), 28–35.

Tobin, G. W., & Brocklehurst, J. C. (1986). Faecal incontinence in residential homes for the elderly: Prevalence, aetiology and management. *Age and Ageing*, 15, 41–46.

Warshaw, G. A., Moore, J. T., Friedman, W., Currie, C. T., Kennie, D. C., Kane, W. J., & Mears, P. A. (1982). Functional disability in the hospitalized elderly. *Journal of the American Medical Association*, 248, 847–850.

Wells, T. J., & Brink, C. A. (1981). Urinary continence: Assessment and management. In I. M. Burnside (Ed.), *Nursing and the aged* (pp. 519–548). New York: McGraw-Hill.

Chapter 7

Mobility and Safety

Jean F. Wyman

INTRODUCTION

Mobility, the ability to move freely in one's environment, is essential to the health and well being of older adults. Limitations in mobility directly affect the independence and safety of the elderly, and place them at high risk for a host of negative physical, psychological, and social consequences, including institutionalization. Imagine being unable to bend over and tie your shoes or being unable to climb stairs. Think of yourself with a walker or confined to a wheelchair, and how you would shop for groceries, cook a meal, clean house, or attend social activities outside your home. What if you were restrained in a chair and were unable to get to the bathroom? How would you get yourself out of a burning house if you were not mobile?

This chapter discusses the concept of mobility and its relevance for the health and safety of the elderly population. Specifically, this chapter will describe nursing assessment, diagnoses associated with mobility alterations, and interventions useful in health promotion with aging adults, as well as strategies for enhancing mobility. This discussion also includes falls, a significant consequence of impaired mobility in older people.

MOBILITY AND THE ELDERLY

Mobility is a complex function that depends on the integration of multiple physical, cognitive, and affective factors (see Table 7.1) in interaction with the environment. Although ambulation is a major component of mobility, the concept of mobility is broader than strictly walking. A person in a wheelchair who is unable to walk may be more mobile than the individual who ambulates with a walker. Mobility influences the ability to perform activities of daily living, but is not synonymous with them.

Many elders define their health status in terms of their mobility, that is, whether they can move in their usual ways or carry out their activities of daily living. Even though multiple chronic diseases may be present, many elders only define themselves as "ill" when they can no longer carry on regular activities, such as climbing steps, walking to the park, or driving to the store (Schwartz, Heneley, & Zeitz, 1964).

Thus, mobility is a critical component of functional health in the elderly influencing both activities of daily living (ADL, e.g., bathing, dressing, grooming, toileting, eating) and instrumental activities of daily living (IADL, e.g., cooking, shopping, cleaning, traveling beyond one's immediate environment). Hogue (1984) described a model for enhancement of mobility in institutional populations (Figure 7.1) that also has applicability to the elderly in the community. The model proposes that individual and environmental factors interact with each other and result in mobility. According to Hogue's model, a person with diminished competence may not interact with the environment in ways that maximize adaptive behavior. The model also explains how environ-

TABLE 7.1 Factors Contributing to Mobility and Safety

Cognitive/affective	Neurological
Level of consciousness	Balance
Mental status	Gait
Mood	Coordination
Motivation	Dexterity
Confidence in ability to prevent falls	Righting reflexes
	Response time
Sensory	Musculoskeletal
Vision	Posture
Hearing	Absence of deformities
Proprioception	Flexibility (range of motion)
Touch	Strength
Cardiovascular/respiratory	
Endurance	

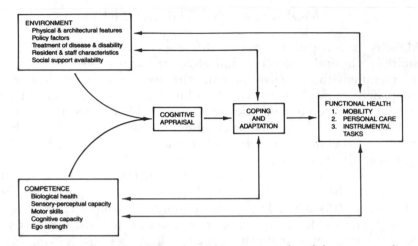

FIGURE 7.1 Hogue's model for the enhancement of mobility, personal care, and instrumental tasks in an institutionalized population. Reprinted with permission from the American Geriatrics Society, Falls and mobility in late life: An ecological model, Hogue, C. C. (1984). *Journal of the American Geriatrics Society, 32,* 859.

mental factors can help minimize diminished competence to maintain mobility. A person who is wheelchair bound living at home can maintain independence because of the social support provided by the family, excellent community resources such as Meals on Wheels, and a senior citizen transportation service with vans equipped for wheelchairs.

NORMAL AGE-RELATED CHANGES AFFECTING MOBILITY

Old age is associated with a modest decline in all body systems. Although this is usually benign, complications from chronic disease superimposed upon normal aging changes can result in significant functional impairments. However, most elders with modest changes in their functional abilities are able to maintain an active and independent lifestyle despite the presence of chronic disease. Bortz (1982) postulated that many normal aging changes result from physical inactivity or disuse, and could be corrected by regular physical exercise.

Changes in the musculoskeletal, neurological, cardiovascular, and sensory systems greatly influence the mobility and independence of older adults. Although there is wide variation in the range of normal, some generalizations can be made. For example, posture tends to become more flexed giving a hunchbacked appearance. This results from the wedging of the vertebrae with thinning of the intervertebral disks.

This new posture shifts the body's center of gravity forward necessitating changes in stance and gait. Stance becomes wider, feet are not picked up as high with each step, steps become shorter, and movement becomes slower and more cautious. Men tend to develop wide-based, small-stepped gait, whereas women develop a narrow-based, waddling gait.

Musculoskeletal changes include loss of muscle mass and tone resulting in decreased strength. Connective tissue tends to become stiff and less elastic, thus, limiting joint range of motion and flexibility.

Changes in the central nervous system alter the integration of sensory inputs and the coordination of motor activity, thereby affecting the ability to correct unstable movements. Age-associated changes include: a general slowing of motor behavior resulting in a decreased reaction time and slower righting reflexes; decreased proprioception and vibratory sense particularly in the lower extremities; and altered vestibular function. Postural sway (side-to-side movement), a measure of postural control, increases with age and is associated with a risk of falls. Changes in short-term memory increase the potential for elders to trip over forgotten objects as they walk.

Sensory function is critical in the maintenance of safety as well as mobility. Visual changes include decreased acuity, restricted visual fields, increased susceptibility to glare, and poor depth perception. Presbycusis, the alteration in hearing that occurs with aging, affects the ability to hear high-frequency sounds. In these ways, the ability to see obstacles while walking or to hear warning signals is impaired.

Cardiovascular changes that affect mobility relate to a decreased cardiac response to stress. The aging heart is less effective in pumping blood during high demand periods, such as exercise or other physical exertion, and takes longer to recover. Thus, activity tolerance is directly affected. With age, there is a decline in baroreceptor sensitivity, so that older people may experience lightheadedness when arising from a bed or chair too quickly and possibly experience a fall.

MOBILITY ALTERATIONS

Mobility alterations are probably the most important problem for older people. Women are more likely to be affected than men. Institutionalized elderly populations have greater mobility impairments than the aged living in the community. A national survey (National Center for Health Statistics [NCHS], 1987) indicated that in nursing homes, only 28% of residents could walk independently, 26% could walk with assistance, 40% were chairbound, and 7% were bedfast. Of the elderly living in the community, 19% have difficulty walking, 8% have difficulty transferring, and 10% are restricted in their ability to get outside their home. Elders are more likely to have problems with walking than any other personal care activity.

The likelihood of mobility problems increases with advancing age, usually as a result of multiple chronic diseases. At age 65 to 74 years, 14% of the elderly have mobility restrictions, increasing to 23% at ages 75 to 84 years, and 40% for those who are 85 years and over (NCHS, 1987).

Mobility may be altered in three ways: (1) it is lost or becomes inactive through disease or trauma; (2) it is externally restricted through prescribed bedrest or mechanical devices (e.g., physical restraints, casts, indwelling catheters); or (3) it is voluntarily curtailed to conserve energy or to maintain equilibrium (Mitchell, 1981).

Although immobility is usually conceived as a limitation in ability to perform independent physical movement, it actually is a much broader concept. Carnevali and Brueckner (1970, p. 1502) defined immobilization as "the prescribed or unavoidable restriction of movement in any area of the patient's life." Areas of a person's life that could be affected include physical, emotional, intellectual, and social. In addition, the ability to move beyond a person's immediate environment through some form of transportation (e.g., bus, car, taxi) is also affected. Restriction of movement occurs on a continuum varying from decreased to absolute lack of movement.

Causes of Immobility

Immobility can have physical, psychological, environmental, and iatrogenic origins. The most common causes include disorders in the musculoskeletal, neurological, cardiovascular, and respiratory systems. The motor system may be affected directly by disease processes, such as a cerebrovascular accident, or indirectly by conditions such as severe congestive heart disease which affects activity tolerance and reduces mobility.

Pain and stiffness associated with osteoporosis, joint diseases such as osteoarthritis and rheumatoid arthritis, and hip fractures are the most common causes of mobility limitations in the elderly. Individuals may limit their activity because of fear of pain. Obesity can be a complicating factor further impairing joint mobility. Severe kyphosis or scoliosis limits spine flexibility, and can impair cardiac and pulmonary function, thus limiting activity tolerance. Foot problems such as bunions, corns, callouses, ulcers, and nail deformities not only cause pain but also limit the desire to walk.

Neurological disorders such as transient ischemic attacks (TIAs), cerebrovascular accidents (CVAs), vestibular dysfunctions, and Parkinson's disease occur more frequently in the elderly leading to mobility impairments. TIAs can cause syncope and subsequent falls. CVAs may result in residual deficits such as muscle spasticity or flaccidity and impaired proprioception. Vestibular dysfunctions cause dizziness and balance problems. Parkinson's disease creates bradykinesia, muscle rigidity, and tremors. Postural instability and the fear of falling restricts many older persons' mobility. If a serious fracture has resulted from a fall, it is particularly difficult to remobilize the person to the prefracture status. Sensory impairments, such as hearing and visual deficits, may also limit physical activity.

Cardiovascular disorders, such as severe congestive heart disease or coronary artery disease with severe angina, as well as chronic obstructive lung disease, limit activity tolerance, and thus mobility in older adults. Peripheral vascular disease with claudication decreases ambulation, and, if severe, may result in lower extremity amputations which further impair mobility.

Urinary incontinence, a major health problem in the elderly (see Chapter 6), can have a serious impact on mobility. Individuals suffering with incontinence or related symptoms such as urinary urgency and frequency will often restrict their activities to be near a bathroom.

Psychological causes of mobility limitations include depression and dementia. Depression, common in the elderly due to multiple losses, can result in decreased interest in one's surroundings and lack of motivation to move. Dementia in mild to moderate stages can lead to inattentiveness to the environment, thus increasing the risk of falls. In addition, balance and gait mechanisms may be affected. In severe stages, dementia results in apraxia or the inability to move or manipulate objects purposefully.

Iatrogenic causes of immobility result from the effect of prescribed tests of medical therapies. Drug side effects are the most common cause of iatrogenesis. Sedatives, hypnotics, tranquilizers, antidepressants, and narcotic analgesics may cause drowsiness, confusion, and ataxia, thus increasing fall risk. Antipsychotic drugs, such as the phenothiazines, can lead to extrapyramidal effects causing muscle rigidity which impairs mobility. Tricyclic antidepressants, diuretics, vasodilators, beta blockers, and other antihypertensives increase the risk of orthostatic hypotension which can result in falls when arising from a bed or chair. Prescribed bedrest as a result of surgery or acute medical illness can have serious adverse reactions particularly in the elderly who may already have compromised functioning due to chronic disease complications.

Various mechanical devices used in medical therapies, such as splints, casts, traction, indwelling catheters, intravenous lines, and oxygen tanks, can limit physical activity. Physical restraints commonly used to protect elderly patients in institutional settings significantly limit mobility. Restraint use can often be unsafe by precipitating or exacerbating disorientation, sensory deprivation, loss of self-image, and dependency (Gerdes, 1968), regressive behavior and withdrawal (Rose, 1987), anxiety, agitation (Strumpf & Evans, 1988), and even falls—for which they are commonly used to protect against (Innes & Turman, 1983; Lund & Sheafor, 1985; Walshe & Rosen, 1979).

Environmental change is an important cause of immobility in the elderly. Relocation into a hospital or nursing home may cause depression or confusion in older adults which restricts physical activity or may lead to a decrease in ambulation due to an unfamiliar environment.

Consequence of Immobility

All body systems are affected to some extent by immobilization (Kottke, 1966; Miller, 1975). The extent of changes that occur depends on the duration, degree, and type of activity limitation. A consequence of immobility can turn into a cause of further activity restriction, thus creating a more serious problem. Treatment of adverse effects of immobility can also lead to further complications. The elderly are at high risk for consequences of immobility because of altered body functioning from pathologic changes from chronic disease superimposed on normal aging changes. If immobilized, older people have a more rapid deterioration and slower recovery from the adverse effects of immobilization.

The effects of immobility result primarily from deconditioning, which is defined as a loss of functional capacity secondary to lack of use. There are three aspects of deconditioning: (1) diminished maximum range of response usually evoked in physiological activity; (2) decreased endurance for activity; and (3) changes in regular adjustment during transient states, such as position change (Spencer, Vallbona, & Carter, 1965). Although these phenomena are described for loss of physiological function, Mitchell (1981) pointed out that these same concepts can be applied to loss of psychological functioning. For example, being confined to bed or at home restricts a person's social environment. Disuse of communication skills may make it difficult for the individual to interact normally.

Physiological Consequences

Prolonged physical inactivity affects the functioning of each organ resulting in delayed recovery and possibly permanent disability. The most dramatic effect is seen in the musculoskeletal system with loss of muscle mass and strength. Muscles lose 10 to 15% of initial strength per week for the first 4 to 5 weeks, with a slightly lower rate of loss in subsequent weeks (Washburn, 1981). This loss of strength decreases endurance or activity tolerance. Muscle and joint mobility is decreased through a process of fibrosis. The dense collagen network which forms may occur in as few as five days of immobilization, with movement being restricted within a week (Kottke, 1966). Gradually progressive shortening of the muscle will occur, creating a joint contracture. Contractures are more likely to occur when the immobility is caused by paralysis or other conditions affecting motor ability than by bedrest alone. However, severe contractures have formed in persons confined to wheelchairs who do not exercise hip joints. Osteoporosis or the loss of bone occurs because of the lack of muscle tension on the bones. Once mobilization occurs, there is a higher risk of fracture.

Cardiovascular and respiratory consequences of immobility can be life-threatening, particularly in the elderly. Physical inactivity results in cardiovascular deconditioning impairing activity tolerance. Orthostatic hypotension, venous thrombosis, and pulmonary embolus formation can occur. Altered pulmonary function results in a decreased tidal volume, increasing the potential for atelectasis and even aspiration pneumonia.

Prolonged inactivity, whether it be in bed or sitting in a chair or wheelchair, can predispose toward the development of pressure sores. Gastrointestinal complications may result, including anorexia, malnutrition, constipation, and fecal impaction. Genitourinary problems, such as stones and infections, can arise. Both urinary and fecal incontinence may develop because of inability to get to the bathroom in time or the inaccessibility of caregivers to assist with toileting.

Metabolic consequences of immobilization include dehydration, electrolyte imbalances, negative nitrogen and calcium balance, altered glucose tolerance, and altered pharmacokinetic response to drugs. Hematopoietic alterations, such as decreased blood volume and red blood cell mass, may also occur.

Psychological Consequences

The behavioral consequences of immobility are variable and include: anger, hostility, aggression, withdrawal, passivity, and anxiety. Sleep disturbances can result. Body image and self-concept can be altered, having a serious effect on mood.

Depression frequently occurs with the loss of any aspect of mobility function. Having to sell one's car or surrender a driver's license is difficult for most older people. Loss of the ability to transport oneself independently can create an increased dependence on others which may be intolerable. Depression also results from not having the ability to pursue long-enjoyed social, recreational, and leisure activities because of mobility limitations. Often a vicious cycle occurs, beginning with decreased mobility which leads to social withdrawal and isolation, it is followed by altered self-concept and esteem, and finally results in depression.

Depression also can act as a cause of immobility. Depressed individuals who have decreased energy and interest in their surroundings will further limit mobility. This is a significant cause of immobility for the institutionalized elderly. In addition, depression has been linked to falls because the depressed person is inattentive to the immediate environment and may trip over obstacles.

Fear is another psychological consequence of mobility alterations, particularly for those older adults who have fallen. The fear of falling further restricts activity (Vellas, et al., 1987).

Social Consequences

Immobilization contributes to the gradual breakdown of social relationships with withdrawal of the person from participating in social activities. Increasing dependence on others to meet activities of daily living can eventually result in institutionalization, especially if there are few social supports available. Institutionalization further tends to promote immobility. Residents tend to become apathetic or depressed and give up their will to move.

Family members and other caregivers must also cope with the older adult's loss of mobility. Caring for an impaired family member can be physically taxing as well as emotionally stressful. Depending on the severity of the mobility impairment and the availability of social support, nursing home placement may be sought.

FALLS

Falls are a major cause and consequence of mobility restrictions, with a high rate of morbidity and mortality among the elderly. The highest incidence of falls and injury with falls occurs in the institutionalized elderly. More than half of nursing home residents fall during a year, with serious injury occurring in 10 to 15%. Only half of those hospitalized will be alive a year later (Margulec, Librach, & Schadel, 1970). Approximately one-third of elders in the community will fall during a year, with this figure rising to almost one-half of persons 80 years and older (Campbell, et al., 1981). While most falls will not be life-threatening, they often result in a reduction of functional ability either due to complications associated with an injury or a psychological impairment from the fear of falling contributing to self-imposed mobility restrictions.

The etiology of falls is multifactorial and is not clearly understood. Advanced age, age-associated changes previously described, chronic conditions, medications, and environmental factors have all been implicated as causative factors in falls. Table 7.2 highlights causes of falls in the elderly. In a review of fall studies, Rubenstein and his associates (1988) found that 55% of all falls were related to medical conditions, with 37% related to environmental hazards. Characteristics associated with a high risk of falling include: advanced age, female gender, poor health status, impaired gait and balance, prior history of falls, and multiple chronic diseases.

ASSESSMENT

Nursing assessment of mobility alterations focuses on the individual within the context of his or her own environment. The purposes of the assessment are to: (1) describe the nature and degree of the mobility alteration; (2) identify possible reversible causes; and (3) identify potential adverse consequences. Important components of this assessment are summarized in Table 7.3.

Subjective Data

Assessment of mobility usually begins with subjective data when nurses interview older persons to learn about their mobility and related problems such as pain, stiffness, fatigue, shortness of breath, visual deficits, dizziness, etc. Nurses should also assess adaptations made to any impairments, including use of assistive devices; the impact of mobility on normal activities, including self-care activities and instrumental activities of daily living, recreational or leisure activities, and social activities. It is also important to determine each individual's perception of how his or her mobility affects the ability to carry out desired roles and to identify personal goals for mobility function.

A history of falls and other accidents caused by mobility impairments should be noted. If falls have occurred, nurses should elicit information on their frequency, circumstances surrounding the fall, associated symptoms, and events following the fall.

A review of current and past medical problems including medication use (both prescription and over-the-counter preparations) will provide valuable information on conditions that may be contributing to mobility impairment and falls if they are occurring. Neurological disorders, such as a stroke with residual paresis or paralysis and Parkinson's disease, directly affect the motor system. Cardiovascular diseases, such as severe congestive heart failure, coronary artery disease with angina, and peripheral arterial disease, affect activity tolerance. Pulmonary disease, such as emphysema, also influences exercise tolerance. Musculoskeletal disorders, such as osteoporosis, degenerative joint disease

TABLE 7.2 Causes of Falls

Environmental
    Hazards: Unstable furniture, throw rugs, loose carpets, loose wires and
       cord, slippery surfaces, uneven surfaces, cluttered environment, beds and
       toilets of inappropriate height, poor lighting
    Unfamiliar surroundings
    Restraint use

Psychological
    Stress
    Depression
    Fear of falling
    Confusion

Sensory
    Impaired visual acuity
    Impaired visual perception
    Vestibular dysfunctions

Neurological
    Syncope (transient ischemic attacks)
    Stroke
    Seizure
    Parkinson's disease
    Gait disorders
    Balance disorders
    Peripheral neuropathies
    Dementia

Cardiovascular
    Syncope (heart block, arrhythmias, aortic stenosis, carotid sinus syndrome)
    Congestive heart failure
    Impaired venous return
    Orthostatic hypotension

Metabolic
    Hypoxia
    Hypoglycemia
    Hyperventilation
    Hypercalcemia
    Hypovolemia
    Thyroid disease
    Acute illness

Musculoskeletal
    Cervical spondylosis
    Myopathies
    Fractures/dislocations
    Joint pain and stiffness
    Muscle weakness

Idiopathic (use of drugs, psychotropics, sedatives/hypnotics, vasodilators, anti-
    hypertensives, diuretics, hypoglycemics, alcohol)

TABLE 7.3 Nursing Assessment of Mobility and Safety in the Elderly

Subjective data

Mobility status (independent; requires use of cane, walker, wheelchair; requires help from another person for assistance, supervision, or teaching; requires help from another person and mobility aid; dependent)

Symptoms affecting mobility
 Weakness and fatigue
 Joint stiffness
 Pain
 Paralysis or paresis
 Urinary frequency, urgency, or incontinence

Dizziness
Chest pain
Shortness of breath
Claudication

Psychological response to mobility impairment
 Perception of cause and severity
 Interference with activities
 Goals

Fall history (if applicable)
 Number of falls
 Injury associated with falls
 Fear of falling
 Circumstances surrounding fall (location, time of day, relationship to posture, turning, cough, aware of fall or unexpected, cause if known, aura preceding fall, ability to get up after fall)
 Associated symptoms (lightheadedness, dizziness, or vertigo; palpitations; chest pain; dyspnea; sudden focal neurological symptoms, i.e., weakness, sensory disturbance, speech difficulty, ataxia, confusion; incontinence; loss of consciousness)

Relevant medical history
 Recent acute illness, surgery, or trauma
 Malignancy
 Depression
 Musculoskeletal disease (osteoarthritis, gout, rheumatoid arthritis, osteoporosis, fractures especially hip)
 Neurologic disease (transient ischemic attacks, stroke, Parkinson's disease, dementia, vestibular dysfunction, vertebrobasilar disease)
 Cardiovascular disease (congestive heart failure, coronary artery disease, peripheral arterial disease)
 Respiratory disease (chronic obstructive lung disease)
 Gastrointestinal disorders (malnutrition, dehydration, electrolyte disturbance)
 Hematopoietic (severe anemia)

Medications (including nonprescription drugs)

Caregiver's perceptions/response to mobility impairment

The following data can be obtained by self-report. However, direct observation is preferred.

Functional abilities
 Self-care activities (bathing, grooming, dressing, toileting, eating)
 Instrumental activities of daily living (cooking, cleaning, shopping, laundry, paying bills, taking medications, transporting self)
 Driving skill

Environment
 Architectural features and physical design (stairs, ramps, location of rooms, etc.)

(continued)

TABLE 7.3 (continued)

Lighting (glare-free, adequate illumination)
Accessibility of bathroom
Use of safety features in bathroom (raised toilet seat, grab bars, shower or tub chair, rubber mats)
Hazards (clutter, loose wires, cords or carpets, throw rugs, slippery surfaces)
Furniture safety (height of chairs and bed; armrests on chairs)
Accessibility of telephones (reachable from floor)
Use of assistive devices (toileting, dressing, grooming, eating, cooking, cleaning)

Objective data

Use of mechanical devices or medical therapies that restrict activity
Vital signs
   Blood pressure (supine, sitting, standing)
   Weight (obesity)
Musculoskeletal
   Posture (normal, kyphosis, kyphoscoliosis)
   Dominant hand
   Muscle: Atrophy, tone, strength testing
   Joints: Contractures or other deformity
             Signs of inflammation: redness, warmth, swelling
             Range of motion in degrees (active and passive)
             Pain or tenderness on movement
   Foot: Type and fit of shoes and painful conditions (calluses, corns, bunions, ulcers, nail deformities)
Neurologic
   Cognitive function
      Level of consciousness
      Mental status
      Mood
   Gait and station
      Use of assistive devices
      Balance: Sitting, arising and sitting down, standing, turning, reaching, bending
      Walking ability (ability to initiate gait, speed, step length, step width, height foot lifted from floor, step symmetry, turning ability, need to hold onto objects)
      Stair climbing ability
      Transfer ability (wheelchair bound patients: wheelchair to bed and commode; bedbound patient: roll from side to side, sitting balance, transfer onto bedpan)
      Motor: Abnormal movements or tremors, paralysis, rigidity or flaccidity, spasms, bradykinesia
   Coordination and dexterity
      Fine motor (ability to button or zip clothing, writing skill)
      Gross motor
   Sensory
      Hearing (use of hearing aid and in proper working condition)
      Vision (near and distant, use of corrective lenses)
      Light touch
      Pain
      Proprioception
      Vibratory sense

including osteoarthritis, gout, and rheumatoid arthritis, directly alter mobility.

If family caregivers are involved, nurses should interview them to determine their perceptions of the individual's mobility function and how it interferes with activities of daily living, as well as the impact of caring for the family member on them.

Environmental factors are important to consider. If a home evaluation cannot be conducted (see Table 7.4), nurses can inquire about physical features of the home, including accident hazards and safety modifications.

Objective Data

Mobility assessment focuses on four types of activities: bed mobility, transfers, wheelchair mobility, and ambulation. Wherever possible, nurses should quantify the degree of impairment and assistance needed during activities. Use of mobility aids should be noted. In addition, mechanical devices that restrict movement, such as restraints, casts, splints, indwelling catheters, oxygen tanks, and intravenous lines, or medical therapies that limit activity should be documented.

Nurses can obtain significant objective data from careful observation of a person's ability to move during performance of daily activities. Valuable information on muscle strength, range of motion, dexterity, balance, gait, and judgment can be obtained through casual observation of the individual within his or her own environment. It is important to observe ambulation directly even in those who seem confined to a wheelchair. Many elders in hospitals and nursing homes who are capable of independent walking have voluntarily chosen to use wheelchairs for mobility (Pawlson, Goodwin, & Keith, 1986).

Physical mobility depends on gait and balance. Tinetti (1986) devised a performance-oriented instrument that is useful in mobility assessment in the elderly. The balance portion of the instrument consists of 13 balance maneuvers, such as sitting, arising and sitting down on a chair, standing, turning, bending, and reaching. The gait portion of the instrument consists of nine observations while a person is walking, such as ability to initiate gait, step height, step length, step symmetry, step continuity, path deviation, trunk stability, walking stance, and turning ability.

Bedbound patients should also be observed for their mobility. The ability to turn from side to side, transfer onto a bedpan, move self by use of a trapeze, and maintain independent sitting balance should be evaluated. Wheelchair patients should be observed for their ability to transfer from bed to wheelchair and from wheelchair to toilet.

A musculoskeletal examination should be performed to detect any signs of joint inflammation and abnormalities in posture, as well as

TABLE 7.4 Home Assessment Checklist for Fall Hazards

Exterior
  Are step surfaces nonslip?
  Are step edges visually marked to avoid tripping?
  Are steps in good repair?
  Are stairway handrails present? Are handrails securely fastened to fittings?
  Are walkways covered with a nonslip surface and free of objects that could be tripped over?
  Is there sufficient outdoor lighting to provide safe ambulation at night?

Interior
  Are lights bright enough to compensate for limited vision?
  Are light switches accessible to the person before entering rooms?
  Are lights glare free?
  Are stairways adequately lighted?
  Are handrails present on both sides of staircases?
  Are handrails securely fastened to walls?
  Are step edges outlined with colored adhesive tape and slip resistant?
  Are throw rugs secured with nonslip backing?
  Are carpet edges taped or tacked down?
  Are rooms uncluttered to permit unobstructed mobility?
  Are chairs throughout home strong enough to provide support during transfers? Are armrests present on chairs to provide assistance while transferring?
  Are tables (dining room, kitchen, etc.) secure enough to provide support if leaned on?
  Do low-lying objects (coffee tables, step stools, etc.) present a tripping hazard?
  Are telephones accessible?

Kitchen
  Are storage areas easily reached without having to stand on tiptoe or a chair?
  Are linoleum floors slippery?
  Is there a nonslip mat in the sink area to soak up spilled water?
  Are chairs wheelfree, armrest equipped, and of proper height to allow for safe transfers?
  If the pilot light goes out on the gas stove, is the gas odor strong enough to alert the person?
  Are step stools strong enough to provide support? Are stool treads in good repair and slip resistant?

Bathroom
  Are doors wide enough to provide unobstructed entering with or without a device?
  Do door thresholds present tripping hazards?
  Are floors slippery, especially when wet?
  Are skid-proof strips or mats in place in the tub or shower?
  Are tub and toilet grab bars available? Are grab bars securely fastened to the walls?
  Are toilets low in height? Is an elevated toilet seat available to assist in toilet transfers?
  Is there sufficient, accessible, and glare-free light available?

(continued)

TABLE 7.4 (continued)

Bedroom
  Is there adequate and accessible lighting available? Are nightlights and/or
    bedside lamps available for nighttime bathroom trips?
  Is the pathway from the bed to the bathroom clear to provide unob-
    structed mobility (especially at night)?
  Are beds of appropriate height to allow for safe on and off transfers?
  Are floors covered with a nonslip surface and free of objects that could be
    tripped over?
  Can the person reach objects from closet shelves without standing on tip-
    toe or a chair?

Source: Tideiksaar, R. (1987). Fall prevention in the home. Reprinted from *Topics in Geriatric Rehabilitation*, Vol. 3, No. 1, p. 59, with permission of Aspen Publishers, Inc., © October 1987.

amputations, contractures, and significant muscle atrophy. Muscle strength and tone should be tested. All joints should be put through full active and passive range of motion with pain or tenderness noted. A foot examination to assess type of shoes worn and presence of painful conditions that may interfere with walking should also be conducted.

Because mobility is closely linked to cognitive and emotional factors, assessment of level of consciousness, mental status, mood, and motivation toward becoming more mobile should be conducted. A brief neurological examination is helpful in detecting abnormal or slowed movements, tremors, difficulties in fine and gross motor coordination, rigidity or flaccidity, and spasms. Assessment of the ability to perceive light touch and painful stimuli provides valuable information on the person's ability to detect possible safety hazards. Vision and hearing deficits should be noted because of their role in maintaining safety.

Assessment for orthostatic hypotension in which blood pressure is checked in the supine, sitting, and standing position three minutes after each change in position should be conducted because it is a significant cause of falls. Drops of 20mm/Hg systolic blood pressure indicate orthostatic hypotension.

NURSING DIAGNOSIS

The main nursing diagnostic category related to the topics of this chapter is *impaired physical mobility*. Specific nursing diagnoses within this category identified by NANDA (Duespohl, 1986) arise from the following etiologies, and thus relate impaired physical mobility to intolerance to activity/decreased strength and endurance; pain/discomfort; perceptual/cognitive impairment; neuromuscular impairment; musculoskeletal impairment; and depression/severe anxiety. The challenge to the nurse is to identify specific nursing diagnoses and etiologies that apply to a particular person.

Mobility affects the whole person including physical, psychological, and social functioning. Alterations in mobility can arise from a variety of causes. Complications from being immobilized are numerous, and can lead to further impairments in several body systems. Thus, considerable overlap exists among the nursing diagnoses that may be appropriate in a particular patient situation. Although the primary diagnosis may be *impaired physical mobility*, there are many associated diagnoses that could also be relevant, such as potential for injury, self-care deficits, powerlessness, activity intolerance, sensory/perceptual alterations, functional urinary incontinence, impaired skin integrity, impaired role performance, and social isolation. Therefore, elderly individuals will often have several nursing diagnoses that apply. The key to selecting the appropriate diagnosis(es) will be based on identifying the primary problem(s) through a thorough nursing assessment.

PLANNING

The management of mobility alterations is based on a thorough nursing assessment which quantifies the type of mobility problem and identifies its underlying etiology. Planning takes account of the individual's strengths and goals. Realistic goal-setting done jointly between the nurse, client, and/or family caregiver is essential.

Four general goals describe client behaviors related to mobility. The client will: (1) achieve optimal mobility; (2) prevent further impairment and adverse consequences of immobility; (3) remove cause(s) of immobility if possible; and (4) promote adaptation to the mobility alteration, if necessary. Specific objectives and time frames—for example, ambulate with walker 50 feet or increase hip flexion to 90° within one week—indicate measurable outcomes to determine whether and/or in what degree these goals have been or are being achieved.

INTERVENTION

The primary nursing interventions for mobility alterations involve (1) body positioning; (2) physical exercise for strength, flexibility, and endurance; and (3) environmental modifications for safety. Body positioning, along with active and passive range of motion exercises, has been well-described in basic nursing textbooks and will not be discussed here.

Positive attitudes of caregivers are critical in the promotion of mobility with older adults. Enthusiasm, patience, and perseverance are important traits in working with the elderly who have mobility impairments. For example, it is difficult to motivate depressed nursing home residents who are complaining of pain and fatigue to realize that they must get out of bed and walk several times a day.

Therapeutic Exercise

The importance of physical activity in slowing the rate of the aging process and preventing complications in the immobilized person cannot be overemphasized. Exercise programs have demonstrated positive effects on muscle strength, flexibility, cardiovascular conditioning, and the respiratory system. In addition, exercise can have significant social and psychological benefits leading to a sense of well being while decreasing anxiety and depression (Benison & Hogstel, 1986).

Most older people, despite mobility status (i.e., bed bound, wheelchair bound, or ambulatory) can participate in an exercise intervention that is designed to maintain joint and muscle function. Individuals with acute inflammatory joint disease may need to rest their joints until the acute phase is over. Persons with painful noninflammatory joint diseases or recovering from fractures will benefit from an exercise regimen but may need analgesia prior to physical activity.

Prior to beginning any exercise program, activity tolerance should be assessed. This includes checking baseline heart rate, respirations, and blood pressure. Ambulatory older adults who wish to engage in a strenuous aerobic program for cardiovascular conditioning should be checked by their physician, particularly if they have cardiovascular or pulmonary disease. As a general rule, people age 70 years and older should not exceed exercising heart rates of 120–125 beats per minute. Other exercise warning signs include heart rate that does not return to normal after five minutes of rest, arrythmia, irregular heart rate, dyspnea, increase of systolic blood pressure greater than 20mm/Hg or diastolic increase of more than 10mm/Hg, faintness, lightheadedness or dizziness, aggravation of musculoskeletal problems, nausea, vomiting or severe discomfort, chest pain or pain referred to arm, jaw, teeth or ear, loss of coordination, or persistent fatigue (Gordon, 1976).

The components of an exercise regimen should include exercises for muscle strength, joint flexibility, and endurance. Muscle strength is maintained by contracting the muscle against resistance. Strength will be maintained by at least two contractions of 20% maximal tension held for a few seconds (Washburn, 1981). Although both isotonic or isometric muscle contractions will maintain strength, isometric contractions should be minimized or avoided in older adults because of their effect on decreasing blood flow especially to the myocardium. Isometric contractions are those in which force is exerted without change in the length of the muscle, such as flexing the feet against a foot board.

These contractions may be necessary for individuals on bedrest or who have casts. In contrast, isotonic contractions occur when the length of the muscle changes with joint function as with range of motion. They are preferred in the elderly, producing a training effect both on skeletal muscle and the heart.

Joint flexibility is improved or maintained by basic range of motion exercises. Each joint should be moved three to five consecutive full range of motion at least twice daily either through active or passive exercise (Vallbona, 1982). Persons with painful joint conditions should move the joint only to the point of resistance or pain. Individuals should be encouraged to perform daily self-care activities to the fullest extent possible. For example, brushing hair exercises the shoulder joint. Putting on socks promotes hip flexion. Any exercise that fixes or stiffens the joints, such as toe touches with locked knees, should be avoided. Also, avoid exercises that use jerking or bouncing against joint resistance.

Endurance is improved or maintained by gradually increasing the number of repetitions of each exercise. For ambulatory individuals, walking is an excellent exercise for overall conditioning. Individuals should start slowly, perhaps at 15 minutes of walking, and gradually build up to an hour of walking (approximately three miles) three times per week.

The frequency of the exercise program depends on the mobility status. Daily range of motion exercises are necessary for immobilized patients. In general, older adults should exercise at least three times per week lasting 15 to 30 minutes at a minimum.

Motivation is a significant problem that nurses will experience in trying to implement an exercise intervention. Interventions should be individually tailored to the needs of the older adult. Creative approaches using music, recreational methods such as dancing or playing games, and reinforcement techniques such as certificates for levels of achievement are helpful. For some people, a structured group program that has peer support will be an excellent approach. For others, particularly those with cognitive and sensory-perceptual deficits, a one-to-one program may be necessary.

Environmental Modifications

The environment plays an important role in the mobility and safety of the older adult. Modifications to the environment are based on a careful assessment of accident hazards. In addition, mobility aids can be useful in stabilizing balance and gait or extending the capabilities of the person who is unable to walk but has good upper extremity strength and function. An important consideration in recommending a mobility aid is the meaning of the aid to the individual. Many older adults feel that a cane or walker carries a stigma marking them as old and infirm. Even though they may acknowledge the necessity of these aids, many elders will refuse to use them.

Mobility aids such as canes, walkers, and wheelchairs need to be properly fitted to each person. Physical or occupational therapists can be helpful in selecting and fitting appropriate aids. Older adults should be cautioned about borrowing used equipment which can produce new problems if improperly fitted.

Interventions Related to Falls

Management of the person who falls is directed toward treating the underlying medical condition(s) and risk factors, and minimizing environmental hazards. Vision and hearing deficits should be corrected. Drugs should be carefully monitored to reduce polypharmacy and inappropriate use of psychotropic medications, as well as to assess for adverse effects affecting both cognitive and mobility function. Cognitive function should be maximized using reality orientation, sensory stimulation, and other techniques incorporating one-to-one therapeutic interaction or group approaches. Physical therapy for gait retraining or muscle strengthening can be beneficial for individuals with stroke, hip fractures, or Parkinson's disease. Exercise programs for flexibility and strength should be implemented. Assistive devices are recommended for persons with gait and balance disturbances. Transfer techniques for chair or wheelchair bound patients should be taught.

Nurses play a significant role in educating elderly persons and their caregivers about the cause(s) of falls. Nurses can promote adaptive behaviors to compensate for functional changes that are contributing to falls and can modify the environment for maximum safety.

In institutional settings, nursing interventions are designed around early identification of the patient who is at high risk for falls, and implementing fall prevention programs. On-going staff education is important in increasing the attention and participation of nursing personnel in fall prevention. Restraints or other protective devices for patients at risk for falling should only be used with caution and care. Often, they have the opposite effect and contribute to falls. Some researchers (e.g., Morrison, et al., 1987; Strumpf & Evans, 1988) have pointed out potential short- and long-term harmful effects of inappropriate use of restraints, leading to the suggestion that their use should be avoided in every case but the most serious, short-term emergency (Evans & Strumpf, 1989). In many instances, restraints are used without adequate assessment and follow-up. As a general rule, restraints should only be used as a last resort after other alternatives have failed. Careful supervision of restrained patients should be conducted.

EVALUATION

Expected outcomes for care of an older adult with impaired mobility are derived from goals and objectives established in the planning phase of the nursing process. Quantitative criteria should be used to measure these outcomes, such as graded muscle strength, degrees of joint range of motion, and levels of independence in physical function. In general, outcomes for impaired physical mobility indicate that the patient has:

1. Maintained independence in mobility to the fullest extent possible with assistive devices if necessary.
2. Maintained independence in self-care activities and instrumental activities of daily living to fullest extent possible.
3. Maintained full range of motion in all joints.
4. Maintained or increased muscle strength.
5. Prevented adverse effects of immobility, i.e., no pressure sores, incontinence, thrombus or embolus formation, contractures, etc.
6. Identified, as early as possible, potential adverse effects of immobility.
7. Avoided falls or had a decreased frequency of falls without injury.

HEALTH PROMOTION AND WELLNESS

The goals of health promotion are to promote optimal mobility within the capabilities of the individual and to prevent falls. The following list provides interventions useful in health promotion with aging adults (Craven & Bruno, 1986; Gibson, et al., 1987).

1. Provide client education
    *   Use low-heeled, well-fitting shoes with non-slip surfaces and good support. Avoid leather shoes.
    *   Visit the podiatrist on a regular basis for treatment of painful foot conditions, e.g., bunions, corns, calluses.
    *   Obtain regular eye examinations. Wear glasses if prescribed, keep glasses clean, and repair broken frames.
    *   Use walking aids (cane, walker) if necessary. If a cane is used, it should be held on the good side opposite the side with weakness or
    *   Avoid walking in crowds or use cane for increased balance.

- Use adaptive behaviors:
    slowly get up from lying or sitting position, waiting
        until dizziness disappears;
    pause for eyes to adjust when going from light to dark
        environments;
    steady self by holding contact with furniture when
        walking at home;
    use caution at curbs and uneven sidewalks;
    do not wear long robes that can be tripped upon;
    avoid carrying large and bulky packages.
- If living alone, establish a telephone support system for
  checking in daily with a friend or family member. Alternatively, use an electronic alarm device that signals when one
  is ill or injured in the home.

2. Alter environment to promote optimal mobility and safety.

3. Establish a regular time for exercise at least 3 to 5 times per
   week. Prior to beginning any strenuous exercise program, be
   evaluated by a physician. Start slowly and gradually build up to
   30–45 minutes of exercises. Begin a walking program; build up to
   1–3 miles per week.

CASE STUDY

The following case illustrates the multifactorial nature of mobility
alterations in the elderly. An 88-year-old woman who lives alone was
seen in the Emergency Room because of a fall which resulted in a
fractured humerus of her dominant arm. She reported that she fell
while trying to get out of a chair and that she experienced dizziness
prior to the fall. She also admitted to having fallen at least two other
times in the past month, with both falls occurring while walking in her
apartment without the use of her cane. Her medical diagnoses included
degenerative joint disease affecting the hip joint, primary hypertension,
bilateral cataracts, and noninsulin-dependent diabetes mellitus. Her
only medication was hydrochlorthiazide.

On examination, the woman appeared underweight, withdrawn, and
sad. When questioned about her mood, she began crying and stated
that her husband had died three months earlier, and that she had no
family or friends left. Her blood pressure dropped from 152/80 in the
supine position to 132/84 in the standing position, with light-headedness persisting after she stood. She had difficulty reading newsprint as
well as seeing the Snellen eye chart. Her gait was unsteady with a
slowed walking speed, short irregular steps, and difficulty arising and
sitting down in a chair. However, balance was intact. Mental status was

normal but a screening questionnaire indicated depression. Other than generalized weakness, the rest of her physical examination was unremarkable. Laboratory tests were also negative.

After the woman received medical treatment, which involved arm casting and a prescription for analgesic medication, the emergency room nurse referred her to the visiting nurse for further evaluation. A home assessment revealed a messy environment with stacks of magazines and newspapers throughout the apartment. In addition, the nurse noted the use of throw rugs on hardwood floors, and the fact that the woman was wearing slippers which slid easily.

The nursing diagnosis included: impaired physical mobility related to hip pain; potential for injury related to gait instability, history of falls, cluttered and unsafe environment, and orthostatic hypertension; self-care deficits in bathing, grooming, and dressing related to the arm cast; sensory-perceptual alteration—vision; altered nutrition—less than body requirements related to disinterest in eating; ineffective coping related to bereavement over husband's death.

The nursing care plan involved the use of community resources to provide support during the period the cast was worn—Meals on Wheels and a home health aide for assistance with bathing, dressing, and light housecleaning. Referral to an opthalmologist resulted in a new eyeglass prescription which helped resolve the visual problem. Ambulation was improved with the decrease in hip pain secondary to analgesic use. A four-legged cane and athletic shoes provided improved stability in walking, with use of a walker planned following cast removal. Environmental modifications included the installation of grab bars by the tub and a raised toilet seat with armrests. Throw rugs, newspapers, and other clutter were removed from the apartment. The woman was instructed to arise slowly from a lying or sitting position and not to move until any light-headedness disappeared. Her depression improved with weekly visits by the nurse who provided support and bereavement counseling. The woman agreed to attend a weekly support group for widows at the senior center after her cast was removed. Following cast removal, she received physical therapy and resumed full range of motion in her arm. Six months later, she had made friends at the senior center and was attending events at least three times a week including a light exercise program. Her morale had improved, and she had no further falls.

CONCLUSION

Mobility is essential in the psychological and physical well-being of older adults. The elderly are more likely to have problems with mobility than any other physical or cognitive function, placing them at higher on the aging system, and ad-

normal processes of aging are
early adulthood. Except for acci-
gressive disease conditions occur-
, these changes are generally not
Because age-related changes occur
t aging persons have adapted and

er 75 is expected to show the greatest
attributed to aging. However, chrono-
st indicator of physiological age or of
tenuto & Bullock, 1980). While sensory
s and organ systems, they do not neces-
older persons as they sense and perceive
4). Nevertheless, when losses do occur in
he potential for risk increases and altera-
can become more difficult (Gioiella & Bevil,
aging is the tendency on the part of society
mselves to consider alterations in sensory
itants of growing old, thus deferring consul-
this basis.

RISTICS OF THE AGING SENSES

ies of taste and smell are interactive; that is, the
predominantly dependent upon the acuity of smell
ste buds. Smell and taste belong to the chemical
the "chemosenses" (Flynn & Heffron, 1987). In
complex mechanisms, triggered by environmental
he nerve cells in the nose, mouth, or throat, which, in
e sense center of the brain to identify specific smells or
impulses travel shorter distances and leave more last-
s in the brain than do those of other senses (Davis,

lated Changes

ue accommodates approximately 245 tastebuds which
by approximately two-thirds in the latter part of life.
of bitter and sour are found on the posterior one-third
while the anterior two-thirds produces sensations of

risk for falls and injuries. Nursing management of the person with a mobility alteration is based on a thorough nursing assessment which identifies the type and degree of mobility alteration, its underlying etiology, and possible adverse effects of immobilization. The hallmarks of effective nursing intervention include body positioning, therapeutic exercise, and environmental modifications.

REFERENCES

Benison, B., & Hogstel, M. O. (1986). Aging and movement therapy: Essential interventions for the immobile elderly. *Journal of Gerontological Nursing, 12*(12), 8–16.

Bortz, W. M. (1982). Disuse and aging. *Journal of the American Medical Academy, 248*(10), 1203–1208.

Campbell, A. J., Reinken, J., Allan, B. C., & Martinez, G. S. (1981). Falls in old age: A study of frequency and related clinical factors. *Age and Ageing, 10,* 264–270.

Carnevali, D., & Brueckner, S. (1970). Immobilization: Assessment of a concept. *American Journal of Nursing, 70,* 1502–1507.

Craven, R., & Bruno, P. (1986). Teach the elderly to prevent falls. *Journal of Gerontological Nursing, 12*(8), 27–33.

Duespohl, T. A. (1986). *Nursing diagnosis manual for the well and ill client.* Philadelphia: W. B. Saunders.

Evans, L. K., & Strumpf, N. E. (1989). Tying down the elderly: A review of the literature on physical restraint. *Journal of the American Geriatrics Society, 37,* 65–74.

Gerdes, L. (1968). The confused or delirious patient. *American Journal of Nursing, 68,* 1228–1233.

Gibson, M. J., Andres, R. O., Isaacs, B., Radebaugh, T., & Worm Peterson, J. (1987). The prevention of falls in later life. *Danish Medical Bulletin, 34* (Supplement 4), 1–24.

Gordon, M. (1976). Assessing activity tolerance. *American Journal of Nursing, 76,* 72–75.

Hogue, C. C. (1984). Falls and mobility in late life: An ecological model. *Journal of the American Geriatrics Society, 32,* 858–861.

Innes, E., & Turman, W. (1983). Evolution of patient falls. *Quality Review Bulletin, 9*(2), 30–35.

Kottke, F. J. (1966). The effects of limitation of activity upon the human body. *Journal of the American Medical Academy, 196*(10), 825–830.

Lund, C., & Sheafor, M. L. (1985). Is your patient about to fall? *Journal of Gerontological Nursing, 11*(4), 37–41.

Margulec, I., Librach, G., & Schadel, M. (1970). Epidemiological study of accidents among residents of homes for the aged. *Journal of Gerontology, 25,* 342–346.

Miller, M. B. (1975). Iatrogenic and nurisgenic effects of prolonged immobilization of the ill aged. *Journal of the American Geriatrics Society, 23,* 360–369.

Mitchell, P. H. (1981). Motor status. In P. H. Mitchell & A. Loustau (Eds.), *Concepts basic to nursing* (3rd ed.; pp. 343–391). New York: McGraw-Hill.

Morrison, J., Crinklaw-Wiancko, D., King, D., Thibeault, S., & Wells, D. L. (1987). Formulating a restraint use policy. *The Journal of Nursing Administration, 17*(3), 39–42.

National Center for Health Statistics [NCHS] (1987). Health statistics on older persons: United States, 1986. *Vital and health statistics*, Series 3, No. 25. DHHS Pub. No. (PHS) 88-1409. Hyattsville, MD: Public Health Service.

Pawlson, L. G., Goodwin, M., & Keith, K. (1986). Wheelchair use by ambulatory nursing home residents. *Journal of the American Geriatrics Society, 34*, 860–864.

Rose, J. (1987). When the care plan says restrain. *Geriatric Nursing, 8*, 20–21.

Rubenstein, L. Z., Robbins, A. S., Schulman, B. L., Rosado, J., Osterweil, D., & Josephson, K. R. (1988). Falls and instability in the elderly. *Journal of the American Geriatrics Society, 36*, 266–278.

Schwartz, D., Heneley, B., & Zeitz, L. (1964). *The elderly ambulatory patient*. New York: Macmillan.

Spencer, W. A., Vallbona, C., & Carter, R. E. (1965). Physiologic concepts of immobilization. *Archives of Physical Medicine and Rehabilitation, 46*, 89–100.

Strumpf, N. E., & Evans, L. K. (1988). Physical restraint of the hospitalized elderly: Perceptions of patients and nurses. *Nursing Research, 37*, 132–136.

Tideiksaar, R. (1987). Fall prevention in the home. *Topics in Geriatric Rehabilitation, 3*(1), 57–64.

Tinetti, M. E. (1986). Performance-oriented assessment of mobility problems in elderly patients. *Journal of the American Geriatrics Society, 34*, 119–126.

Vallbona, C. (1982). Bodily responses to immobilization. In F. J. Kottke, G. K. Stillwell, & J. F. Lehmann (Eds.), *Krusen's handbook of physical medicine and rehabilitation* (3rd ed.; pp. 963–976). Philadelphia: W. B. Saunders.

Vellas, B., Cayla, F., Bocquet, H., de Pemille, F., Albarede, J. L. (1987). Prospective study of restriction of activity in old people after falls. *Age and Ageing, 16*, 189–193.

Walshe, A., & Rosen, H. (1979). A study of patient falls from bed. *Journal of Nursing Administration, 9*(5), 31–35.

Washburn, K. B. (1981). *Physical medicine and rehabilitation: Essentials of primary care* (2nd ed.). Garden City, NY: Medical Examination Publishing Co.

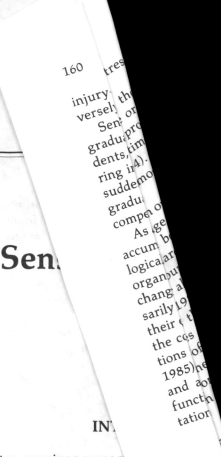

This chapter examines sensory
the impact of the normal agi
Normal and abnormal physiolo
to sensory functioning for taste
hearing (audition), and touch (tac
tics of the aging senses are discu
changes, alterations in health statu

The human body interacts with
sory system and its complex mechar
process stimuli into meaningful inform
tant to the sensory process are recepti
received through the sensory organs (
nerve pathways to the cortex of the bra
processed, organized, and interpreted or
mal adaptation in a constantly changing e
these sensory-neural processes (Flynn &
receiving and perceiving stimuli through t
nervous system can adversely affect adaptatio
functioning—which include normal age-relate
cial changes, the impact of various illnesses an

risk for falls and injuries. Nursing management of the person with a mobility alteration is based on a thorough nursing assessment which identifies the type and degree of mobility alteration, its underlying etiology, and possible adverse effects of immobilization. The hallmarks of effective nursing intervention include body positioning, therapeutic exercise, and environmental modifications.

REFERENCES

Benison, B., & Hogstel, M. O. (1986). Aging and movement therapy: Essential interventions for the immobile elderly. *Journal of Gerontological Nursing,* *12*(12), 8–16.

Bortz, W. M. (1982). Disuse and aging. *Journal of the American Medical Academy,* *248*(10), 1203–1208.

Campbell, A. J., Reinken, J., Allan, B. C., & Martinez, G. S. (1981). Falls in old age: A study of frequency and related clinical factors. *Age and Ageing, 10,* 264–270.

Carnevali, D., & Brueckner, S. (1970). Immobilization: Assessment of a concept. *American Journal of Nursing, 70,* 1502–1507.

Craven, R., & Bruno, P. (1986). Teach the elderly to prevent falls. *Journal of Gerontological Nursing, 12*(8), 27–33.

Duespohl, T. A. (1986). *Nursing diagnosis manual for the well and ill client.* Philadelphia: W. B. Saunders.

Evans, L. K., & Strumpf, N. E. (1989). Tying down the elderly: A review of the literature on physical restraint. *Journal of the American Geriatrics Society, 37,* 65–74.

Gerdes, L. (1968). The confused or delirious patient. *American Journal of Nursing, 68,* 1228–1233.

Gibson, M. J., Andres, R. O., Isaacs, B., Radebaugh, T., & Worm Peterson, J. (1987). The prevention of falls in later life. *Danish Medical Bulletin, 34* (Supplement 4), 1–24.

Gordon, M. (1976). Assessing activity tolerance. *American Journal of Nursing, 76,* 72–75.

Hogue, C. C. (1984). Falls and mobility in late life: An ecological model. *Journal of the American Geriatrics Society, 32,* 858–861.

Innes, E., & Turman, W. (1983). Evolution of patient falls. *Quality Review Bulletin, 9*(2), 30–35.

Kottke, F. J. (1966). The effects of limitation of activity upon the human body. *Journal of the American Medical Academy, 196*(10), 825–830.

Lund, C., & Sheafor, M. L. (1985). Is your patient about to fall? *Journal of Gerontological Nursing, 11*(4), 37–41.

Margulec, I., Librach, G., & Schadel, M. (1970). Epidemiological study of accidents among residents of homes for the aged. *Journal of Gerontology, 25,* 342–346.

Miller, M. B. (1975). Iatrogenic and nurisgenic effects of prolonged immobilization of the ill aged. *Journal of the American Geriatrics Society, 23,* 360–369.

Mitchell, P. H. (1981). Motor status. In P. H. Mitchell & A. Loustau (Eds.), *Concepts basic to nursing* (3rd ed.; pp. 343–391). New York: McGraw-Hill.

Morrison, J., Crinklaw-Wiancko, D., King, D., Thibeault, S., & Wells, D. L. (1987). Formulating a restraint use policy. *The Journal of Nursing Administration, 17*(3), 39–42.

National Center for Health Statistics [NCHS] (1987). Health statistics on older persons: United States, 1986. *Vital and health statistics,* Series 3, No. 25. DHHS Pub. No. (PHS) 88–1409. Hyattsville, MD: Public Health Service.

Pawlson, L. G., Goodwin, M., & Keith, K. (1986). Wheelchair use by ambulatory nursing home residents. *Journal of the American Geriatrics Society, 34,* 860–864.

Rose, J. (1987). When the care plan says restrain. *Geriatric Nursing, 8,* 20–21.

Rubenstein, L. Z., Robbins, A. S., Schulman, B. L., Rosado, J., Osterweil, D., & Josephson, K. R. (1988). Falls and instability in the elderly. *Journal of the American Geriatrics Society, 36,* 266–278.

Schwartz, D., Heneley, B., & Zeitz, L. (1964). *The elderly ambulatory patient.* New York: Macmillan.

Spencer, W. A., Vallbona, C., & Carter, R. E. (1965). Physiologic concepts of immobilization. *Archives of Physical Medicine and Rehabilitation, 46,* 89–100.

Strumpf, N. E., & Evans, L. K. (1988). Physical restraint of the hospitalized elderly: Perceptions of patients and nurses. *Nursing Research, 37,* 132–136.

Tideiksaar, R. (1987). Fall prevention in the home. *Topics in Geriatric Rehabilitation, 3*(1), 57–64.

Tinetti, M. E. (1986). Performance-oriented assessment of mobility problems in elderly patients. *Journal of the American Geriatrics Society, 34,* 119–126.

Vallbona, C. (1982). Bodily responses to immobilization. In F. J. Kottke, G. K. Stillwell, & J. F. Lehmann (Eds.), *Krusen's handbook of physical medicine and rehabilitation* (3rd ed.; pp. 963–976). Philadelphia: W. B. Saunders.

Vellas, B., Cayla, F., Bocquet, H., de Pemille, F., Albarede, J. L. (1987). Prospective study of restriction of activity in old people after falls. *Age and Ageing, 16,* 189–193.

Walshe, A., & Rosen, H. (1979). A study of patient falls from bed. *Journal of Nursing Administration, 9*(5), 31–35.

Washburn, K. B. (1981). *Physical medicine and rehabilitation: Essentials of primary care* (2nd ed.). Garden City, NY: Medical Examination Publishing Co.

Chapter 8

Sensory Functioning

Barbara A. Brant

INTRODUCTION

This chapter examines sensory functioning in the elderly and discusses the impact of the normal aging process on each sensory modality. Normal and abnormal physiological and psychological changes related to sensory functioning for taste (gustation), smell (olfaction), vision, hearing (audition), and touch (tactile sense) are described. Characteristics of the aging senses are discussed relative to normal age-related changes, alterations in health status, and potential risk factors.

The human body interacts with the environment through the sensory system and its complex mechanisms which activate the brain to process stimuli into meaningful information. The two functions important to the sensory process are reception and perception. Information received through the sensory organs (reception) is transmitted along nerve pathways to the cortex of the brain where sensory stimuli are processed, organized, and interpreted or perceived (perception). Optimal adaptation in a constantly changing environment occurs through these sensory-neural processes (Flynn & Heffron, 1984). Barriers to receiving and perceiving stimuli through the sense organs and the nervous system can adversely affect adaptation. Alterations in sensory functioning—which include normal age-related physical and psychosocial changes, the impact of various illnesses and disease processes, and injury—can and do create undue stress on the aging system, and adversely affect adaptation.

Sensory changes attributed to the normal processes of aging are gradual, beginning in adolescence or early adulthood. Except for accidents, serious illness, or certain progressive disease conditions occurring in most aging adults over time, these changes are generally not sudden happenings (Steffl, 1984). Because age-related changes occur gradually over the life span, most aging persons have adapted and compensated successfully.

As a general rule, the person over 75 is expected to show the greatest accumulation of sensory change attributed to aging. However, chronological age is not always the best indicator of physiological age or of organ system functioning (Carotenuto & Bullock, 1980). While sensory changes vary among age groups and organ systems, they do not necessarily imply dysfunction for all older persons as they sense and perceive their environment (Steffl, 1984). Nevertheless, when losses do occur in the compensatory senses, the potential for risk increases and alterations in adaptive responses can become more difficult (Gioiella & Bevil, 1985). One complication of aging is the tendency on the part of society and aging individuals themselves to consider alterations in sensory function as normal concomitants of growing old, thus deferring consultation and treatment on this basis.

CHARACTERISTICS OF THE AGING SENSES

Taste and Smell

The sensory modalities of taste and smell are interactive; that is, the sensation of taste is predominantly dependent upon the acuity of smell to stimulate the taste buds. Smell and taste belong to the chemical sensing system or the "chemosenses" (Flynn & Heffron, 1987). In healthy persons, complex mechanisms, triggered by environmental stimuli, activate the nerve cells in the nose, mouth, or throat, which, in turn, activate the sense center of the brain to identify specific smells or tastes. Ofactory impulses travel shorter distances and leave more lasting impressions in the brain than do those of other senses (Davis, 1984).

Normal Age-Related Changes

The adult tongue accommodates approximately 245 tastebuds which tend to diminish by approximately two-thirds in the latter part of life. Taste sensations of bitter and sour are found on the posterior one-third of the tongue, while the anterior two-thirds produces sensations of sweet and salty. Taste sensitivity increases, particularly when stimulation occurs over a large area of the tongue (Davis, 1984). Salivary secretions serve to break down food elements which stimulate nerve endings to discriminate taste. Because taste activates many digestive processes, a malfunction or alteration may impede normal digestion and appetite. Combinations of sweet, salty, bitter, and sour sensations, in concert with odors, textures, temperatures, and other chemosensory stimuli, produce flavors that are recognized mainly through the sense of smell (Flynn & Heffron, 1987).

Alterations in Health Status

Diminished smell acuity (hyposmia) resulting from a reduction in the number of olfactory nerve fibers occurs in approximately 30% of elderly persons 75 years and older (Colavita, 1978). Conditions other than those of normal aging can alter taste and smell responses. Head trauma, injury to the tissues of the nose or mouth, nerve damage, illness, disease processes, surgery on the mouth, nose, or throat, certain drugs, cigarette smoking, noxious environmental stimuli, and genetic influences contribute significantly (Whitbourne, 1985; Yen, 1982).

Risk Factors

Elders are at risk for hazards to their health resulting from aging changes or from other alterations in taste and smell. Inability to detect smoke and gas leaks, food spoilage, and poisonous or harmful chemicals all affect the safety and health of older adults. Serious burns may be an outcome. Undetected changes in nutritional status, eating patterns, and weight loss can lead to malnutrition. Loss or change in taste and smell are integral to assessment and identification of risk factors in elderly persons.

Vision

Contrary to societal beliefs, vision loss is not an inevitable outcome of aging, but one that is most feared by elderly persons. Interestingly, most older adults have moderate to excellent vision and will probably retain more than adequate visual acuity into old age (Marmor, 1981). As Kornsweig (1984) asserted, the human eye is so constructed that it is expected to function normally well beyond the owner's lifetime.

To activate vision, light passes through the cornea, the aqueous humor, a clear viscid fluid in the eye itself, the pupil, lens, and a gelatin-like substance, the vitreous humor. It then continues to the retinal area in the inner eye, where visual receptors, the cones and rods, provide the "crucial link" in making contact with the environment (Belsky, 1984).

Light waves, transformed as impulses by the cones and rods, are transmitted to the brain by neurons in the optic nerve (Whitbourne, 1985).

Vision is an integral part of effective communication and learning, and is highly valued. Visual function enables elders to carry out activities of daily living safely and independently. Generally, by the time one reaches 75 years of age, adaptation to aging changes in visual acuity has occurred through the increased use of other senses to manage the environment.

Normal Age-Related Changes

Structural changes in the aging eye affecting visual accommodation usually begin in the second or third decade of life. Both heredity and environment can influence structural and functional changes. *Presbyopia* ("presby"= old; "opia" = eyes), the inability to focus on near objects, resulting from loss of elasticity in the aging lens, is present in most older adults before 60 years of age. Loss of lens elasticity accompanies gradual loss of accommodation and decreased depth perception (Buseck, 1980). Distances from which one can see clearly slowly recede with age.

Senile miosis, the tendency of pupils to become smaller, is thought to begin at high school age (Cohen & Lessell, 1984). Pupil size affects the amount of light reaching the retina, thereby reducing the ability to see darkened objects in dimmed lighting. Because older persons usually have smaller pupils, they may react poorly to light and glare. Glare, the sensory response produced by the scattering of light as it enters the aging eye, inhibits distant vision (Hatton, 1977). Increased lens opacity also contributes to increased glare. *"Senile yellowing"* of the optic lens causes low tone colors, such as blues, greens, violet, and pastels to fade, while reds and yellows tend to be seen best (Buseck, 1980).

Decreased peripheral vision, often referred to as "side" or "tunnel" vision, reduces the ability to see objects in the peripheral fields, thereby altering the extent or range of vision. *Corneal thickening* results in decreased transparency and inability to discriminate the fine details of objects within a visual field (Buseck, 1980). *Decreased lacrimal secretions*, especially post-menopausal, lead to dryness of the eyes, discomfort, and often damage to the corneal surface. The older person's orientation and level of independence are often affected by these changes.

Many older persons do not realize the extent of their visual limitations because the onset has been gradual. However, when disease impacts normal aging, it increases the potential to severely limit activities of older adults. Awareness of normal physiological changes occurring with age will assist health care providers to recognize abnormal, pathological eye disorders common to the elderly. Eye dysfunction in older persons, including failing vision, can often be prevented with regular eye examinations, and should not be dismissed as an expected outcome of aging (National Society to Prevent Blindness [NSPB], 1983).

Alterations in Health Status

There are an estimated 1.7 million visually handicapped Americans unable to read the newspaper even with the aid of glasses. Sixty-five percent of these persons are over 65, and approximately two-thirds are women (National Center for Health Statistics [NCHS], 1982). Decreased visual acuity in older adults is attributed mainly to local diseases of the eye, rather than to optic nerve or nervous system disease (Eliopoulos, 1984).

A wide range of sight is affected by various sensory alterations. Four leading causes of low vision and blindness in elders are cataracts, glaucoma, senile macular degeneration, and diabetic retinopathy (NSPB, 1983). *Cataracts*, the most prevalent of the eye diseases in old age, are the most easily and successfully remedied through advanced surgical procedures that shorten hospital stays. Cataract formation on the lens of the eye begins in nearly everyone over the age of 30, progressing at varying rates in different individuals (Bennett & Eklund, 1983; Kollarits, 1986). Symptoms of cataract formation include distorted perception, haziness, a dimming of vision, intolerance for glare, or inability to accommodate sudden changes from lighted to darkened areas. However, what the older person presumes to be early cataract formation may be related to other visual difficulties that require immediate medical intervention; therefore, early detection is essential.

"Chronic glaucoma," "the sneak-thief of sight" (NSPB, 1983), is the second most common eye disorder among the elderly. Glaucoma, a slow, progressive, and painless disease, gradually causes damage to the optic nerve as a result of elevated pressure within the eye (Marmor, 1981). All forms of glaucoma involve some impairment in normal drainage of the aqueous humor. Diminished peripheral (side) vision can become irreversible if pressure is not controlled. Other symptoms include blurred vision and inability to adjust to dark and light. In *acute* glaucoma, colored rings or halos may be perceived around lights.

Laser technology as a treatment modality is frequently used for iridectomies to promote improved drainage of aqueous humor. Regular use of ocular drops such as pilocarpine, or other prescribed medication, is very important to treatment and control (Marmor, 1981). An important control measure is to reduce stress situations that stimulate the autonomic nervous system to dilate the pupil. Annual intra-ocular pressure monitoring is recommended for people over 40 years of age.

Macular degeneration, often referred to as "senile" macular degeneration, is the progressive loss of central vision, "the most perfect spot for seeing" (Ferraro, 1983, p. 11). Peripheral vision is usually retained so that blindness is not complete. The macula is most vulnerable to age-related and sclerotic changes, but the exact cause of its deterioration is not fully understood. Hemorrhages from the vessels around the macular site may cause the sudden onset of visual loss (Marmor, 1981). Although laser therapy is currently being used with some success (Dickman, 1982), macular degeneration remains a major cause of visual disability in the older adult. Since rapid loss of vision may also indicate acute glaucoma or retinal detachment, both treatable conditions, any symptom(s) of rapid visual loss requires immediate opthalmologic attention.

Diabetic retinopathy is another leading cause of blindness in people who have been diabetic for more than 10 years (Marmor, 1981). In this condition, small hemorrhages from neovascular vessels leak into the vitreous humor causing visual alterations. Older adults diagnosed with vascular disease are frequently prone to retinal hemorrhage, with scarring and loss of vision. Any visual change, sudden redness, or pain requires immediate medical attention. Periodic examinations are a MUST for the client. Assessing the need for health education is essential.

A common visual interference in the elderly, known as ectropion, results from diminished muscle tone, with sagging and eversion or rolling out of the lower lid. Entropion, the inrolling or inversion of the lower lid and lashes, often causes corneal irritation. Both conditions respond favorably to surgical intervention (Carotenuto & Bullock, 1980). Other causes of eye trauma can easily occur from injury, rubbing, scratching, or introducing foreign objects onto the corneal surface.

Risk Factors

Impaired vision can render the aging person less mobile, more prone to injury or falls (Tobis, Nyak, & Hoehler, 1981), and more apt to make mistakes in identifying medication and household cleaners. Isolation and sensory deprivation (Chodil & Williams, 1970) are always a concern "in a world that is already marginally tolerant of the elderly person" (Marmor, 1981, p. 18). The toxicological effects of hypervitaminosis, especially Vitamins A and D, are a potential threat to vision (Buseck, 1980). The emotional effects of reduced or total vision loss can be devastating. Depression may result.

Inteference with visual function can change the way in which older persons perceive (interpret) and interact with their world. Thus early detection and prompt treatment are imperative since "more than half of all cases of blindness can be prevented" (NSPB, 1983, p. xx). A risk factor worthy of consideration is Sullivan's (1985) assertion that "as long as the elderly believe that nothing can be done to assist them [in correcting failing eyesight] . . . they will do nothing" (p. 233).

Hearing

"Hearing is a function that governs the individual's ability to exchange communication with others and to appreciate the variety of natural and artificial sounds that form the essential matrix of everyday life" (Whitbourne, 1985, p. 175). Sound is created by sound waves which are directed through the auditory canal to the middle ear, exerting pressure against the tympanic membrane to set the ossicles and windows in motion. The cochlea and other structures of the inner ear are activated to convert sound waves into electrical signals or impulses to relay to the auditory nerve and the brain (Larsen, 1986). Although the majority of older adults retain sufficient hearing for normal living (Anderson & Meyerhoff, 1986), some loss of hearing usually becomes evident by age 50.

Normal Age-Related Changes

Sensorineural and conductive hearing is affected by normal aging. Sensorineural changes in the aging auditory system involving the cochlea, the diminution of sensory or hair cells, and the brain itself may produce change in the two functions of the human ear, hearing and balance (Goode, 1981).

Presbycusis, a progressive hearing disorder of the inner ear is the most common cause of bilateral sensorineural hearing dysfunction among older adults. Hearing is diminished for high frequency sounds, speech processing and discrimination, and pure tone. The decreased ability of higher brain centers to process auditory stimuli may contribute to poor speech perception (Kane, Ouslander, & Abrass, 1984). Speech perception may be further hampered by background noise in the environment. A reduction in sound volume and inability to discriminate frequency sounds made by the consonants s, sh, f, and th, may result in a partial loss of words, sentences, and meaning for what has been verbally communicated (Belsky, 1984; Kopac, 1983). Tinnitus or ringing in the ears is one common disruption to the interpretation of incoming stimuli.

In conduction, the transmission of sound to the inner ear is channeled through the external and middle ear structures. Noise and excess cerumen accumulation are major factors which impede this transmission. Longer, thicker hair growth, and a thinning of the tissues of the ear canal may contribute to excess cerumen (Whitbourne, 1985).

Cerumen impaction in the ear canal results from a reduction in the moisture supply to aging tissues and an increase in keratin production.

Alterations in Health Status

Impairment of hearing ranks third among the five most common chronic conditions affecting the health of older adults (NCHS, 1981). Of those persons 65 and older, 28% experience hearing dysfunction. Nearly 50% of elderly men and 30% of elderly women are affected (NCHS, 1981).

Sensorineural impairment of the inner ear is usually attributed to damage from the eighth cranial nerve (Goode, 1981). Other factors include vascular changes and exposure to middle ear disease in early life. Functional hearing deficits affect loss of performance in perceiving signals, binaural listening, speech understanding, and language communication. For persons who have experienced a stroke, deficits or alterations can be magnified.

Risk Factors

Communication may be difficult because of the energy and effort required to understand others and to be understood. Intolerance may prompt the older adult's exclusion from activities and meaningful interaction. With alterations in emotional balance and harmony in external and internal environments, hearing-impaired elderly persons can experience hallucinations, mistrust, loss of self-esteem, depression, and periodic paranoia (Whitbourne, 1985). There is a tendency for these elders to become "out of sync" with their environment if the condition is not or cannot be corrected. Under such conditions, isolation often becomes a major problem (Bolin, 1974). Because depression is a major factor in older persons who attempt and commit suicide (Osgood, Brant, & Lipman, 1988), hearing-impaired elderly are potentially at risk. It is important to keep in mind that hearing impairment in elderly persons usually has a treatable cause.

Tactile Senses

"The 'somesthetic' or 'tactile' senses provide information about touch, pressure, pain, and external temperatures which enable the individual to experience pleasure, discomfort, and sensitivity to environmental threats" (Whitbourne, 1985, p. 191). Multiple touch receptors in the skin or in tissues beneath the skin are very sensitive to even the lightest stimulation. Hair growth and receptors in the hands, soles of the feet, fingertips, tongue, and lips are particularly responsive to local stimuli. Shifts in the intensity of stimuli or abrupt changes in sensory signals are rapidly transmitted to the central nervous system and brain through the spinal cord (Whitbourne, 1985).

Normal Age-Related Changes

While certain receptors cells and corpuscles (e.g., Merkel's and free nerve endings) responding to touch stimulation may not be affected by the aging process, other cells (e.g., Meissner's and Pacinian) are thought to be significantly reduced or impaired by aging (Colavita, 1978; Whitbourne, 1985). A gradual dulling of tactile sensitivity is presumed to begin near the fiftieth year. Not all elderly will experience tactile changes, but for those who do, the range of sensitivity is expected to vary (Kenshalo, 1977). Areas most commonly affected in older adults are the hands, soles of the feet, and fingertips. Elders often express frustration in attempting to pick up small objects or managing the fasteners and their clothing because they have "no feeling" in their fingertips. Pressure sensitivity, pain, and thermal response may also be affected.

Alterations in Health Status

Generally, alterations in tactile sensitivity result mainly from injury, central nervous system disorders, neuropathies often found in diabetes mellitus or cardiovascular disease, and arthritic conditions (Gioiella & Bevil, 1985).

Risk Factors

Because studies of touch sensitivity in aging are sparse (Kenshalo, 1977), limited information is available to indicate clearly those factors which place older adults at risk. However, the literature does reflect a need for elders to take safety precautions when manipulating objects, cooking, applying heat, exerting pressure, or during exposure to extremes of heat and cold. For this reason, assessment is extremely important in recognizing strengths and deficits in sensory functioning.

ASSESSMENT

The goal of assessment with elderly persons is twofold: (1) to determine adequate levels of functioning relative to daily living needs and activities, resources, and life style; and (2) to establish baseline data. A thorough and systematic nursing assessment of older adults is a prime requisite to determining the need for health promotion, protection (Pender, 1987), restoration, and rehabilitation in achieving optimal sensory functioning. Well-developed observation, communication, and interview skills are particularly essential to the success of the data-gathering process with older adults. A comprehensive assessment of sensory function would include the health history, and functional, nutritional, psychosocial, environmental, and physical parameters as highlighted below.

Health history involves assessing sensory functioning through questions about the older adult's last visit to a specialist in the senses; familial history of sensory dysfunction; occupation and workplace; recent changes in sensory acuity; current or past history of allergies, illnesses, diseases, surgery, or injury, which may affect sensory function; prescribed, over-the counter, illicit, or illegal drugs currently used; changes in medication; use of assistive devices or prostheses; stimulus tolerance; changes in behavior; and falls.

Functional assessment determines how well older adults function in and negotiate the environment of their worlds. Functional capability is validated with a demonstration of performance in *activities of daily living* (ADL, e.g., bathing, mobility, or eating) and *instrumental activities of daily living* (IADL, e.g., shopping, answering the telephone, or paying bills) in each sensory modality. When a sensory group is unable to function at its optimal level, a "weak link" in the receptive and perceptive processes creates a functional deficit (Belsky, 1984; Whitbourne, 1985). Thus, functional assessment explores the older adult's ability to respond to environmental cues in each of the senses.

Nutritional assessment explores individual food preferences, daily meal patterns, financial and social resources, use of dental prostheses, and the ability of individuals to feed themselves. A nutritional assessment can also disclose whether or not food has lost its palatability and attractiveness for older adults with a sensory deficit. Often the elderly person has little knowledge of the necessity for adequate food intake that will enhance health and adequate resources for maintaining nutritional balance. Many elders are especially prone to vitamin deficiencies and to excessive accumulations of Vitamins A and D.

Psychosocial assessment may reveal situations in which loss of sensory functioning interferes with normal lifestyle, appearance, coping abilities, and cognitive or affective responses, thus contributing to fear of living with less than normal sensory functioning. Changes in behavior, mood, or mental status, and inability to orient to place and time, as in sensory-perceptual alteration (Chodil & Williams, 1970), are important indicators. Behaviors need to be observed and described accurately, without labels and assumptions. Past patterns and quality of social interaction, family relationships, and usual lifestyle are essential areas to explore in the assessment process.

Environmental assessment considers the significance of the environment and the degree and intensity of environmental stimuli as they affect sensory functioning. Assessment can begin with the initial interview, but ideally it is best conducted in the person's home. Reliable tools and sharp observational skills are invaluable in detecting clues to the elderly person's ability to negotiate the daily living environment. Inability to perceive the environment through the senses tends to increase the older adult's vulnerability to diminished functional health. Assuring safety and freedom from barriers in the environment is a key factor in reducing this vulnerability.

Physical assessment of taste, smell, vision, hearing, and the tactile senses can provide important data bearing on normal and abnormal changes which impact sensory function. Assessment of these particular areas is always well worth the screening effort if a deficit is suspected. Physical assessment is integral to the promotion and maintenance of health and well-being of older adults. Health assessment texts (e.g., Bellack & Bamford, 1984) geared to the examination of older adults can provide the tools necessary to complete a comprehensive assessment of sensory function.

Astute assessment is crucial to improvement, preservation, or restoration of optimal sensory functioning and quality of life for older adults.

NURSING DIAGNOSIS

The principal nursing diagnostic category for this chapter is *sensory-perceptual alteration*, defined as "a condition in which the individual experiences a change in therapeutic and/or social stimuli" (Duespohl, 1986, p. 269). In each case, nurses must specify whether the alteration is visual, auditory, kinesthetic, gustatory, tactile, or olfactory. NANDA etiologies also indicate that these diagnoses are related to one or more of the following: environmental factors; altered sensory reception, transmission, and/or integration; chemical alteration; or psychological stress.

PLANNING

Planning results from a thorough and on-going nursing assessment to identify areas for nursing intervention. The process involves setting priorities based on the nursing diagnosis, and the establishment of mutual, long-term client goals and objectives or outcomes with the older adult. Behavioral outcomes should be stated in terms of client behaviors that are clear, measurable, timely, reachable, and reasonable for the elder. Prescribed nursing actions to meet the elderly person's needs are based on scientific rationales for action.

Since the overall goal is to preserve, improve, or restore sensory function to optimal wellness levels, client goals and objectives must take account of the older person's particular health alterations related to sensory functioning. Because of the multiple and complex needs of many aging persons, the written care plan is communicated to the older adult, the family or significant other, and the nursing staff to provide continuity and direction in the care planning process. Planning requires on-going assessment to determine appropriateness and effectiveness of the action plan. Documentation of progress and outcomes is essential.

INTERVENTION

Four broad intervention categories introduced by Sullivan (1983) can easily be adapted as helpful guides to all of the sensory modalities discussed in this chapter: (1) enhance sensory functioning through environmental modification or "engineering" (Burnside, 1988); (2) increase awareness of information provided by other senses through sensory stimulation; (3) provide improved emotional coping through social support systems, resources, practical knowledge, and application; and (4) increase the sensitivity and knowledge of persons who work with the elderly through education, community involvement, and casefinding.

To complement these categories, focus interventions on the involvement of the elderly client in decision making, reinforcement of health-promoting behaviors, health teaching, education about normal aging changes, and strategies to preserve, improve, or restore sensory function. Particular emphasis should be placed on psychosocial needs and adjustment, assisting the person and family to understand the need for independence and continuance of life goals, fostering independence, developing communication-enhancing approaches, supportive involvement of the family, and spiritual support. Other equally important interventions focus on environmental modification, prevention of hazards and promotion of safety, assistance in negotiating the health care system, resource availability, and sensory stimulation and retraining to improve interactions with the environment through the senses (Weiner, Brok, & Snadowsky, 1987).

Examples of nursing interventions specific to taste, smell, vision, hearing, and tactile senses follow.

Taste and Smell

To maintain and improve nutritional status, develop strategies for enhancing appetite and dietary intake, assure weight maintenance equal to nutritional requirements, and consult with a nutritionist, if appropriate. In addition, suggest substitutes for salt and sugar, and add a variety of textures in food. Establish a schedule for disposal of outdated foods (Yen, 1982). To modify the environment in a positive manner, remove noxious odors and add familiar fragrances and smells, such as those of flowers and cooking. Maintain a clean, safe environment (Hayter, 1983). Add smoke detectors to the home.

Vision

To promote functional independence in elders with poor vision or total loss of visual function, support and reinforce the use of low vision aids, such as hand magnification, telescopic aids, and large print (McGrath, 1984). Arrange for orientation and mobility training (Hill & Hartley, 1984). Offer suitable leisure and recreational substitutes, using braille and talking books, radios, and closed circuit television (Pesci, 1986). Provide sensory stimulation and training for those persons who may have psychologically withdrawn from the environment (Scott & Crawhurst, 1975; Weiner, Brok, & Sandowsky, 1987; Wiggins, 1978).

To provide assistive intervention, place medications in the client's hands, not on the table or bedside stand. Use the "clock" method to introduce the client to the position of the food on the plate at meal times. Offer *your elbow* as a guide for mobility in the environment (note: the client should not be left standing alone in an unfamiliar area) (Pesci, 1986). Provide assistive intervention with activities of daily living. Encourage independence.

To enhance communication and establish rapport, allow the client to recognize your voice. Speak to the person directly, not to others in the surroundings. Inform the client why you are there and what you intend to do. Orient the client to the environment (Pesci, 1986).

To modify the environment, acquaint the older person with unfamiliar areas. Reduce glare, check lighting, and use red and yellow color combinations. Keep furniture in place to assist in mobility. Teach use of touch to locate doorways and furniture (Bernardini, 1985). Document falls, if any have occurred.

Hearing

To foster functional independence with the person who has a hearing deficit or total loss of hearing function, support and reinforce the use of an ear horn or hearing aid if the older client owns one. Demonstrate the care and fitting of a prosthesis (Clark & Mills, 1979; Holder, 1982). Seek auditory training, rehabilitation, and counseling for the elder with impaired hearing (Larsen, 1986; Ventura, 1978). Encourage the individual to learn sign language and speech reading, if appropriate. Arrange for a speech evaluation.

To facilitate communication, encourage the use of sign language or speed reading (if known). Communicate through the written word, as necessary. Use spectacles to enhance the ability to see visual cues (Bernardini, 1985). Approach the person face-to-face, address the elder by his or her surname, use a low voice tone without shouting, and rephrase words or sentences if not clearly understood. Use normal—not exaggerated—gestures, facial expressions, and speech.

To modify the environment, use drapes, furnishings, or rugs to absorb sound and reduce background noises. If necessary, relocate the person away from noisy distractions (Snyder, 1978).

Tactile Senses

Pain, touch, and temperature receptors shield the body from potential trauma or injury in the environment. Check and document the elderly person's response to light touch, pain sensation, vibratory stimuli, heat and cold, deep pressure, and kinesthetic sensations. Promote awareness of touch through self-contact (Snyder, 1978). Encourage and/or assist older persons to button and unbutton clothing, pick up small objects, and lift weighted objects.

To promote tactile sensitivity, modify the environment using, for example, textured surfaces. Encourage foot tapping and hand clapping. Promote the use of hands and feet in meaningful activity for as long as possible. Employ sensory stimulation techniques. Introduce domestic or stuffed animals into the environment to encourage touching (Francis & Munjas, 1988). Use touch and hug therapy to enhance communication between caregivers and clients, and teach clients and families about conditions that would prompt tactile deprivation. Promote safety and avoid injury. Initiate health teaching.

EVALUATION

The older adult's progress and the quality of care are measured by the success of the prescribed nursing interventions as implemented through planning and the achievement of stated client goals and objectives. Examples of outcome or evaluation criteria based on the work of Wolanin and Phillips (1981) are:

EXAMPLE ONE: *Vision.* "Reports and demonstrates comfortable interaction in an unseen environment; reports and demonstrates reduction in anxiety level; is successful in the environment 85% of the time; can discuss comfortably visual perceptions of the environment" (p. 238).

EXAMPLE TWO: *Hearing*. "Communicates in a successful and comfortable manner; uses hearing prosthesis to best advantage; reports and demonstrates reduction in anxiety level" (p. 254).

EXAMPLE THREE: *Tactile*. "Reports decrease in anxiety level; reports, and is observed to be comfortable with the amount of affective touching used; level of awareness is increased by the use of tactile input" (p. 215).

Evaluation as a process measurement assures effective nursing care with aging adults. Modifications in the elderly person's behavior and in environmental adaptation are the hallmarks of success. The importance of the implementation of the nursing process and continuous re-evaluation cannot be underestimated in this population.

HEALTH PROMOTION AND WELLNESS

Health promotion with the elderly is defined by Pender (1987) as the active, purposeful evolving of change in health behavior necessary for optimal functioning and well being. Older persons are interested in their health, are interested in learning, and are self-directed. This group provides a ready access for health promotion activities. However, it is important to note that older individuals participate best when they can also make a contribution, when a program is suited to their particular interests, and when the activity is meaningful (FallCreek & Mettler, 1984). Aging and health promotion carries its own set of values.

For planning and implementation purposes, identify specialized professionals in the community to determine their availability as resources in a health promotion program to enhance sensory functioning. Contact the local AARP (American Association of Retired Persons), the State Department for the Blind, the Talking Book Library, and various audiologic agencies. Write to national organizations (see Table 8.1) to obtain pamphlets, handouts, and other information. Survey community organizations and agencies to determine programs already in existence and within reach for the elderly. Establish linkages. Network with potential community and organizational resources.

Health promotion strategies to enhance sensory functioning in the elderly might include: establishing a vision and hearing clinic in long-term care facilities; conducting sensory retraining groups in adult homes and senior centers; and implementing a health education program around normal and abnormal sensory changes in aging at local high-rise housing facilities for elders. Mahoney (1987) designed a program for cerumen screening and removal which was well received by older adults. A health maintenance project developed by Sanderson

TABLE 8.1 Helpful Organizational Resources

<u>Vision</u>

American Academy of Opthalmology
P.O. Box 7424
San Francisco, CA 94120
Tel. 415-561-8500

Food and Drug Administration
5600 Fishers Lane
Rockville, MD 20857
Tel. 301-443-1544

American Foundation for the Blind
15 West 16th Street
New York, NY 10011
Tel. 1-800-232-5463
  or 212-620-2000

National Society to Prevent
  Blindness
500 East Remington Road
Schaumburg, IL 60173
Tel. 312-843-2020

American Optometric Association
243 N. Lindbergh Boulevard
St. Louis, MO 63141
Tel. 314-991-4100

National Eye Institute
Information Office
Building 31, Room 6A32
Bethesda, MD 20892
Tel. 301-496-5248

<u>Hearing</u>

American Academy of
  Otolaryngologists
1101 Vermont Avenue, NW
Washington, DC 20005
Tel. 202-289-4607

Office of Scientific Health Reports
National Institute of Neurological
  and Communication Disorders
  and Stroke
Building 31, Room 8A16
9000 Rockville Pike
Bethesda, MD 20892
Tel. 301-496-4000

American Speech-Language-
  Hearing Association
10801 Rockville Pike
Rockville, MD 20852
Tel. 1-800-638-8255

(1986) and her colleagues was designed to perform ocular screening for older persons, including screening for glaucoma and cataracts. Health promotion programs such as these serve as vehicles for enhancing the functional and independent capabilities of elders.

CONCLUSION

The impact of normal and abnormal physiological, psychological, and social changes related to sensory function has been examined within the framework of the nursing process. Knowledge of these changes in the aging senses is essential to the planning and management of nursing care with older adults. Health promotion and wellness programs are integral to developing self-help and self-care attributes. Assisting elders to recognize their own strengths and areas for development in sensory function is crucial to preserving, restoring, and improving functional health and optimal wellness in the senses. This is the challenge to nursing.

REFERENCES

Anderson, R. G., & Meyerhoff, W. L. (1986). Otologic disorders. In E. Calkins, P. J. Davis, & A. B. Ford (Eds.), *The practice of geriatrics* (pp. 259–271). Philadelphia: W. B. Saunders.

Bellack, J. P., & Bamford, P. A. (1984). *Nursing assessment: A multidimensional approach.* Monterey, CA: Wadsworth.

Belsky, J. K. (1984). *The psychology of aging: Theory, research, and practice.* Monterey, CA: Brooks/Cole.

Bennett, E. S., & Eklund, S. J. (1983). Vision changes, intelligence, and aging: Parts I & II. *Educational Gerontology, 9,* 225–278, 435–442.

Bernardini, L. (1985). Effective communication as an intervention for sensory deprivation in the elderly client. *Topics in Clinical Nursing, 6*(4), 72–78.

Bolin, R. H. (1974). Sensory deprivation: An overview. *Nursing Forum, 13,* 240–258.

Burnside, I. M. (1988). *Nursing and the aged: A self-care approach* (3rd ed.). New York: McGraw-Hill.

Buseck, S. (1980). Visual changes in the elderly. In E. M. Stilwell (Ed.), *Readings in gerontological nursing* (pp. 67–73). Thorofare, NJ: Slack.

Carotenuto, R., & Bullock, J. (1980). *Physical assessment of the gerontological client.* Philadelphia: Davis.

Chodil, J., & Williams, B. (1970). The concept of sensory deprivation. *Nursing Clinics of North America, 5,* 453–465.

Clark, C. C., & Mills, G. C. (1979). Communicating with hearing impaired elderly adults. *Journal of Gerontological Nursing, 5*(3), 41–44.

Cohen, M. M., & Lessell, S. (1984). The neuro-opthalmology of aging. In M. L. Albert (Ed.), *Clinical neurology of aging* (pp. 313–344). New York: Oxford University Press.

Colavita, F. B. (1978). *Sensory changes in the elderly.* Springfield, IL: Charles C Thomas.

Davis, A. J. (1984). *Listening and responding.* St. Louis: C. V. Mosby.

Dickman, I. R. (1982). *A vision impairment of the later years: Macular degeneration.* New York: American Foundation for the Blind, Public Affairs Pamphlet, Number 610.

Duespohl, T. A. (1986). *Nursing diagnosis manual for the well and ill client.* Philadelphia: W. B. Saunders.

Eliopoulos, C. (Ed.) (1984). *Health assessment of the older adult.* Menlo Park, CA: Addison-Wesley.

FallCreek, S., & Mettler, M. (1984). *A healthy old age: A sourcebook for health promotion with older adults* (rev. ed.). New York: Haworth Press.

Ferraro, G. B. (1983). Like a fist before your eye. *Your life and health, 98,* 10–11.

Flynn, J-B. Mc., & Heffron, P. B. (1984). *Nursing from concept to practice.* Bowie, MD: Brady.

Flynn, J-B. Mc., & Heffron, P. B. (1987). Focus: Smell and taste disorders. *AAOHN Journal*, *35*, 463–464.

Francis, G. M., & Munjas, B. A. (1988). Plush animals and the elderly. *Journal of Applied Geriatrics*, *7*, 161–172.

Gioiella, E. C., & Bevil, C. W. (1985). *Nursing care of the aging client*. Norwalk, CT: Appleton-Century-Crofts.

Goode, R. L. (1981). The effects of the aging ear. In F. G. Ebaugh (Ed.), *Management of common problems in geriatric medicine* (pp. 45–61). Menlo Park, CA: Addison-Wesley.

Hatton, J. (1977). Aging and the glare problem. *Journal of Gerontological Nursing*, *3*(5), 18–44.

Hayter, J. (1983). Modifying the environment to help older persons. *Nursing & Health Care*, *4*, 265–269.

Hill, M. M., & Hartley, R. K. (1984). Orientation and mobility for aged visually impaired persons. *Journal of Visual Impairment & Blindness*, *78*(2), 49–54.

Holder, L. (1982). Hearing aids. *Nursing '82*, *12*, 64–67.

Kane, R. L., Ouslander, J. G., & Abrass, I. B. (1984). *Essentials of clinical geriatrics*. New York: McGraw-Hill.

Kenshalo, D. R. (1977). Age changes in touch, vibration, temperature, kinesthesis, and pain sensitivity. In J. E. Birren & K. W. Schaie (Eds.), *Handbook of the psychology of aging* (pp. 562–579). New York: Van Nostrand Reinhold.

Kollarits, C. R. (1986). The aging eye. In E. Calkins, P. J. Davis, & A. B. Ford (Eds.), *The practice of geriatrics* (pp. 248–258). Philadelphia: W. B. Saunders.

Kopac, C. A. (1983). Sensory loss in the aged; the role of the nurse and the family. *Nursing Clinics of North America*, *18*, 373–384.

Kornsweig, A. L. (1984). Rehabilitation in opthalmology for the aged. In T. F. Williams (Ed.), *Rehabilitation in the aging* (pp. 229–234). New York: Raven Press.

Larsen, G. (1986). Hearling loss. In D. L. Carnevali & M. Patrick (Eds.), *Nursing management for the elderly* (2nd ed.; pp. 467–477). Philadelphia: W. B. Saunders.

Mahoney, D. F. (1987). One simple solution to hearing impairment. *Geriatric Nursing*, *8*, 242–245.

Marmor, M. F. (1981). Management of elderly patients with impaired vision. In F. G. Ebaugh (Ed.), *Management of common problems in geriatric medicine* (pp. 17–44). Menlo Park, CA: Addison-Wesley.

McGrath, L. A. (1983). Functional low vision assessment. *Physical & Occupational Therapy in Geriatrics*, *3*(1), 55–61.

National Center for Health Statistics [NCHS]. (1982). *Current estimates from the National Health Interview Survey: United States, 1981*. DHHS Publ. No. (PHS) 82-1569, Series 10, No. 141. Hyattsville, MD: DHHS, Public Health Service.

National Society to Prevent Blindness [NSPB]. (1983). *The aging eye: Facts on eye care for older persons*. New York: Author.

Osgood, N. J., Brant, B. A., & Lipman, A. A. (1988). Patterns of suicidal behavior in long-term care facilities: A preliminary report on an on-going study. *Omega*, *19*, 69–77.

Pender, N. J. (1987). *Health promotion in nursing practice* (2nd ed.). Norwalk, CT: Appleton & Lange.

Pesci, B. R. (1986). When the patient's problem is really poor vision. *RN*, *49*(10), 22–25.

Sanderson, D. (1986). Ocular screening for the elderly. *Canadian Nurse, 82*(1), 19–20.

Scott, D., & Crowhurst, J. (1975). Reawakening senses in the elderly. *Canadian Nurse, 71*(1), 21–22.

Snyder, L. H. (1978). Environmental changes for socialization. *Journal of Nursing Administration, 8*(1), 44–50.

Steffl, B. M. (Ed.) (1984). *Handbook of gerontological nursing.* New York: Van Nostrand Reinhold.

Sullivan, N. (1983). Vision in the elderly: Declining visual function in old age, Part I. *Journal of Gerontological Nursing, 9*(4), 228–233.

Tobis, J., Nayak, L., & Hoehler, F. (1981). Visual perception of verticality and horizontality among elderly fallers. *Archives of Physical & Medical Rehabilitation, 62,* 619–622.

Ventura, F. P. (1978). Counselling the hearing-impaired geriatric patient. *Patient Counseling & Health Education, 1*(1), 22–25.

Weiner, M. B., Brok, A. J., & Snadowsky, A. M. (1987). *Working with the aged: Practical approaches in the institution and community.* Norwalk, CT: Appleton-Century-Crofts.

Whitbourne, S. K. (1985). *The aging body: Physiological changes and psychological consequences.* New York: Springer-Verlag.

Wiggins, R. (1978). The importance of sensory stimulation in caring for the elderly. *The Journal of Practical Nursing, 28*(1), 24–25.

Wolanin, M. O., & Phillips, L. R. F. (1981). *Confusion: Prevention and care.* St. Louis: C. V. Mosby.

Yen, P. L. (1982). Taste, smell, and appetite—They go together. *Geriatric Nursing, 3,* 56–57.

Chapter 9

Cognitive Functioning

Stephanie J. Nagley

INTRODUCTION

As individuals grow older there are changes in cognitive functioning, but it is not accurate within the nursing perspective to think of these changes as necessarily involving decrements in cognitive functioning. Instead, the cognitive changes that occur reflect new patterns of thinking more useful to the needs of older adults. Cognitive function has usually been measured by comparing older adults to younger adults, which skews understanding of elders (Leabouvie-Vief, 1985). The changes that occur in elders involve movement to cognitive functioning that uses knowledge gained with experience to assist older persons in developing a broader understanding of the world around them. As older adults continue in their development, they become less concerned with processing details and more concerned with developing abstract understanding; they are less interested in the "whats" and more interested in the "whys" (Reed, 1983). If nurses think of the changes that occur through the aging process as simply differences rather than decrements, health promotion becomes a much more meaningful task. As Hesse (1974, p. 269) so eloquently reminds us, "Old age is a stage in our lives, and like all other stages it has a face of its own, its own atmosphere, and temperature, its own joy and miseries."

There are, of course, problems that can occur which threaten the mental status of older adults. One of the common problems associated with aging, especially in the very old, is that of changes in cognitive functioning as a result of physical and psychological insults. These changes can be classified as either acute brain syndrome or chronic brain syndrome (dementia). In an acute process the changes observed are usually reversible if recognized promptly and treated appropriately. To date there is little that can be done to reverse the course of chronic brain syndrome (usually referred to as senile dementia in the elderly), but there are interventions that can ameliorate the difficulties that this syndrome presents to the individual and to caregivers.

COGNITIVE IMPAIRMENT: CONFUSION

All negative manifestations of cognitive changes can be categorized under the general label of "confusion." Most nurses in their practice use the term "confused" or the terms "confused and disoriented" to describe a client's behavior, although research has not yet helped us fully to explicate the meaning of that language. Labeling of behavior in this general way suggests the value of initiating a more careful assessment to determine the type of confusion present, possible causes, and appropriate interventions.

"Confusion" is a term used to describe a constellation of behaviors that indicate impairments in cognitive functioning. Elderly persons who are confused not only show changes in thinking, but also demonstrate changes in ways in which they interact with others. Confusion, therefore, describes both cognitive and behavioral changes. Usually there are indications of impairment in one or more of the following cognitive functions: orientation, memory, abstract thinking, attention/concentration, and interpretation of the environment. Confused individuals may be combative, belligerent, and suspicious. They may have difficulty engaging in purposive interactions, which inhibits effective care. Table 9.1 lists predictors that nurses can use to identify confusional states in the elderly, while Table 9.2 contrasts differences between acute and chronic confusional states.

ACUTE BRAIN SYNDROME

Confusion can be the result of a sudden, reversible insult to the brain referred to as "acute brain syndrome." In the nursing literature, these may also be called "acute confusional states." Such states are rapid in onset, occurring within a matter of hours or days. The degree of confusion may fluctuate throughout the episode. Individuals are often aware, in moments of mental clarity, that they have been confused. In contrast, most irreversible brain syndromes tend to have a more pro-

TABLE 9.1 Predictors of Confusion in the Elderly

1. Loss of sense of self (depersonalization)
2. Loss of continuity with life history
3. Distortion of time and space cues (the hospital condition)
    a. Restricted space
    b. Lack of familiar objects
    c. Distortion of light and darkness
    d. Disruption of sleep cycle
    e. Period of amnesia (drugs and surgery)
4. Loss of control
    a. Sensory deficits
    b. Sensory overload
    c. Sensory deprivation
    d. Intubation (parenteral, suction, and oxygen)
    e. Urinary problems (bladder emptying, catheters, infection, and incontinence)
    f. Restraints
    g. Disruption of patterns of daily living (sleep, food intake, mobility, and orientation cues)
    h. Pain
5. Age (80 and over very vulnerable)
6. Sex (older men more prone to confusion)
7. Living alone
8. Physiologic problems that interfere with cerebral support
    a. Hyperthermia
    b. Hypothermia
    c. Dehydration or excessive hydration (edema)
    d. Hypoxia
    e. Hypotension
9. Physiologic action of drugs

Reprinted with permission from M. O. Wolanin & L. R. F. Phillips (1981). *Confusion: Prevention and care.* St. Louis, MO: C. V. Mosby, p. 56.

tracted onset and an unremitting course of cognitive decline over a period of years. Psychomotor behavior in acute brain syndrome may range from hyperactivity to hypoactivity. The sleep-wake cycle is disturbed, usually with greater lethargy during the day and fragmented sleep at night. Individuals misinterpret the environment, experiencing illusions, delusions, and hallucinations.

Acute brain syndrome is thought to occur as a result of physiological and/or psychosocial changes. There are a number of physiological alterations that appear to place elderly persons at risk for the development of acute confusional states, such as fluid and electrolyte imbalances, hypo/hyperthermia, drug toxicity, and metabolic disturbances. Psychosocial changes that might lead to these states include sudden environmental changes, disruptions in daily routine, loss of a loved one, stress,

TABLE 9.2 A Comparison of Clinical Features Between Acute Confusional States (ACS) and Dementia

Feature	ACS	Dementia
Essential feature	A clouded state of consciousness	Not based on disordered consciousness; based on loss of intellectual functions of sufficient severity to interfere with social and occupational functioning
Associated features	Variable affective changes with fear, apprehension, and bewilderment predominating Symptoms of autonomic hyperarousal Some degree of disorientation	Affect tends to be superficial, inappropriate, and labile and includes apathy, depression, and euphoria with some degree of personality change Attempts to conceal deficits in intellect
Onset	Acute/subacute, depends on cause	Chronic, generally insidious, depends on cause
Course	Short, diurnal fluctuations in symptoms, worse at night, dark, and on awakening	Long, no diurnal effects, symptoms progressive yet relatively stable over time
Duration	Hours to less than 1 month	Month to years
Awareness	Fluctuates, generally impaired	Generally normal
Alertness	Fluctuates, reduced or increased	Generally normal
Orientation	Fluctuates in severity, generally impaired	May be impaired
Memory	Recent and immediate impaired, unable to register new information or recall recent events	Recent and remote impaired, loss of recent 1st sign, some loss of common knowledge
Thinking	Disorganized, distorted, fragmented, slow, or accelerated	Difficulty with abstraction
Perception	Distorted, based on state of arousal or mood, illusions, delusions, and hallucinations	Misperceptions often absent
Sleep-wake cycle	Disturbed, cycle reversed	Fragmented
EEG	Predominance of slow or fast cycles related to state of arousal	Normal or slow

response to pain, and depression (Foreman, 1986; Wolanin & Phillips, 1981). Sensory-perceptual alterations, which would fall into a different nursing diagnostic category (see Chapter 8) than alterations in thought processes, are also thought to render older adults vulnerable to confusion. Nurse researchers in this area of investigation generally agree that acute confusion is often the result not just of one factor but a number of factors (Foreman, 1986; Nagley, 1986; Vermeersch, 1986; Wolanin & Holloway, 1980; Wolanin & Phillips, 1981).

While nurses use the label "acute confusional states," which increases the scope of possible causative factors, or the nursing diagnostic category, "alteration in thought process," physicians are more likely to use the term "delirium." Lipowski (1983) described delirium as a transient global cognitive disorder that is determined to be of *organic* etiology; "pseudodelirium" is his term (p. 1433) for delirium-like states for which no organic cause can be identified, a situation for 5 to 20% of hospitalized elderly. The *DSM-III-R* (American Psychiatric Association, 1987) provides the criteria for determining the medical diagnosis of delerium.

It is estimated that 30 to 50% of elderly hospitalized patients experience acute confusional states (Foreman, 1986). This is but a rough estimate. One study of 99 patients 60 years old and over found a daily prevalence rate of acute confusion that ranged from 0 to 13% (Chisholm, et al., 1982). In another study of elderly patients admitted for surgical care of hip fracture, the incidence ranged from 24 to 53% (Williams, et al., 1979). Important to the practicing nurse is the fact that elderly hospitalized patients do appear to be at greater risk for the development of acute confusional states which are known to be associated with higher mortality and longer hospital stays (Lipowski, 1983; Weddington, 1982).

CHRONIC BRAIN SYNDROME

Chronic brain syndrome, or long-term cognitive dysfunction which is not reversible, is most commonly represented in the elderly by Alzheimer's disease (AD) or senile dementia of the Alzheimer's type (SDAT) (Abraham, Buckwalter, & Neundorfer, 1988). But as we acknowledge that the elderly are subject to senile dementia, it is important to note that this problem only occurs in a minority of older persons. Thus, it is estimated that only 10 to 20% of elders living in the community suffer from significant cognitive impairment (Dodson, 1985), even though the majority of elderly persons living in institutional settings are reported to suffer disabling cognitive changes (Gurland & Cross, 1982; Rovner & Rabins, 1985).

   Alzheimer's disease (AD) or senile dementia of the Alzheimer's type (SDAT) is a disabling condition for the individual, family, friends, and the health care system. It is estimated that 5 to 7% of individuals over the age of 65 years and 20% over the age of 80 years have SDAT (Terry, 1978). Senile dementia can be the result of other causes, such as multiple infarctions, chemical abuse, brain trauma, and the consequences of Pick's and Huntington's diseases, but the most common disease is of the Alzheimer's type.

   Hall (1988) has organized the manifestations of alteration in thought processes resulting from AD into four dimensions: cognitive or intellectual losses, affective or personality losses, planning losses, and progressively lowered stress threshold. Within these categories, the behaviors noted in the person with an irreversible or chronic brain syndrome include problems with memory, abstraction, poor judgment, and deficiencies in communication. The personality of the individual also changes over time, which can be especially difficult for family and friends. The individual may lose affect, withdraw socially, become inappropriate in social settings, or lose recognition of others, the environment, and eventually self. The effect of AD on thinking eventually includes an inability to plan activities. Usually, what is first affected is the ability to carry out the instrumental activities of daily living, such as managing finances, shopping, planning meals, and performing household chores. As the disease progresses, the basic activities of daily living, such as dressing, bathing, and eating are affected (Hall, 1988; Hayter, 1974; Reisberg, 1984).

   The course of SDAT is specific to each individual, but there are stages elderly persons with this condition seem to follow. In the *early stage*, perhaps over a period of two to four years, there is the manifestation of forgetfulness. In the *forgetful stage* (Hall, 1988), the older adult is usually aware of the forgetfulness and will attempt to compensate. The *second* or **confused stage** is characterized by increased confusion. The instrumental activities of daily living, such as banking, shopping, home maintenance, and driving, become harder to carry out. Decrease in social activities is noted; the person finds that it is much more manageable to remain in the familiar environment of the home. At the confused stage there often is a need to arrange for some type of minimal supervised care.

   The *third stage* of this process has been termed **ambulatory dementia** (Hall, 1988). It involves loss of the ability to carry out basic activities of daily living without assistance. The individual loses the ability to plan and carry out a task, and has difficulty with verbal and written communication. Misperceptions of visual stimuli occur. For example, what is seen on television is confused with what is actually occurring in the environment. Dependence on the primary caregiver increases to the point that to have any other persons but that person give care is resisted by the individual. At this stage, caregivers tend to feel a tremendous burden of care.

In the *end* or *terminal stage* of the disease, individuals lose the ability to ambulate and engage in volitional activity. Recognition of others is lost, for the most part, as is recognition of self. The individual loses the ability to eat, forgetting how to swallow and chew. There may be a tendency to scream spontaneously or the person may become mute. The person eventually enters a vegetative state and dies of complications usually related to immobility and poor nutritional intake.

For a small number of older adults, SDAT is the result of cerebrovascular disorder, such as multiple infarctions. In these cases, manifestations of the disease in its early stages tend to fluctuate. There are periods of confusion and then temporary remissions. As the vascular insults continue, more ischemic damage occurs and the symptoms increase and remain.

The outward manifestations of SDAT are readily apparent to the caregiver; why the disease occurs remains unknown. SDAT is a progressive disorder with a somewhat unpredictable course. Some individuals will experience rapid deterioration, while others may have a slow steady decline or seem to plateau for a lengthy period. On autopsy, the brain of an individual with AD is found to have characteristic morphological changes: neurofibrillary tangles, granulovascular degeneration, reduction in dendrite branching, and neuritic plaques (Terry, 1978). There is also evidence of areas of regional brain cell loss, neurochemical alterations, and changes in circulatory, metabolic, and electrical activity (Burns & Buckwalter, 1988).

Three hypotheses have been suggested as to the cause of SDAT: (1) an environmental origin, which may be a slow virus; (2) an immunological response; and (3) a genetic factor of origin, since there is evidence that AD does have a familial pattern, particularly in more early onset AD (Burns & Buckwalter, 1988). Whatever the cause, the challenge to the nurse is to assist the individual to live out his or her life as fully as possible and to assist those who care for the individual.

ASSESSMENT

Confusion and Functional Health Patterns

Assessment of the cognitive status of elderly persons depends on nursing observations, developing an understanding of the individual through interaction, and the use of measurement tools. Altered thought processes will be evident in nearly all functional health patterns, but particularly in cognitive-perceptual, activity-exercise, health maintenance, sleep/rest, and coping patterns. Role-relationship patterns are also affected. What distinguishes an acute from a chronic process are potential precipitating factors described above as characteristic of acute vs. chronic brain syndrome and the length of time the alteration has been present.

Cognitive-Perceptual

In assessing older adults, it is important to make observations about cognitive and perceptual status. In both acute and chronic brain syndrome, individuals will have difficulty communicating effectively. For example, they may be unable to articulate a clear response to questions, or may be unable to understand verbal or written communication. One way to determine this is to ask the individual to follow commands, such as to undress or dress. The cognitive ability to plan and organize activities, such as dressing, is often affected. The status of memory and orientation (time, person, place) is assessed through questioning and the use of mental assessment tools. Abstract reasoning can be tested through the use of proverb interpretation and performance of simple math tasks which are incorporated in the mental status tools. The ability to name items is often impaired and nurses can ask the individual to name common items in pictures or by displaying objects like paper, a watch, or a pencil.

Assessment includes observing the person's behavior. Both acute and chronic brain syndromes manifest in the general behavior of individuals. Inability to attend to situations may cause the individual to appear distracted or not engaged in what is going on in the surroundings. The person may seem overly anxious and become hyperactive. This is especially true in individuals with chronic brain syndrome who are feeling stressed, and is indicative of progressively lowered stress threshold. In the later stages of this condition, individuals tend to develop a flat affect.

Even though they may need to deny the problem, family members or others are brought into the assessment process to provide additional information. To break through denial, nurses may ask questions more than once or rephrase questions to make sure that the assessment is complete. Nurses can inquire about the individual's ability to engage in activities of daily living and general behavior. Questions might include: Is the individual able to dress without help? Does he or she bathe without reminding? Who takes care of the cooking (housekeeping, banking, shopping, etc.)? Have you noticed changes in behavior, such as increased irritability, suspiciousness, decreased desire to leave the house, or inability to make decisions?

Activity-Exercise

Difficulty with cognitive function can be identified in self-care practices. If the individual does not have assistance and suffers from planning losses associated with dementia, there will be difficulty with activities of daily living. Because of difficulty with tasks such as bathing and dressing, the individual may appear poorly groomed or may have dressed inappropriately. Poor grooming and mismatched clothes are not diagnostic of cognitive dysfunction, but they can indicate that additional assessment is warranted. Further, being well groomed and having social skills is not indicative of cognitive function. Clinicians often miss cognitive dysfunction in older adults who are socially skilled (Williams, Ward, & Campbell, 1988).

Health-Maintenance

The ability of individuals to protect themselves from harm is a matter of particular concern. If the person has an acute brain syndrome while not hospitalized, it may be the failure to make safe judgments that leads to injury and admission to the hospital. If the acute process occurs while hospitalized, nursing interventions are designed to protect the patient. Determination of the potential for injury of the person with dementia is usually assessed through interview of family members. The nursing assessment probes the family for their sense of concern about the individual's safety. Common areas for inquiry are whether the family is concerned about the individual's ability to drive or be independent in activities. Is the family concerned about the safety of the person in the home, e.g., have doors been left unlocked or pots left on a burner?

Sleep-Rest

The sleep-rest pattern of individuals with acute brain syndrome will be disrupted, with fragmented sleep during the night and often lethargy during the day. Persons with chronic brain syndrome also experience diurnal variation in sleep pattern, but because they are usually unable to provide assessment data, nurses rely on the family or others for this information. Characteristic of persons with dementia is the tendency to become fatigued as the day wears on and to be up during the night.

Coping-Stress Tolerance

Persons with chronic brain syndrome do not tolerate excessive stimuli; their intolerance manifests in catastrophic reactions, such as combativeness, agitation, or wandering. It is not clear if the coping-stress pattern of the person with acute brain syndrome is affected similarly.

Again, the family or others are asked about the person's response to stress. Indications of this intolerance incude the individual's avoidance of or inability to tolerate new environments or social functions, and when disruptions in daily routine seem to lead to increased difficulty.

Role-Relationship

For the family or others supporting the individual with chronic brain syndrome, the experience is very stressful. Assessment of the functional pattern of coping-stress tolerance includes assessment of the status of the significant others in the system. Areas to consider are the ways in which the situation is affecting the financial, emotional, and physical health of each individual. In addition, data need to be collected with regard to the effect of the situation on the health of the family system.

Assessment of the family or support system also includes identification of the primary caregiver, that is, the person who is providing the bulk of care for the individual. Often the family or friends of the individual will parcel out these responsibilities, that is, one person may take care of financial or legal aspects of care, while another attends to day-to-day care needs.

Most often the caregivers are the spouse or children. Spouses who provide care are very committed to the care of their husband or wife. Still, the burden of increasing care demands often leaves the spouse physically and emotionally exhausted. The demands of the situation, along with the loss of the partner to the disease process, arouse feelings of anger and resentment. These are normal and expected feelings that need to be expressed. When the caregiver is a child, again there are special losses occurring that must be expressed. Assessment includes questions that allow these feelings to emerge.

The aim of all nursing care is to promote and maintain the strengths of each individual. Both psychosocial and physiological variables need to be considered in the assessment process to determine if the alteration in thought processes is reversible. Failure to recognize and treat reversible causes of confusion can lead to chronic brain syndrome. Nurses explore psychosocial factors that may underlie confusional states, such as sudden relocation, loss of control, loss of significant others, or changes in daily routine. In addition, it is important to work with the health care team to determine if physiological status is optimal. Laboratory tests are essential in identifying possible reversible causes of the confusion. Most geriatricians will recommend blood chemistry analyses, including a routine blood panel, thyroid studies, vitamin B12 studies, and folate studies. In some situations, a CAT scan will be done, as well as chest X-ray and EKG.

Mental Status Assessment Tools

For the sake of completeness in the data base, it is essential to conduct an initial mental status assessment of all clients. This is especially critical when caring for older adults. For the elderly hospitalized patient, a mental status assessment should be a component of the initial assessment and then should be repeated as appropriate throughout the hospital stay. Similarly, elderly residents in nursing homes or other long-term care facilities should have their mental status assessed in a systematic way on admission and then on a routine basis every four to six months. Finally, mental status assessments should be incorporated into the care of elderly persons in the community. Systematic mental status assessments provide all members of the health team with a consistent profile of the individual's cognitive functioning.

Research indicates that neither clinical assessments alone nor the use of mental status assessment tools on their own will provide sufficient data on which to build a system of interventions (Williams, Ward, & Campbell, 1988). Both are needed together to lay the foundation for a complete data base.

Formal assessment tools are not foolproof; they provide only one strategy in understanding individuals. Tools are subject to a high rate of false negatives (Williams, Ward, & Campbell, 1988), so that some confused individuals may receive scores that do not support difficulty in cognitive functioning. Because most tools require verbal responses, some individuals cannot be assessed in this way. To complement the tool, nursing research (Nagley & Byers, 1987; Williams, et al., 1985) has consistently emphasized the importance of careful observation in making an accurate diagnosis of altered thought processes.

There are a number of tools for the measurement of mental status. These tools were developed, for the most part, to provide ways for clinicians to screen for problems in cognitive functioning. The Short Portable Mental Status Questionnaire (SPMSQ), developed by Pfeiffer (1975), is a tool that is frequently used to determine cognitive status. It is a 10-item questionnaire which asks individuals to respond to questions that determine their orientation to person, place, and time, as well as the status of their memory and ability to engage in abstract reasoning through mathematical calculations.

Another tool widely used is the Mini-Mental State Examination (MMSE), developed by Folstein, Folstein, and McHugh (1975). This 30-item test assesses orientation, recall, short-term memory, serial subtractions, registration, and language. The tool is short and easy to administer.

Two other tools less often mentioned in the literature are the Cognitive Capacity Screening Examination (CCSE) and the Dementia Rating Scale (DRS), both of which are considered to be very reliable and valid measures of cognitive functioning in the elderly.

Foreman (1987) reported the results of a study to determine the reliability and validity of the SPMSQ, MMSE, CCSE, and DRS when used with elderly hospitalized patients. In his conclusions, Foreman stated that the CCSE was found to be the most reliable and valid measure of mental status in this population. He went on to say, however, that this 30-item questionnaire may not be clinically desirable for use with individuals who have limited cognitive abilities, since it may be too stressful for the individual to tolerate. Foreman therefore recommended that the MMSE may be a better choice for those individuals who have limitations in cognitive functioning.

The choice about which mental assessment tool to use depends on the following: (1) How precise does the information about the person's mental status need to be at this time?; (2) What do clinical observations suggest about the status of cognitive functioning in this individual?; (3) What do clinical observations suggest about the individual's ability to tolerate a more-extensive versus less-extensive interview? If the individual gives indications of moderate to severe difficulty in cognition and/or appears very anxious, or is physically very ill, the suggestion would be to choose a tool that permits easy and quick responses. For the beginning nurse clinician, whose service setting does not already use a standard measure, the suggestion is to begin with one tool, such as the SPMSQ, and then work toward increasing familiarity with other tools.

A Note about Additional Complexity

Acute and chronic brain syndromes can occur together. When nurses have cared for chronically confused individuals over a long period of time, there is a tendency to accept the confusion and not to recognize alterations until the confusion pattern changes. But elderly residents in a nursing home who become restless or combative when that is not their pattern may be experiencing a urinary tract infection or a respiratory infection, or may have been upset by having a new nurse. Similarly, the person with senile dementia who is hospitalized for illness may have an exacerbation of confusion as a result of physiological and environmental changes. Also, there is an interesting form of acute confusion, called *Sundown Syndrome*, which is seen at bedtime but clears by the next day (Evans, 1987). This is a specific form of alteration in thought processes which may occur in those with chronic brain syndrome or in individuals who do not show signs of altered thought processes at other times. Fatigue and lack of visual stimuli because of darkness may be the cause of sundowning. If a formal assessment of mental status has been obtained earlier in all of these circumstances, nurses have a baseline from which to determine if change has indeed occurred and to what degree.

Experienced gerontological nurses working in long-term care settings usually look for signs of physical illness when the resident develops acute confusion. As a part of the detective work, the nurse may first assess whether or not there is any evidence of an infectious process. Urinary tract infections and respiratory infections are not uncommon. Commercial products are available to test urine to determine if there may be a urinary tract infection. This testing is similar to that for glucose in the urine. Testing of this sort, along with attention to increased frequency or odor, can help the nurse to determine an appropriate course of action. With respiratory infections there may be a slight increase in temperature along with changes in breath sounds. Sometimes the clues are subtle, which makes the nursing care of the older adult particularly challenging.

NURSING DIAGNOSIS

The primary nursing diagnostic category identified for those with acute and chronic brain syndrome is *alteration in thought processes* (Duespohl, 1986). The NANDA-approved identified etiologies that lead to a nursing diagnosis of "Thought Processes, Alteration in, Related to" are: physiological changes; psychological conflicts; loss of memory; impaired judgment; and sleep deprivation.

Since optimal cognitive functioning is essential to most health patterns, there are a number of actual or potential problems secondary to the primary diagnosis that are considered: potential for injury, sleep pattern disturbance, alteration in nutrition, self-care deficit, impaired communication, alterations in elimination, health maintenance alteration, alterations in coping (family or individual), and alterations in family processes.

The definition of alteration in thought processes states that the individual has a disruption of mental status in such activities as conscious thought, reality orientation, problem-solving, judgment, and comprehension related to coping (Carpenito, 1987). The major defining characteristic is inaccurate interpretation of stimuli, be they internal or external. Also present may be deficits in memory, suspiciousness, disorientation, delusions, hallucinations, poor attention/concentration, and difficulty communicating.

The pathological risk factor category for alteration in thought processes includes the process of dementia and physiological alterations. Situational factors are also included, such as depression, anxiety, loss, and environmental change.

Alteration in thought processes due to acute brain syndrome may result from the following changes in physiological status: hypo/hyperthermia, decreased cardiac output, airway obstruction or other factors that lead to poor oxygenation, fluid and electrolyte imbalances, metabolic disturbances, such as hypo/hyperthyroidism, hypo/hyperglycemia, increased intracranial pressure, and blood dyscrasias. Acute brain syndrome may also be related to factors considered more psychosocial such as environmental change, pain, fatigue, stress, loss of any kind, depression, and anxiety.

PLANNING

The aim of nursing care for all elderly persons who are experiencing actual or potential alterations in thought processes is to restore, maintain, and promote optimal cognitive functioning. Planning takes into account many potential problems related to alterations in physiological and psychosocial status that can lead to acute or chronic confusional states. Planning is expressed in terms of client goals and objectives, and objectives are expressed in terms of measurable behaviors and time frames. Time frames for individual behaviors are stated in hours, days, weeks, etc.

Examples of long-term goals for planning in relationship to acute confusion might include that the elderly person will:

1. Maintain optimal physiological status.
2. Maintain optimal psychosocial status.
3. Maintain orientation to person, place, and time.
4. Prevent physical injury to self and others.

Specific measurable objectives for planning in relationship to acute confusion might include that the elderly person will, within 24 hours:

1. Have gradual improvement of and/or demonstrate beginning adaptation to alterations in thought processes through:
   a. improved level of orientation;
   b. improved attention span and problem-solving abilities;
   c. decreased irritability and aggressiveness;
   d. utilization of techniques to aid memory.
2. Prevent physical injury to self and others.
3. Have gradual reduction in anxiety or stress.
4. Have gradual realistic and constructive interpretation of reality.
5. Have gradually increased ability to relate with family and staff positively.
6. Have gradually increased responsibility for self care.
7. Show no decline in scores obtained on a mental assessment tool.

When the elderly person has a chronic brain syndrome or dementia, the aim of nursing care addresses both the chronic process and the potential for alteration in thought processes due to an acute process that may arise from physiological or psychosocial changes. The goals and objectives given above are included, as appropriate, in planning, together with those that follow. Examples of long-term goals in planning related to chronic confusion might include that the elderly person will (time dependent on individual):

1. Experience independence within the capacity of the individual.
2. Experience self-esteem through activities and promotion of self-care abilities.
3. Experience a calm and supportive environment.

Specific measurable objectives in planning related to chronic confusion might include that the elderly person will (time dependent on individual):

1. Carry out activities of daily living with appropriate supervision.
2. Evidence no episodes of disruptive behavior.
3. Maintain optimal physical health and sense of well-being.
4. Interact with others effectively within the constraints of the effects of the chronic brain syndrome.

Examples of measurable objectives for the elderly person without or with dementia who evidences an acute confusion might include that he or she will:

1. Demonstrate improvement in cognitive function as evidenced by:
   a. improved orientation to person, place, and time;
   b. ability to exercise safe judgment and follow instructions;
   c. improvement on tests of mental status.
2. Resume responsibility for self care at previous level of functioning.
3. Interact with others at previous level of functioning.

In addition, nurses work with the family assisting them to:

1. Recognize the signs and symptoms of acute confusion.
2. Maintain and promote optimal health of the elderly person, with attention to nutrition, personal hygiene, sleep, and exercise.

3. Monitor the health needs of the family.

4. Obtain access to support services available in the community.

INTERVENTION

Before moving into the specifics of physical and psychosocial interventions for confused elderly persons, it is important that nurses are present to the wholeness of the human being who is confused. How does one approach the individual who is confused? What are some basic guidelines for interactions? The first rule is to remember that these are persons with their own individual life stories, and that their confusion is a way of communicating to the caregiver what is happening with them. Confused persons need to be treated with respect, concern, and compassion. Often they are not only confused, they are also quite frightened, perhaps of the caregiver, their surroundings, or simply their awareness that they are not functioning quite properly.

It is usually more effective to approach agitated confused individuals one-on-one, unless they are a clear danger to themselves or others because of their potential for violence if not subdued immediately. Most confused elderly persons will respond to a calm, quiet approach, with one person gently inquiring about the problem as the individual is perceiving it. Restraints, be they chemical or mechanical, are *not* initial interventions of choice. In fact, chemical and mechanical restraints will only aggravate alterations in thought processes. Distraction and humor are usually very effective ways to help individuals through a very agitated confused state (Nagley & Dever, 1988).

Nursing interventions required for alterations in thought processes require consideration of physical and psychosocial factors which may cause the alteration and exacerbate confused states. In the case of acute confusion, the alteration is considered to be multifactorial in nature. Most often the interventions are designed first to address a physiological cause of the confusion, such as hypoxia, alteration in fluid and electrolytes, or alterations in body temperature. The idea is to look first for the simplest and most rectifiable cause of the confusion. This suggests starting with physical rather than psychosocial antecedents, since the latter are usually more complex.

Nursing Interventions for Acute Brain Syndrome

What one learns in care of adults who are ill, regardless of age, can be incorporated into the care of the confused elderly as a foundation for appropriate responses to confusion resulting from alterations in physiological status. The difference is that nurses, when caring for the

elderly, are sensitive to the tendency of older persons to exhibit alterations in thought processes as a result even of slight physiological
deviations. Because of changes concomitant with growing older, elderly
persons are less able to tolerate deviations in physiological status. For
example, a slightly febrile state in older adults may show itself in
confusion, whereas in younger adults this tends to occur only with very
high body temperature. Elderly persons experiencing myocardial infarction may not complain of pain but instead may become confused.

Nurses should anticipate that older adults may be more sensitive to
physical and psychosocial changes than younger persons. Thus, nurses
should anticipate that all elderly clients have the potential for the
development of alterations in thought processes. The most vulnerable
persons will be the oldest old, those 75 years of age and older, and those
patients who are already physically and/or mentally challenged.

Because of physiological differences, older patients will react to medications differently than younger patients. Often one of the adverse
responses to drugs will be confusion. Medications that can lead to
confused states include not only those that affect the central nervous
system, but also cardiovascular drugs, steroids, and antihistamines, or
drugs like cimetidine (Kane, Ouslander, & Abrass, 1984). Effective drug
therapy requires that nurses be familiar with acceptable medications
for use in the elderly and proper dosage for older patients. Nurses must
also continually reassess for signs of changes in cognitive functioning.

The nursing diagnosis of potential for injury needs to be included in
the plan for elderly patients. Falls are a common problem for confused
elderly patients in the acute care environment. A fall can often be traced
to the combination of a strange environment, effects of physical illness,
and perhaps the use of hypnotics, sedatives, or drugs that induce
postural hypotension. Frequent checks on patients throughout the day
and night are helpful. Avoiding use of medications that can lead to
development of confusion will assist in preventing falls. Most acute
care institutions encourage use of siderails. If elderly patients are confused and want to get out of bed, the danger of even greater injury
exists when they attempt to crawl around or over siderails.

Falls can happen even with the best preventive programs. Thus, the
second line of defense is to make the environment conducive to preventing serious injury. For example, beds for elderly patients should be
kept as low to the floor as possible. In addition, the nurse can maintain
an environment free of objects that elderly patients could trip or fall
over should they wander at night. In these ways, trauma may be
lessened should elderly patients get out of bed and fall.

Alterations in body temperature, either hypothermia or hyperther-
mia, can lead to confusion. Hypothermia often occurs in surgical environments. In such settings, elderly patients may not tolerate low am-

bient temperature, often becoming "confused and disoriented." In situations where hypothermia is a possibility, extra blankets should be provided and ambient temperature adjusted if possible. The elderly patient who is sedated, moving very little, or recovering from surgery is the patient who is prone to the development of confusion due to hypothermia. Similarly, the elderly patient with even slight increases in body temperature may develop confusion. The potential for confusion in this situation can be anticipated and interventions undertaken to reduce fever, such as tepid sponge baths and medications.

Elderly patients whose intake is poor or who are not receiving fluids for diagnostic or therapeutic reasons are also at risk for developing confusion. Careful monitoring of intake and output should be maintained on these patients. Because of changes in renal functions, elderly patients do not tolerate fluid underload easily. In addition, careful monitoring of intake and output can allow for early detection of fluid overload, another familiar precursor to the development of confusion (Wolanin & Phillips, 1981).

The NANDA taxonomy includes the diagnosis of "sensory perceptual alteration." This diagnosis takes on meaning for hospitalized older adults with respect to the challenge that the hospital environment can present to the cognitive functioning of such elderly persons and for those individuals who have alterations in sensory processes. Roslaniec and Fitzpatrick (1979) found changes in cognitive functioning of older adults hospitalized for four days. They inferred that the reason for changes in mental status was environmental.

When older adults are hospitalized, especially if the hospitalization was sudden, they are thrust into a strange and seemingly chaotic world. It is an environment of unfamiliar sights, sounds, and people. Wolanin and Holloway (1980) have used the phrase "traumatic relocation" to capture the force of this experience. The presence of familiar possessions is believed to help older patients adjust to the changes. Large clocks and calendars are useful in helping individuals maintain a sense of time orientation.

As simple as it may seem, one of the problems that often occurs in the initial hospitalization is the failure to make sure that patients have the use of sensory aids, such as eye glasses and hearing aids. If the environment is confusing just by the mere fact of its unfamiliarity, it will be even more difficult when patients cannot see or hear well. Seeing, hearing, and mobility are primary ways in which individuals make sense of their experiences. In a study of elderly persons who had surgical repair of hip fracture, the use of hearing aids and glasses, as well as increased mobility, were noted in those whose mental status was reported better in the postoperative period (Williams, et al. 1979).

Nursing Interventions for Chronic Brain Syndrome

Nursing care of persons with chronic brain syndrome, whether they reside at home or in an institutional setting, begins with the intent of promoting and maintaining optimal wellness. Planning and subsequent interventions start with consideration for self-care needs and the activities of daily living, such as eating, bathing, toileting, and dressing. The environment also needs to be structured to provide a balance of stimulation and periods of rest. Finally, nursing interventions are presented within the value framework of accepting the individual as a person who has dignity and worth.

Activities of Daily Living

Any activity that requires accomplishing several tasks, such as dressing and bathing, is easier when the task is broken down into smaller units. Individuals may experience ideational apraxia which prevents them from sequencing actions. The nurse needs to organize the activity for them, for example, by placing the clothes out in the sequence in which they will be put on. If there is ideomotor apraxia, the individual will know what to do but be unable to carry out the activity without physical assistance, such as sitting on the toilet (Beck & Heacock, 1988).

Maintaining nutritional intake in chronically confused older adults can be very challenging. As the confusion becomes more severe, individuals lose the ability to feed themselves and require increasing amounts of assistance. Nurses are alert to signs of increasing difficulty and may want to record intake and output for one to two days to determine more accurately intake patterns of each individual. Often, if confused individuals are presented one food at a time, they will be able to feed themselves. Presenting an entire meal to confused individuals is overwhelming. It requires them to evaluate what is before them, plan how they will consume the meal, and make choices about what to eat. This is a process which may exceed the cognitive ability of individuals with chronic brain syndrome.

There also are individuals with chronic brain syndrome whose memory loss includes a failure to remember that they have eaten. In order not to get into a struggle about overeating, it is helpful to portion out foods throughout the day. In this way, snacks are available so that the person maintains an appropriate caloric intake and does not become either obese or undernourished. It usually does matter that elderly persons stay at optimal weight, since many of these individuals have other medical problems that excess weight would exacerbate, such as arthritis and cardiovascular problems.

Another factor to consider with residents in long-term care facilities who are experiencing difficulty eating is the problem of congregate dining. As Hall (1988) pointed out, the inability to tolerate and make sense of multiple stimuli presents a stressful situation. Individuals may have more success in eating meals if they are allowed to eat alone or with one or two people, as opposed to a group dining room. The dining environment should be quiet and calm in order to avoid distractions from eating.

Environmental Concerns

The concept of "progressively lowered stress threshold" (PLST), as developed by Hall (1988), offers a promising perspective from which to understand the experience of persons with chronic brain syndrome and their care needs. PLST takes account of catastrophic behaviors, since it recognizes that persons with chronic brain syndrome, when pushed beyond their stress tolerance, may respond by violent, agitated, or anxious behavior, wandering, purposeless behavior, belligerence, and other behaviors which render them socially and cognitively inaccessible.

In order to prevent catastrophic events, the environment of elderly persons with chronic brain syndrome is an important consideration in the implementation of care. Since those with chronic brain syndrome have difficulty understanding and responding to stimuli, the environment should be kept as calm and consistent as possible. In an institutional setting, a balance must be maintained so that individuals do not become victims of too much or too little stimuli. Activities should be planned for small groups and should depend upon cognitive skills that are within the limits of each individual. Art projects, such as working with clay or paints, are a good way to provide stimulation while giving individuals a vehicle for self-expression. Many individuals enjoy cooking and, with supervision, can bake or even prepare meals. Nature walks can be another excellent experience and an opportunity to have periods of exercise. Nurses should work closely with recreational therapists in various projects of this sort for chronically confused elderly persons.

Because elders with dementia have their own unique interpretations of the world around them, care must be taken to structure the environment to match their perceptions and needs. For example, many persons with dementia wander. A safe environment that can allow for wandering is much more constructive than one which imposes restrictions on that activity. The colors used in the environment should be soothing and landscape scenes for art work are usually good choices. Judicious use should be made of television or radios. If television is used at all, the nurse should introduce and if possible watch with the individual to explain whatever needs to be explained (e.g., type of program, season of year). Sometimes elderly individuals will incorporate aspects of a television event into a later experience. If the nurse knows what has been viewed, it is easier to understand the content of such thoughts and behavior.

Sleep and Rest

Individuals with dementia need an opportunity to rest during the day. These persons tend to exhibit distinctive diurnal rhythms and sleep-wake cycles. They also tend to wake frequently at night, and to exhibit loss of rapid eye movement (REM) or dream sleep which can cause restlessness and irritability (Norris, 1986). Because of their PLST, morning naps are useful for those with loss of REM sleep and afternoon naps are helpful for those whose restlessness is associated with fatigue (Norris, 1986).

Communication

Time should be allotted so that the nurse can spend part of each day in an individual relationship with the person who has chronic brain syndrome. If the nurse listens carefully, even the most confused person has a story to tell. Active listening is a process of hearing the person from the point of view of his or her own perspective and understanding the individual's unique experience. It is a process of listening with the ears to hear the verbal clues and listening with the eyes to recognize the nonverbal clues. In listening, the nurse will discover what the concerns of the person are, what gives the individual comfort, and how the nurse can help most effectively. Spending individual time with each person is an act that affirms his or her worth and dignity.

There is a tendency to try to confront the person's confusion or disorientation by correcting it. In those with chronic brain syndrome, this often leads to a struggle. The most effective communication involves the nurse entering into the world of the confused person rather than trying to force that individual to come into the nurse's world. This is not a process of agreeing with or pretending to understand all that is said or done. Rather, this is a process of listening and talking with the person in order to provide clarification and validation so that the message and meaning are understood. Respecting confused persons as individual human beings, addressing them by their surnames, and employing some form of gentle touch usually conveys a sense of security and well being.

Individuals with dementia do not lose their ability to feel. They have feelings of anxiety, anger, happiness, and sadness like any other human being. They also seem to be particularly sensitive to the feelings of those around them. When the caregiver is rushed, anxious, or irritable, the confused individual will tend to respond. The response may be in the form of increased restlessness, irritability, or physical aggression. Changes in mood or an increase in physical activity are warnings that something is upsetting the person. Anticipating these changes or attending to them promptly will usually prevent a catastrophic reaction later.

EVALUATION

For elderly individuals with acute brain syndrome, addressing the causes of confusion will result in improvement of cognitive function and resolution of the problem. This progress can be determined through continuous reassessment of cognitive status and through interaction with the older adult and family. Elderly persons who have an acute process together with chronic brain syndrome will return to the previous level of functioning if the acute process is resolved. Improvement in cognitive functioning is not possible for persons with chronic brain syndrome. For such individuals, the aim of nursing care is to maintain independence as long as possible, keeping the demands of daily living within the person's ability to perform such activities. The effectiveness of these nursing interventions is best indicated by the absence of catastrophic behaviors. That is, if the demands of the environment do not exceed the ability of the individual, the elderly person will function well with appropriate supervision. Knowing how much or how little supervision is needed is determined through diligent and ongoing assessment by nurses and other caregivers. Protecting the person from injury is the fundamental concern of all care and one important indicator of successful care.

CONCLUSION

The aim of nursing in caring for elderly persons with alterations in thought processes is to help those persons remain as independent as possible. Woven into every act of care is the intention of maintaining the individual's sense of worth and dignity. Caring for confused elders is an opportunity for nurses to be challenged to enter into the confusion and to create a plan of care that will make the most of the strengths of each individual. The tapestry of older adults is rich in colors of lived experience. If nurses embrace the opportunity to work with elders with cognitive impairment, they can add much to the quality of their own lives.

REFERENCES

Abraham, I. L., Buckwalter, K. C., & Neundorfer, M. N. (Eds.) (1988). Alzheimer's disease. *Nursing Clinics of North America, 23*, 1–133.

American Psychiatric Association (1987). *Diagnostic and statistical manual of mental disorders* (3rd ed., revised). Washington, DC: Author.

Beck, C., & Heacock, P. (1988). Nursing interventions for patients with Alzheimer's disease. *Nursing Clinics of North America, 23*, 95–123.

Burns, E. M., & Buckwalter, K. C. (1988). Pathophysiology and etiology of Alzheimer's disease. *Nursing Clinics of North America, 23*, 11–29.

Carpenito, L. J. (1987). *Handbook of nursing diagnosis* (2nd ed.) Philadelphia: Lippincott.

Chisholm, S. E., Deniston, O. L., Igrisan, R. M., & Barbus, A. J. (1982). Prevalence of confusion in elderly hospitalized patients. *Journal of Gerontological Nursing, 8*(2), 87–96.

Dodson, J. (1985). Recognizing early senility. *Occupational Health Nursing, 33*, 199–201.

Duespohl, T. A. (1986). *Nursing diagnosis manual for the well and ill client.* Philadelphia: W. B. Saunders.

Evans, L. K. (1987). Sundown syndrome in institutionalized elderly. *Journal of the American Geriatrics Society, 35*, 101–108.

Folstein, M. F., Folstein, S. E., & McHugh, P. R. (1975). Mini-mental state: A practice method for grading the cognitive state of patients for the clinician. *Journal of Psychiatric Research, 12*, 189–198.

Foreman, M. D. (1986). Acute confusional states in hospitalized elderly: A research dilemma. *Nursing Research, 35*, 34–38.

Foreman, M. D. (1987). Reliability and validity of mental status questionnaires in elderly hospitalized patients. *Nursing Research, 36*, 216–220.

Gurland, B. J., & Cross, P. S. (1982). Epidemiology of psychopathology in old age: Some implications for clinical services. *Psychiatric Clinics of North America, 5*, 11–26.

Hall, G. R. (1988). Care of the patient with Alzheimer's disease living at home. *Nursing Clinics of North America, 23*, 31–45.

Hayter, J. (1974). Patients who have Alzheimer's disease. *American Journal of Nursing, 74*, 1460–1462.

Hesse, H. (1974). *My belief: Essays on art and life.* New York: Farrar, Strauss and Giroux.

Kane, R. L., Ouslander, J. G., & Abrass, I. B. (1984). *Essentials of geriatric medicine.* New York: McGraw-Hill.

Leabouvie-Vief, G. (1985). Intelligence and cognition, In J. E. Birren & K. W. Schaie (Eds.), *Handbook of the psychology of aging* (pp. 500–525). New York: Van Nostrand Reinhold.

Lipowski, Z. J. (1983). Transient cognitive disorders in the elderly. *American Journal of Psychiatry, 140*, 1426–1436.

Nagley, S. J. (1986). Preventing confusion in your patients. *Journal of Gerontological Nursing, 12*(3), 27–31.

Nagley, S. J., & Byers, P. (1987). Clinical construct validity. *Journal of Advanced Nursing, 12*, 617–619.

Nagley, S. J., & Dever, A. (1988). What we know about treating confusion. *Applied Nursing Research, 1*, 80–83.

Norris, C. M. (1986). Restlessness: A disturbance in rythmicity. *Geriatric Nursing, 1*, 302–306.

Pfeiffer, E. (1975). A short portable mental status questionnaire for assessment of organic brain deficit in elderly patients. *Journal of the American Geriatric Society*, *23*, 433–438.

Reed, P. G. (1983). Implications of the life-span developmental framework for well-being in adulthood and aging. *Advances in Nursing Science*, *6*, 18–25.

Reisberg, B. (1984). Stages of cognitive decline. *American Journal of Nursing*, *84*, 225–232.

Roslaniec, A., & Fitzpatrick, J. J. (1979). Changes in mental status in older adults with four days hospitalization. *Research in Nursing and Health*, *2*, 177–189.

Rovner, B. W., & Rabins, P. V. (1985). Mental illness among nursing home patients. *Hospital and Community Psychiatry*, *36*, 119–120.

Terry, R. D. (1978). Aging, senile dementia, and Alzheimer's disease. In R. Katzman, R. D. Terry, & K. L. Bick (Eds.), *Alzheimer's disease: Senile dementia and related disorders. Aging. Volume 1* (pp. 11–45). New York: Raven Press.

Vermeersch, P. E. H. (1986). *Development of a scale to measure confusion in hospitalized adults*. Cleveland, OH: Case Western Reserve University, unpublished doctoral dissertation.

Weddington, W. W. (1982). The mortality of delerium: An underappreciated problem? *Psychosomatics, 23, 1232–1235.*

Williams, M. A., Campbell, E. B., Raynor, W. J., Mucholt, M. A., Mlynarczk, S. M., & Crane, L. G. (1985). Predictors of acute confusional states in hospitalized elderly patients. *Research in Nursing and Health*, *8*, 31–40.

Williams, M. A., Holloway, J. R., Winn, M. C., Wolanin, M. O., Lawler, M. L., Westwick, C. R., & Chin, M. H. (1979). Nursing activities and acute confusional states in elderly hip-fracture patients. *Nursing Research*, *28*, 25–35.

Williams, M. A., Ward, S. E., & Campbell, E. B. (1988). Confusion: Testing versus observation. *Journal of Gerontological Nursing*, *14*(1), 25–30.

Wolanin, M. O., & Holloway, J. R. (1980). Relocation confusion: Intervention for prevention. In I. M. Burnside (Ed.), *Psychosocial care of the aged* (pp. 179–194). New York: McGraw-Hill.

Wolanin, M. O., & Phillips, L. R. (1981). *Confusion: Prevention and care*. St. Louis: C. V. Mosby.

Part III

Psychosocial Needs
In The Elderly

Following the same structure as the chapters in Part II, the chapters in Part III turn to nursing interventions that are related to psychosocial needs in the elderly. In Chapter 10, Joan Magit examines the central notion of self-concept, and the associated issue of self-esteem. A topic closely related to this is socialization, which is explored by Eleanor Taggart in Chapter 11. Next, Sharon Valente and Joan Sellers consider effective coping, with special reference to threats arising from anxiety, powerlessness, depression, substance abuse, and suicidal behavior. Finally, Sister Karin Dufault takes up issues of loss, grief, and hope as they appear in the lives of elderly persons.

Again, the organizing principles are those of the nursing process and specified nursing diagnoses, leavened with brief practical examples and extended case discussions. In view of our reliance throughout this book upon nursing diagnoses, it may be useful to note that Gordon (1987) has pointed out three problems that underlie current work in establishing nursing diagnostic categories: (1) there may be a lack of clarity in the diagnosis itself; (2) there may be inadequate theoretical knowledge of the problem represented by the diagnosis; and (3) there may be deficiencies in clinical reasoning skills that direct the search for information. All of this is true, even though the North American Nursing Diagnosis Association has striven diligently since its founding in 1973 to improve the quality of and justify the bases for specific nursing diagnoses. Clinical practice cannot come to a halt until some arbitrary degree of perfection is achieved. On the contrary, use of existing diagnostic categories in clinical practice can stimulate the productive thinking and additional research that is required for their improvement.

Gordon, M. (1987). *Nursing diagnosis: Process and application* (2nd ed.). New York: McGraw-Hill.

Chapter 10

Self-Concept

Joan G. Magit

INTRODUCTION

The purpose of this chapter is to define and discuss the meaning of self-concept as it relates to elderly persons. It addresses the importance of self-concept in the elderly and implications this has for the nursing profession. Utilizing the nursing process, this chapter focuses on factors that may have an impact on the elderly and their self-concept, discusses what can be done to alleviate problems associated with disturbances in self-concept, and provides examples of case studies to illustrate problems and effective nursing interventions to minimize or resolve disturbances in self-concept.

Many books and articles have been written about topics related to self-concept (e.g., Gilberts, 1983), but there appears to be a lack of consensus in the literature in distinguishing between the notions of self-concept and self-esteem. Often, these terms are used interchangeably (Elliot & Hybertson, 1982; Stanwyck, 1983). There is also great variation in the definitions of these terms. For example, Driever (1976b, p. 169) defined "self-concept" as "the composite of beliefs and feelings that one holds about oneself at a given time, formed from perceptions particularly of others' reactions, and directing one's behavior," and "self-esteem" as "that pervasive aspect of the self-concept which relates to the worth or value the person has of himself" (Driever, 1976a, p. 233). Similarly, Doenges and Moorhouse (1985, p. 299) defined a disturbance in self-esteem as a "disruption in the individual's perception of own value, worth, and competence." In this chapter, self-concept will be taken as the broader notion having to do with ways in which one understands oneself, while self-esteem will indicate those aspects of self-concept which focus on self-evaluation and feelings about oneself.

In light of definitional and terminological differences, how are nurses working with the elderly in various settings (community, hospital, or long-term care) able to diagnose difficulties with self-concept effectively and employ appropriate interventions? How can nurses promote positive understandings of self-concept in the elderly? Finally, how can nurses enhance self-esteem and assist with overcoming negative feelings about the self or low self-esteem?

It appears that determinants of self-concept can be divided into two categories: external and internal. That is, self-concept arises from reactions to the outside world (external) or from personal thoughts and feelings (internal). It is important to be aware of whether an individual's self-concept and feelings of self-worth are determined by external or internal forces in order to select appropriate nursing interventions. For the purpose of this discussion, self-concept will be defined as the composite result of external forces and forces that emanate from within that influence a person's perception of the self.

When dealing with an aging population, two additional terms must be defined because of their implications for nursing practice:

Sexism is used to describe the negative treatment of women and preferential treatment of men; women perceive that they are treated with less respect, and that perception may extend to the belief that they receive poorer medical care within the health care setting than do men.

Ageism is a term coined by Butler (1969): "Ageism reflects a deep-seated uneasiness on the part of young and middle-aged—a personal revulsion and distaste for growing old, disease, disability; and fear of powerlessness, 'uselessness,' and death" (p. 243). Butler also equates ageism with bigotry: "Ageism can be seen as a process of systematic stereotyping of and discrimination against people because they are old, just as racism and sexism accomplish this with skin color and gender. Ageism allows the younger generation to see older people as different from themselves; thus they subtly cease to identify with their elders as human beings" (Butler, 1977, p. 12).

It is clear that if health-care professionals, particularly nurses, adopt a sexist or ageist attitude, this will only increase the elderly person's problems with self-concept and feelings of worthlessness. Thus, these attitudes will have a negative impact on nursing interventions.

ASSESSMENT

Many factors contributing to disturbances in self-concept seen in the elderly may be associated with physical changes, acute and chronic illnesses, psychological well-being, environment, and societal attitudes. Nurses often overhear or are confronted by elderly persons who say, "I'm too old. Who needs old people? Who cares? No one is interested in me . . . ." These are some verbal cues that indicate difficulties in self-concept and self-esteem.

When taking the older person's present and past history, in the course of a nursing assessment, acute and chronic illnesses, as well as physical, psychological, environmental, and societal factors, are extremely important in terms of evaluating self-concept. During the assessment, it is important to be aware of the nonverbal and verbal clues which are indicative of a problem with self-concept. For example:

Nonverbal clues: poor personal hygiene, unkempt dress, poor posture, sad facial expression, downcast eyes, and sighing.

Verbal clues: "Why is a young person like you working with someone old like me?" "Why should I have my teeth taken care of? I'm too old." "No one looks at me anyway. Who cares what I eat?" "They forced me to leave my house and move here. I hate it." "I can't do anything anymore since I broke my hip. I can't even go to the bathroom myself." "There must be something wrong with me. I still feel sex should be an important part of my life."

From statements of this sort, it is evident that self-concept and self-esteem are closely related to internal and external environmental variables that impact upon the physiological, psychological, and social self (Antonucci & Jackson, 1983; Driever, 1976a). Examples of the relationship between these variables and disruptions in self-concept and self-esteem follow.

Physiological Self

Physical Changes

Normal physiological changes (e.g., grey hair, wrinkles, changes in body structure) may decrease one's sense of self-worth. These changes seem to have the greatest impact on women. Cohen (1985, pp. 15–16) has written: "There is a point in every woman's life at which the physical reality of aging makes its first appearance . . . My punishment will take many different forms, beginning insidiously with advertising and social pressures to wage a serious, concentrated battle against my physical aging. I am told that if I wish to be considered attractive and still desirable, I must hide, cover, or in some way minimize the visible signs of my aging . . . Our aging is both a biological and emotional phenomenon."

Acute and Chronic Illness

Acute and chronic illnesses have a significant impact on self-concept and self-esteem. One or more of these illnesses can bring on an overwhelming sense of powerlessness, lack of autonomy, loss of control over the environment, negative body image, or altered life style. "Health care professionals should be aware of the probability that people with health problems may also have lower levels of self-esteem; low levels of self-esteem may be a major predisposing risk factor for poor health . . ." (Antonucci & Jackson, 1983, p. 8).

Acute illnesses include cardiovascular surgery, mastectomy, prostate surgery, and exacerbations of chronic problems. An example of the impact of an acute illness can be seen in a 65-year-old, successful businessman with a history of diabetes and high blood pressure who found himself in a hospital following a drug interaction. He feared he would lose his job or be forced into early retirement. Because his self-concept and his sense of self-worth were in large part derived from his work, he had an overwhelming sense of powerlessness.

Chronic illnesses or conditions include arthritis, urinary incontinence, colostomy, osteoporosis, coronary artery disease, dental problems, and neurological disorders. An example of the impact of a chronic illness is the case of a 63-year-old woman with a 15-year history of multiple sclerosis. She found herself with decreased ability to walk and occasional bouts of urinary incontinence. She feared embarrassment over losing control of urine in public, and her husband reported that it was difficult to encourage her to leave the house.

Psychological Self

Internal and external forces impact on the psychological well being of an individual. Long-held personal beliefs influence the person's view of the self and the world, and societal attitudes can have a strong influence as well. Older persons often clearly articulate their awareness of prejudicial attitudes of health care personnel and the health system. A typical comment is, "Doctors and nurses have more important things to do than take care of old people." Elderly persons describe health professionals, particularly their physicians, as being "bored with caring for them," or "not wanting to be bothered with them." If an older person accepts society's myths and stereotypes about aging, and/or sexuality, that person's self-concept and coping mechanisms may be adversely affected.

Social Self

Environment

Many environmental factors have an impact on a person's self-concept and well-being, including living conditions, exercise, nutrition, friends, and family. For example, an older woman's husband has recently died and her family lives out of state. Because of the family's concern for her safety and security, they have moved her into a retirement home, forcing her into selling her home and possessions. She feels discarded and powerless.

Societal Factors

How does the role a person plays in society impact on that person's identity and feelings of self-worth? What role does society expect elderly persons to perform? According to Malaznik (1976, p. 247), "role performance . . . is the collection of behaviors observed when an individual with a particular title undertakes those actions which society attributes to that title. Roles are the functional units of society."

Numerous articles have been written about negative attitudes and stereotyping of older persons. Studies focusing on societal attitudes toward the elderly have emphasized negative attitudes, equating the status of the elderly to that of minority groups (Barron, 1953; Drake, 1958).

In a study of students' attitudes toward the elderly, prejudice against the aged was even stronger than prejudice against color (Spence & Feigenbaum, 1968). Additionally, reluctance of therapists to work with the aged is based on stereotyped misconceptions (Kastenbaum, 1963). Clearly, stereotyped views of older persons, combined with a barrier to communication caused by misunderstanding and ignorance, interfere with effective health care and can cause disruptions in self-concept and decreased self-esteem (Whall, 1987).

NURSING DIAGNOSIS

The primary nursing diagnostic category in this content area is *self-concept, disturbance in*, defined as "a disruption in the way one perceives one's body image, self-esteem, role performance, and/or personal identity" (Deuspohl, 1986, pp. 263–264). Each of these four sub-components, in turn, needs its own defining characteristics and etiologies.

Thus, *Disturbance in body image* is defined in terms of verbal or nonverbal responses to actual or perceived changes in structure and/or function, and would be related to one or more of the following etiological factors: biophysical; cognitive-perceptual; psychosocial; cultural or spiritual. *Disturbance in self-esteem* has the following defining characteristics: inability to accept positive reinforcement; lack of follow-through; nonparticipation in therapy; not taking responsibility for self-care (self-neglect); self-destructive behavior; lack of eye contact. Etiology would need to be specified in each individual case.

Disturbance in role performance has the following defining characteristics: change in self-perception of role; denial of role; change in others' perception of role; conflict in roles; change in physical capacity to resume role; lack of knowledge of role change in usual patterns of responsibility. Again, etiology would need to be specified. Finally, *disturbance in personal identity* or inability to distinguish between self and nonself has not yet seen development of defining characteristics and would need to have a specified etiology.

A possible set of nursing diagnoses having to do with disturbance in self-concept in the area of self-esteem for a particular elderly person might involve the following:

1. Loss of self-esteem related to:
    a. Normal physiological changes because of aging
    b. Acute or chronic illnesses
2. Decreased self-esteem related to:
    a. Societal negative attitudes, myths, and stereotypical behaviors toward aging
    b. Concern about sexual attractiveness
    c. Lack of information about the normal physiological changes associated with aging
    d. Lack of education about physical problems and/or medical interventions
3. Feelings of worthlessness or loss of autonomy secondary to:
    a. Placement in a long-term care setting
    b. Forced retirement
4. Lack of self-acceptance secondary to body image changes

PLANNING

Planning establishes priorities, goals, and objectives, along with time frames, for nursing intervention in designing a program of care for elderly persons. It is important that goals and objectives be stated in terms of client behaviors. Also, goals and objectives that are mutually agreed upon by the elderly person, his or her family, and the nurse are the most effective.

Short-Term Goals

The nurse and the elderly person will discuss and develop agreed-upon goals depending upon the clinical setting. The time frame must be individualized and may be stated in terms of hours, days, weeks, or months. Short-term goals might include that the client will:

1. Develop positive feelings about self.
2. Partake in self-hygienic activites of daily living.
3. Participate in decision-making activities and plans for each day.

Measureable objectives for these short-term goals are that the client will:

1. Verbalize two positive feelings about self, family, and friends, within 48 hours.
2. Perform oral care and shower self each day.
3. Make plans for visits with friends and family, and decisions regarding recreational activities for each day.

Long-Term Goals

Long-term goals are those that will be permanently incorporated into a person's life style. As related to self-concept, examples of long-term goals might include that the client will:

1. Recognize self-worth.
2. Have an increase in interdependent behavior.
3. Express feelings of well being.

Measureable objectives for these long-term goals are that the client will:

1. Verbalize statements, such as: "I love myself; I respect myself."
2. Take a more active role within the family, community, and/or nursing home.
3. Verbalize statements, such as: "I'm doing better; I feel better; I'm sleeping better."

INTERVENTION

Ageism can contribute to "one of the greatest losses of old age, that is, choice" (Butler, 1969, p. 246), and this may be reflected unintentionally in the types of intervention that aging persons receive. With this in mind, it is essential that nurses be aware of their own negative attitudes toward aging and recognize their personal values that might cause discomfort in working with the elderly population.

The following specific actions are recommended for nurses to undertake in relationship to care of the elderly. They are divided according to internal and external factors bearing upon self-concept, as previously defined.

Interventions that might help to improve internally caused aspects of self-concept and feelings of self-worth are:

1. Promote the use of life review through discussion, tapes, or writing.

2. Encourage older adults to express their feelings and frustrations regarding the impact of physiological changes and/or illnesses.

3. Assist elderly persons in recognizing positive and negative ageist behaviors in themselves.

4. Direct elderly persons to self-help programs and support groups on such topics as: how to talk to your doctor, stress management, assertiveness training, or building self-esteem.

Interventions that might help to improve externally caused aspects of self-concept and feelings of self-worth are:

1. Counsel the elderly about the importance of preventive health-care measures, e.g., monitoring caloric intake.

2. Provide older adults with available health-care resources.

3. Educate older adults about their medications, toxic effects, and possible interactions; review medications that may cause depression and increase or decrease libido.

4. Educate older men and women about sexuality and aging.

5. When appropriate, encourage elderly persons to volunteer in community organizations.

6. When appropriate, encourage elderly persons to explore new areas of interest, e.g., piano, art, college courses, dance.

7. Refer to health promotion classes offered within hospital or community settings to promote positive self-esteem, e.g., self-esteem, stress management, coping skills, and new directions workshops.

EVALUATION

To evaluate the effectiveness of the nursing interventions specified above, as they relate to self-concept, nurses will evaluate whether planned goals and objectives have been met in the time frames laid down. For example, for interventions related to internally-caused aspects of self-concept: Is the older adult engaging in life review? Is the elderly person expressing feelings and frustrations regarding the impact of physiological changes and/or illnesses? Likewise, for interventions related to externally-caused aspects of self-concept: Is the older adult practicing preventive health-care measures? Which available health-care resources is the elderly person utilizing? In responding to questions of this sort, elderly persons demonstrate whether or not planned goals and objectives have been met, and whether or not nursing interventions have been effective. If not, reassessment is needed.

CASE STUDIES

The following case studies of disturbances in self-concept in elderly persons illustrate the application of the nursing process. These examples are designed so that nurses caring for the elderly will have a better understanding of factors that can impact on self-concept in the elderly and thus be better equipped to address these issues among elderly persons.

Physical contact is a basic lifetime human need. The whole subject of sexuality is generally surrounded by discomfort, embarrassment, misinformation, and, sadly, a lot of unhappiness. This is true for all age groups, but probably more so when we speak about sexuality and aging. Unfortunately, society still imposes strict codes of conduct regarding sexuality for the older adult; an older man interested in sex is described as a "dirty old man," and an older woman as "not acting her age." Butler and Lewis (1976) in their book, *Love and Sex after Sixty*, wrote, "the presumption is that sexual desire automatically ebbs with age— that it begins to decline when one is in one's forties, proceeds relentlessly downward . . . and eventually hits bottom at sometime between sixty and sixty-five" (p. 3).

Case Study #1

Assessment

Mrs. G., is a 64-year-old attractive woman who was seen in the gynecology outpatient clinic following a recent hysterectomy. She was referred to the clinic nurse by the gynecologist because of her expression of negative feelings of being less attractive since the surgery. At the time of the interview with the nurse, Mrs. G voiced her disgust about her greying hair and wrinkling of her skin, and worried that she may become "one of those invisible older women." Mrs. G's health history was negative for any past illnesses, and she considered herself to be a mentally and physically active person who enjoyed a "wonderful" relationship with her husband who had recently retired. They were looking forward to travelling across the country in their camper when following a yearly check-up it was determined that she needed a hysterectomy because of recurring "polyps of the uterus." In addition to the hysterectomy and based on Mrs. G's family history (her mother had died of ovarian cancer), her ovaries were removed. The more extensive surgery necessitated their postponing their trip for six months, adding to Mrs. G's feelings of powerlessness.

During the discussion with the nurse, Mrs. G revealed that she was very surprised to find that she experienced a recurrence of hot flashes since she had not had a period in six years. To counteract this discomfort, her physician had placed her on low-dose estrogen and provera hormonal replacement therapy, and while the hot flashes had lessened she felt a lack of control over her body. Upon further assessment, the nurse discovered Mrs. G experienced occasional loss of urine and vaginal itching, adding to her sense of loss of control over her bodily functions.

Nursing Diagnoses

1. Self-concept, disturbance in body image related to recent surgery, urinary incontinence, and vaginal itching.
2. Self-concept, disturbance in self-esteem related to lack of information about physiological changes associated with surgery.
3. Self-concept, disturbance in self-esteem related to societal devaluation of aging.

Planning

Mutually agreed-upon short-terms goals for client behaviors:

- Explore and identify sociological and psychological sources of negative self-perceptions.
- Demonstrate understanding of psychological and physical changes. associated with hysterectomy.
- Discuss health concerns with health professionals and husband.

Mutually agreed-upon long-term goals for client behaviors:

- Acknowledge self as a vital person as evidenced by verbalizing positive statements about self.
- Participate in women's self-help/self-care groups.

Intervention

- Provide opportunities for Mrs. G to express openly the meaning hysterectomy has for her.
- Provide accurate information as needed about physical changes associated with aging and recent surgery.
- Promote wellness and sense of control over present situation by providing information about vaginal changes, episodes of urinary incontinence, and hormonal replacement therapy.
- Encourage Mrs. G to communicate feelings with her husband.
- Assist Mrs. G in locating women's support groups and/or self-esteem classes within the community.
- Discuss inaccuracies in self-perception with Mrs. G.
- Refer to appropriate counseling therapy if indicated.

Mrs. G determined that her most immediate concern was the physical changes associated with the current situation. Therefore, the following information was provided to her.

1. *Physical Changes.* Following the removal of ovaries and uterus, and after the menopause, there is a decrease in estrogen production which, in turn, can cause changes in the female reproductive system. These changes also affect the vagina; for example, thinning of the tissue occurs around the vaginal opening and within the vagina. The vagina becomes smoother, drier, and less acidic, which may promote infection and inflammation of the vaginal tissue. It was explained to Mrs. G that she may experience symptoms such as vaginal itching and/or discomfort while others may not have any symptoms. In addition to the hormones already prescribed for Mrs. G, a short-term course of estrogen vaginal cream was recommended to strengthen the vaginal walls (in order to prevent inflammation) and to increase control of urine. The nurse also recommended that Mrs. G practice the following self-care exercise to decrease episodes of urinary incontinence.

2. *Kegel Exercises.* Kegel exercises, a set of exercises originally designed to help women control the leakage of urine that sometimes follows menopause and childbirth, have been found to tone and strengthen the vaginal walls in post-menopausal women. The exercises consist of strengthening the pubococcygeal (PC) muscle. To practice this exercise, one needs to locate the PC muscle. This is done by stopping and starting the flow of urine when urinating. This stop/start action is a way of identifying what it feels like to contract the muscles. It also indicates how much control one has. This first step is *only* a means to familiarize the person with the muscle that needs to be

exercised. Once the muscle has been identified, the individual can practice contracting and relaxing it daily, while sitting, while watching television, while waiting for the bus or driving a car. The goal for Mrs. G was to carry out the exercise in sets of 25 three times a day, and to do so for the rest of her life.

Evaluation

A follow-up appointment in the clinic two weeks later found that Mrs. G was practicing the Kegel exercises and applying estrogen vaginal cream as recommended. She stated that the vaginal discomfort and urine loss had subsided, and that she was feeling better about herself. Mrs. G had found a community-based older women's issues group and would be joining it in a few weeks, although she also expressed interest in obtaining individual counseling at a community mental health clinic. The clinic nurse helped Mrs. G with the referral.

Case Study #2

Assessment

Mr. F is a 70-year-old, Caucasian male patient in a Health Maintenance Organization (HMO), who recently had his yearly physical examination and returned for laboratory results. His medical history was negative with the exception of benign prostatic hypertrophy and asthma. At the time of the review of the laboratory results (which were all within normal limits), he discussed his concern about being impotent. Upon further exploration, the nurse discovered that Mr. F had recently begun dating a woman he met while attending a weekly support group for spouses of cancer victims and on one occasion he attempted sexual intercourse without success. He described this experience as being devastating to him and also as being very embarrassing, even though his date was "very understanding." Based on this one experience, Mr. F was certain he was impotent. Although he was interested in dating and ultimately getting remarried, Mr. F felt quite anxious, a little frightened, and a bit guilty about his interest in becoming sexually active because "my daughter thinks I'm too old."

Mr. F had been married for 41 years and had been widowed within the past year. He reported that he and his wife were happily married and enjoyed a wonderful relationship. He described their sex life as being very satisfying for both of them. However, because of his wife's long-term illness with cancer, they did not engage in sexual intercourse for two years prior to her death. Throughout this time, they continued to comfort each other by touching and holding. During this period, Mr. F attempted masturbation on one occasion without success. He attributed this failure to his feelings of guilt: "How could I enjoy sexual release when my wife could not?" Mr. F had not engaged in any sexual experience leading to climax for over two years.

Mr. F reported that in the past he was always able to reach orgasm through intercourse and masturbation with no difficulty. He was very concerned about his inability to have an erection. He denied having early morning erections, or the ability to become aroused by self- or partner stimulation. He wondered if a penile implant might be the answer to his problem.

Nursing Diagnoses

Disturbance in self-concept related to:

1. Loss of self-esteem related to inability to have an erection.
2. Decreased self-esteem related to lack of information and knowledge about normal bodily functions, sexuality, and aging.
3. Low self-esteem related to possible guilt or shame over interest in sex.

Planning

Mutually-agreed-upon short-term goals for client behaviors:

- Rule out any physiologically based cause of impotence.
- Understand normal physiological changes in aging and sex.
- Explore possible psychological and emotional problems associated with sex and aging.

Mutually agreed-upon long-term goals for client behaviors:

- Identify both physical and psychosocial issues related to sexuality and aging.
- Discuss concerns with partner or significant other.
- Explore acceptable sexual practices.
- Achieve ability to have a satisfying sexual relationship.

Intervention

- Made appointment with the clinic's urologist.
- Loaned paperback book to patient about sexuality and aging, *Love and Sex after Sixty*, by Butler and Lewis.
- Arranged for return to outpatient clinic in one week.

Evaluation

Within one week, Mr. F had a complete physical examination by the urologist. At that time, it was confirmed that he had a slightly enlarged prostate gland (benign) and a low testosterone level. His doctor gave him a "shot" of testosterone. No follow-up was indicated, as the urologist did not believe that the enlarged prostate gland or low testosterone level was the cause of his sexual problem.

Mr. F had read the first two chapters of the paperback book. He found them very informative and stimulating, and had many questions. He also wanted information about penile implants. Mr. F was praised for the progress that he had made in one week, yet based on the original goals it was determined that more information was needed. Further assessment was made of Mr. F's use of medication, alcohol intake, smoking habits, and his knowledge of physical and psychological factors associated with aging.

    1.   *Medications*. Medications, whether prescription or nonprescription, can cause serious sexual problems for *both* men and women. All too often, physicians fail to take a thorough medication history from patients.

    2.   *Alcohol*. Most people are surprised to learn that alcohol is a drug. It is a depressant and not a stimulant. Alcohol is notorious for causing nonerection. In small amounts, it usually interferes with sexual performance. According to Castleman (1980), long-term use of alcohol lowers the male sex hormone, testosterone, in the body.

    3.   *Cigarette Smoking*. There is a growing body of research that suggests that there is a correlation between smoking and nonerection, as well as depressed testosterone levels (Castleman, 1980).

Reassessment

Mr. F denied smoking, medication use, and considered himself to be an occasional drinker. Mr. F was lacking important information about factors that can contribute to disruptions in self-concept and self-esteem.

Additional Interventions

The following interventions in terms of discussion, education, and providing specific information took place on two following clinic visits.

    It was important to explain to Mr. F that, as men age, there are some *physiological changes* that occur. It is essential to recognize these changes in order to exclude a physical or emotional cause of an erection problem. About the age of 50, men begin to notice some changes, such as the inability to have an erection upon demand. Also, the erection may not be quite as hard as when they were younger. Finally, it may take longer to have a second erection. (The period of time changes from 10 to 30 minutes as an adolescent to 12 to 24 hours for an older man). In practical terms, this means that a man over 60 usually cannot make love more than twice a day on an average day (Zilbergeld, 1978).

Unfortunately, like many other men, Mr. F viewed these changes as signs of impending impotence rather than changes due to the aging process. Also, like men who worry about their performance and fear impotency, Mr. F tended to create the very problem that he feared most. Further, like other older men, Mr. F required more time and stimulation to obtain an erection than he did in his youth. This may be problematic in a relationship where the man has been the aggressor and his female partner, raised under the influence of Victorian standards, was conditioned to be sexually passive (Butler & Lewis, 1976).

Most elders are unaware that any number of life situations cause stress. This includes both good and bad stressful events. Sexual problems, especially the inability to have an erection, may be caused by the death of a loved one, retirement, marital conflicts, guilt, or new exciting situations, like an upcoming marriage, vacation, or holiday. As Butler and Lewis (1976) have pointed out, "The male penis is a barometer of a man's feelings and quickly reflects his state of mind and his current life situation" (p. 53). Therefore, it was necessary to explain to Mr. F that a sudden attack of impotence was probably associated with his new relationship. Unfortunately, the psychological trauma arising from a single episode of not being able to have an erection appeared to lead Mr. F to additional problems.

There also were a number of *psychological factors* to explore with Mr. F in order to reestablish and enhance his sexual activity. The most important factor was to give Mr. F permission to enjoy intimacy and sexual pleasure (Table 10.1). Many sex therapists and counselors recommend a temporary ban on genital sex. There are two reasons for doing this: first, to remove any pressure to produce an erection; and, second, to allow the client time to become reacquainted with his or her body and that of the partner. During this interim period there are several important nursing actions to consider and to recommend to individuals such as Mr. F.

1. *Massage*. Friendly playful touching is important for both men and women. This helps the person become relaxed. Massage is a very special form of intimacy, which works best in the nude, and in a warm, cozy place that is free of interruption. Mr. F was instructed on following home exercises. In the beginning, start the massages away from the genital areas, concentrating on sensations in other parts of the body. It is important to be able to enjoy giving as well as receiving a massage.

TABLE 10.1 A Conceptual Scheme for Intervention

Annon's model (Annon, 1976) is referred to as the P-LI-SS-IT model. It is a four-level approach that can be used for treating sexual concerns and problems of the aging population. The scheme provides nurses in any setting—hospital, clinic, community—with a guideline for intervention.

1. Permission (P)

    Example: Older married couple admitting they are still sexually active and expressing feelings of guilt.

    Interventions:
    Clients just need to hear that what they are doing is OK, normal.
    Older people do have strong and continued interest in sex.

2. Limited Information (LI)

    Example: 65-year-old woman complains of painful intercourse.

    Interventions:
    Provide information about the use of a lubrication during intercourse and/or Premarin® vaginal cream.
    Provide information about Kegel pelvic muscle exercises.

3. Specific Suggestion (SS)

    Example: A sexually active 80-year-old man complaining of angina during intercourse.

    Interventions:
    At this time, a brief sexual history should be obtained about the problem.
    May need suggestions about different positions to be used in problems with chronic illness.

4. Intensive Therapy (IT)

    Example: 67-year-old man complains of lack of desire for the past five years.

    Intervention:
    When problem involves sexual dysfunctions, refer to certified sex therapist or counselor.

Headings for the above examples adapted from: J. S. Annon (1976). *Behavioral treatment of sexual problems*. Hagerstown, MD: Harper & Row.

Some men have a problem accepting massages, yet sharing and exchanging pleasure is essential in any relationship (Hite, 1976).

2. *Romance.* Whether it is a long-standing or a new relationship, the addition of candlelight, music, flowers, a little wine, or a luxurious bath can set the scene for a most romantic encounter (Barbach, 1984).

3. *Masturbation.* Some therapists consider masturbation to be the single most important way to deal with nonerection. Self-stimulation provides an opportunity to rediscover sexual feelings. Although many

individuals were taught that masturbation is wrong or harmful, it should be considered by those who find it acceptable as one possible healthy form of sexual expression (Butler & Lewis, 1976; Heiman, LoPiccolo, & LoPiccolo, 1976; Zilbergeld, 1978).

4. *Fantasy.* Fantasies can add variety to love making and allow lovers to explore their own feelings while sharing the intimacy of love making with each other (Friday, 1973; Nin, 1969; Zilbergeld, 1978). Remember that sex and pleasure go together—not sex and performance. It is essential for both partners to openly and honestly discuss their feelings, needs, likes, and dislikes with each other. Slow down love making and try to appreciate whole-body sensuality. There are many wonderful books about sexuality now available in libraries and bookstores. Mr. F was encouraged to take time out to explore some of these books and choose the ones that worked best for him.

Re-Evaluation

Within a few weeks, Mr. F resumed his relationship with the woman he had met in the support group and was engaging in satisfactory sexual activity. It was clear that this man benefitted from nursing interventions within an open, nonjudgmental environment that included education, discussion, and information about normal physiological changes associated with aging and about myths relating to sexuality and aging. Follow-up with the urologist and a yearly physical examination were recommended.

CONCLUSION

To a certain extent, many physiological, psychological, and sociological factors identified in this chapter that seem to contribute to disturbances in self-concept are, in fact, within an older person's control, provided that person has an understanding of the relationship between these factors and his or her perception of self. In order to overcome disturbances in self-concept and self-esteem, the role of the nurse is to assist elderly persons to identify those internal and external determinants that have an impact upon them. Within this chapter, two case studies have been described to demonstrate how nursing approaches and actions can assist older persons to overcome disruptions of their perceptions of their own "value, worth, and competence" (Doenges & Moorhouse, 1985).

When working with older persons, nurses need to recognize that their approaches and actions "are shaped by input from many contextual layers of the surrounding society; cultural values filter through social and political systems to affect nursing education, practice, and care delivery" (Lillard, 1982, p. 631).

REFERENCES

Antonucci, T. C., & Jackson, J. S. (1983). Physical health and self-esteem. *Family and Community Health, 9,* 1–9.

Barbach, L. G. (1984). *For each other, sharing sexual intimacy.* New York: Signet New American Library.

Barron, M. L. (1953). Minority group characteristics of the aged in American society. *Journal of Gerontology, 8,* 477–482.

Butler, R. N. (1969). Age-ism: Another form of bigotry. *The Gerontologist, 9,* 243–246.

Butler, R. N. (1977). *Why survive? Being old in America.* New York: Harper & Row.

Butler, R. N., & Lewis, M. I. (1977). *Aging and mental health.* St. Louis: C. V. Mosby.

Butler, R. N., & Lewis, M. I. (1976). *Love and sex after sixty.* New York: Harper & Row.

Castleman, M. (1980). *Sexual solutions.* New York: Simon & Shuster.

Cohen, L. (1985). *Small expectations.* Toronto: McClelland and Stewart.

Doenges, M., & Moorhouse, M. (1985). *Nurse's pocket guide: Nursing diagnoses with interventions* (2nd ed.). Philadelphia: F. A. Davis.

Drake, J. T. (1958). *The aged in American society.* New York: Ronald Press.

Driever, M. J. (1976a). Problems of low self-esteem. In Sr. C. Roy (Ed.), *Introduction to nursing: An adaptation model* (pp. 232–242). Englewood Cliffs, NJ: Prentice-Hall.

Driever, M. J. (1976b). Theory of self-concept. In Sr. C. Roy (Ed.), *Introduction to nursing: An adaptation model* (pp. 169–179). Englewood Cliffs, NJ: Prentice-Hall.

Duespohl, T. A. (1986). *Nursing diagnosis manual for the well and ill client.* Philadelphia: W. B. Saunders.

Elliot, B., & Hybertson, D. (1982). What is it about the elderly that elicits a negative response? *Journal of Gerontological Nursing, 8*(10), 568–571.

Friday, N. (1973). *My secret garden.* New York: Pocket Books.

Gilberts, R. (1983). The evaluation of self-esteem. *Family and Community Health, 29,* 29–40.

Heiman, J., LoPiccolo, L., & LoPiccolo, J. (1976). *Becoming orgasmic: A program of sexual growth for women.* Englewood Cliffs, NJ: Prentice-Hall.

Hite, S. (1976). *The Hite report.* New York: Dell.

Kastenbaum, R. (1963). The reluctant therapist. *Geriatrics, 18*(4), 296–301.

Lillard, J. (1982). A double edge sword: Ageism and sexism. *Journal of Gerontological Nursing, 8*(11), 630–634.

Malaznik, N. (1976). Theory of role function. In Sr. C. Roy (Ed.), *Introduction to nursing: An adaptation model* (pp. 245–255). Englewood Cliffs, NJ: Prentice-Hall.

Nin, A. (1969). *Delta of Venus.* New York: Bantam.

Spence, D. L., & Feigenbaum, E. M. (1968). Medical students' attitudes toward the geriatric patient. *Journal of Gerontology, 16,* 976–983.

Stanwyck, D. J. (1983). Self-esteem through the life span. *Family and Community Health, 9,* 11–28.

Whall, A. L. (1987). Self-esteem and the mental health of older adults. *Journal of Gerontological Nursing, 13*(4), 41–42.

Zilbergeld, B. (1978). *Male sexuality: A guide to sexual fulfillment.* Boston: Little, Brown.

Chapter **11**

Socialization

Eleanor Taggart

INTRODUCTION

Socialization is the natural process through which human beings become competent functioning adults in their social groups and particular societies. As individuals progress through the life cycle, social roles, knowledge, and skills are gained, dropped, or changed. Simultaneously, the sociocultural environment with which individuals interact is also changing. These conditions require continuous socialization if people are to maintain themselves as competent functioning individuals in society.

A major concern in our society, as well as in other developed countries of the world, is whether the elderly are able to maintain socialization with others or whether they experience increasing isolation as they age. The purpose of this chapter is to examine if and why there is cause for concern, and second, who among the elderly are at risk for reduction and absence of socialization. Next, the chapter presents guidelines for assessing the socialization status of elderly persons, and for assessing and diagnosing absence or decrease in social interaction. On that basis, interventions are offered which promote maintenance and/or restoration of socialization, and which prevent loss of social interaction. Finally, outcomes are evaluated and a case study of a socially-isolated elder is introduced to illustrate some of the major points in the chapter.

SOCIALIZATION AND THE ELDERLY

Socialization, as a concept, emerged simultaneously from the disciplines of anthropology, psychology, and sociology. Each of these fields uses this concept to delineate, from its own perspective, how the human person develops within a social and cultural environment. Anthropology, for example, views socialization as an enculturation process in which the individual learns and internalizes cultural rules and content, such as values or beliefs, transmitted by the society of which he or she is a member. By contrast, psychology is concerned with processes of learning and the development of self that occurs as an individual becomes socialized. Finally, sociologists focus on the agencies of socialization (e.g., family, peers, schools, or other social institutions) and processes involved in acquisition of social skills, development of the social self, and training for or development of social roles.

In its early stages of conceptualization, socialization was discussed exclusively within the context of childhood. It was seen as the process by which the child learned how to function as an adult in a given society (Parsons, 1955; Piaget, 1954). In the process, the child learner was seen largely as a passive recipient. Today socialization is considered to be a continuous and cumulative process which extends throughout the life cycle (Clausen, 1968). For example, as elderly individuals in society retire or lose a spouse through death, socialization to new roles and activities is a necessary and important component in helping them adapt to the changes that have taken place.

Increasingly, socialization has come to be viewed as an interactional process which influences all persons who are involved in the process—socializees and socializers alike (Rheingold, 1969). Furthermore, it is recognized that the person becoming socialized is an active participant in his or her own socialization. For example, it is postulated that in learning new social roles the individual improvises his or her performance based on immediate cues from others (Heiss, 1976). Roles are identified and given content through social interaction, for example, self and other roles are created and modified as the process of interaction unfolds. Such interactions can influence the elderly negatively as well as positively. For example, through social interactions, which might occur in a nursing home, some elderly incorporate the stereotypic unfavorable images of the aged held by others in society. Such incorporation contributes to a lowering of their self-esteem.

For purposes of analysis, socialization can be viewed both from the perspective of society and from that of the individual becoming socialized. However, it is important to remember that both perspectives are interrelated as the socialization process unfolds. From the societal perspective, the individual is expected to achieve established standards of the society with respect to physical development, skills and capacities, emotional expression, intellectual and conative activity, and patterning of relations with significant others. From the individual perspective, the process of socialization encompasses the acquisition of language or verbal skills, self-identification, social roles, moral standards and values, and the development of affective and cognitive functioning. Through language acquisition, the individual enters into the social world of shared symbols. The use of shared symbols (e.g., words) facilitates social interaction and socialization.

A widely held assumption in American society is that the elderly are deprived of social interaction with others (Blau, 1981). Obviously, this has implications for the ability to maintain socialization. Rosnow (1974, p. 168) asserted that, "our current institutions do not offer a choice between marginality and integration of the aged but simply between alternate forms of alienation." Given such a statement, there is little wonder that one of the most distinctive social characteristics attributed to America's elderly is that of being socially isolated (Bennett, 1980). The impression that elderly persons are socially isolated was derived in part from modernization theory (Cowgill & Holmes, 1972). This theory postulates that as societies become modernized the elderly find themselves deprived of social contact with others. In modern American society this deprivation is seen to result from mandatory retirement policies which cut elders off from work relationships, mobility of their adult children, and deaths of spouses, relatives, or friends.

However, many research studies (e.g., Jacobsen, 1987; Wentowski, 1978) reveal that the majority of non-institutionalized elderly, both in urban and rural settings, maintain strong social ties with family members and close friends. This is also found to be true for elders in other developed countries of the world (Shanas, et al., 1968). Even inner city Single Room Occupancy (SRO) elderly residents who acknowledge having only infrequent social ties with family, who deny friendship ties, and who label themselves "loners," have been found, through extensive observation of their actual day-to-day activities, to have frequent and diverse meaningful relations (Sokolovsky & Cohen, 1978).

URBAN-RURAL DIMENSIONS

The majority of elderly Americans live in metropolitan areas, and the large cities and suburban fringes that encircle them (Uhlenberg, 1987). In older municipalities, such as New York, Chicago, Pittsburg, and San Francisco, the elderly are likely to be found in ethnic enclaves in the central city area. There they maintain links with members of their ethnic groups (Rudzites, 1984).

Those who study the urban elderly claim that modern urban living fosters intergenerational relations and even interdependence within families, facilitated by telephoning and easy access to mass transportation (Cohler & Grunebaum, 1981). Family help (particularly in time of illness), exchange of services, and regular visits are common among old people, their children, and relatives even when they do not live under a single roof (Jacobsen, 1987; Wentowski, 1978). Elders living under a single roof together with their children and grandchildren are unusual in industrialized societies and are becoming less common in developing societies. Instead, elders wish to maintain close contact with their adult children, but at some physical distance.

As of 1980, about one-third of the aged in the United States live in rural areas (U. S. Bureau of Census, 1984). Most of the rural aged are concentrated in the southeast and north-central regions of the country (Harbert & Wilkinson, 1985). Rural elderly have generally received less attention in the literature than their urban counterparts, although since the late 1970s more has been learned about socialization patterns, special needs, and aging experiences of elderly persons in rural areas.

Rural elderly have frequent contact with friends, neighbors, children, and other relatives. In fact, some researchers (e.g., Lawton, 1980) have contended that contact with others is greater for elderly living in rural areas than for their counterparts in urban environments. However, it has been found that quality of social interaction does not differ by community size. If the rural elderly have greater contact with relatives, this does not translate into a greater desire to live in the same household. Similar to urban elderly, those in rural areas wish to remain independent in their own homes. They obtain considerable emotional support from long attachment to a particular house and neighborhood. Living alone, the elderly remain actively involved in community activities and church affairs.

In summary, both in rural and urban areas in contemporary society people as they age become more involved with their families than with non-kin or with extra-familial activities. The family's kin network becomes an extensive link between elderly parents and adult children, and it functions in indirect economic and social ways, such as the mutual exchange of services, gifts, advice, and financial assistance between the generations in as many as 93% of families. Where elderly persons are relatively healthy and receiving social security or pensions, emotional support by adult children has replaced physical support and care of elderly individuals.

Since family life is so important in maintaining the socialization of the elderly in the United States, a question does arise about the fate of childless marriages and childless unmarrieds. Interestingly, research shows that the most important source of support for those elderly who are both unmarried and childless is their siblings. These elderly are also more active with friends, neighbors, and church activities than married elderly persons. The most socially isolated in terms of number of social contacts with others are childless married elderly persons (Johnson & Catalano, 1981).

SOCIAL ISOLATION AND THE ELDERLY

With approximately 40% of older women and about 15% of older men living alone in 1981 (figures that reflect continuing increases over earlier census surveys), with 5% of the older population living in institutions where depersonalization and estrangement from the outside world are common, and with the existence of childless marrieds with reduced social contacts, it would be foolish to assume that social isolation and loneliness are not potential or actual problems for some elderly persons.

The extent to which social isolation exists in the elderly has been difficult to establish through careful research. This is because there is a lack of consensus in the operationalization of "social isolation" in terms of both definition and measurement. Some researchers have defined this concept as involving the "attenuation of interpersonal relationships" (Clausen & Kohn, 1954). For others, social isolation is defined by a constriction of social roles and activities by comparison with age contemporaries (Townsend, 1957).

Bennett (1980) defined social isolation as the absence of specific role relationships which are generally activated and sustained through direct, personal, face-to-face interaction. Isolation measurement tools that followed directly from this definition are: (1) The Past Month Isolation Index; and (2) The Adulthood Isolation Index. The Past Month Isolation Index measures the number of role relationships, such as relationships with children, siblings, friends, relatives, and active memberships in organizations, in which an individual was involved in the month preceding an assessment interview. The Adulthood Isolation Index is constructed to take into account the number of interpersonal relationships experienced by the individual during adult life.

Within the field of nursing, social isolation has also been defined in a variety of ways and vaguely measured. Gordon (1987) described it as social interaction below the level desired or required for personal integrity. Carpenito (1987) defined social isolation as a subjective experience. That is, isolation is a state in which the individual experiences a need or desire for contact with others but is unable to make that contact. Similarly, the North American Nursing Diagnosis Association's (NANDA) "working definition" is that social isolation is a condition of aloneness experienced by the individual and perceived as imposed by others and as a negative or threatened state.

Two characteristics of social isolation which seem most obvious in these definitions are (1) the absence of or diminished contact with other human beings which can be objectively measured, and (2) feeling deprived of meaningful social content and contacts which can be subjectively measured. In order to develop the concept of social isolation in the elderly, it seems logical to assess for the presence of both of these attributes, not just one or the other as has been the practice in the past.

Despite lack of consensus for a definition of social isolation, research continues on its consequences for the elderly. In these studies, social isolation is operationally defined as having significantly fewer number of role relationships than others of comparable age in the study.

These studies reveal that social isolation can lead to desocialization for the elderly and that this has serious consequences for them in adapting to new places and persons. Desocialization is a process by which older people lose their social skills through disuse. Once such a process is instituted, it is easy to predict that a vicious cycle would be created, with the loss of social skills leading to increased isolation which then leads to greater loss of social skills, etc. Several studies found that elders experiencing social isolation prior to entry (new admission) into old age homes, nursing homes, and apartment residences made poor adjustments to the new setting (e.g., Bennett & Nahemow, 1961; Brand & Smith, 1974). They did not become well integrated into the planned activities in these environments. Additionally, previous presence of social isolation of elderly stroke patients was found to have adverse effects upon their rehabilitation. Isolation rendered these patients less malleable to the influence of a stroke rehabilitation program (Hyman, 1972).

FACTORS WHICH CONTRIBUTE TO SOCIAL ISOLATION

Various factors contribute to a decrease in social contacts which may lead to social isolation for the elderly. Some of these factors relate to *biological changes* associated with the aging process, itself, or to chronic disease processes; others relate to *biopsychosocial phenomena*; and a third group relate to the *sociocultural environment*. It would be unlikely that a single factor alone would cause social isolation. More commonly, one antecedent factor interacting with others leads to a situation in which, barring constructive intervention, elderly persons become socially isolated. A description of the principal factors in each of these three primary categories provides a systematic guide for a purposeful and thorough assessment for social isolation.

Note that contributing or antecedent factors may be present not only in those elderly judged as having inadequate or decreased socialization, but also in those judged as maintaining their socialization. Since these factors predispose to a dysfunctional pattern of socialization, one that potentially could occur in the future, attention to their presence is useful even for those elders whose current socialization pattern is healthy.

Biological Factors

Common biological and sensory changes that accompany aging include diminished hearing and visual functioning, and declines in physical energy and activity. Fortunately, these changes occur gradually so that most individuals are able to compensate for losses and make suitable adjustments. Thus, when nurses assess these functions and find deficits (see Chapters 7 and 8), they must also assess whether or not and how compensation has taken place.

While there is sufficient evidence to support the view that certain visual and hearing deficits are a natural part of the aging process, declines in physical energy and activity are not thought to occur through muscle disuse resulting from a sedentary lifestyle prevalent in our society. Thus, it is important to encourage continued physical activity and exercise for people of all ages. Decreased physical energy and activity which cannot be attributed to disuse are usually associated with an existing chronic disease.

Whatever their origin, these changes often lead to reduced social contact with others through limiting the physical independence of elderly persons. For example, as people grow older the ability to see light after 30 minutes in the dark is diminished. This discourages them from driving at night. Persons who live alone, as most elderly do, and are unable to get around without someone else to drive them, often cannot attend social affairs in the evening. This can narrow a person's social sphere unless meaningful social activities are offered in the morning or afternoon hours. Similarly, elders who fail to recognize and correct declines in hearing often are deserted by others because it is so difficult to communicate with them. Having to repeat statements or receiving responses which indicate that what was said was not heard correctly exasperates even family members who love the elderly person. Such elders require encouragement by family members, friends, and nurses to undergo testing to determine whether vision or hearing aids would help them.

As noted above, elders often compensate for common limitations arising from minor or mild decline in physical activity. However, severe physical incapacitation resulting from painful and contracted arthritic joints, paralysis or paresis from stroke, and decreased energy from congestive heart failure, diabetes, or pulmonary disorders often prevent individuals from venturing outside their homes or even their bedrooms. Such persons are at high risk for social isolation.

Another biological change which contributes to decreased social contact in the elderly is urinary incontinence (see Chapter 6). Many causes of such incontinence are treatable and reversible. But fear of embarrassment in older persons who experience incontinence is often so great that they do not venture out into public places. This interferes with maintaining current or developing new friendships and activities.

Biopsychosocial Factors

The interplay of biological, psychological, and social factors has been widely recognized and is especially evident in the elderly. Older adults often have multiple impairments, and a comprehensive assessment frequently reveals that biological, psychological, and social factors combine to contribute to impairment. This is particularly true of cognitive functioning in elders.

Although some changes in the manner in which people take in information and act upon it occur in most people as they age, a marked decline in this function is not inherent in the aging process. Information processing is the individual's ability to receive, register, process, and respond to stimuli. Perception (the receiving and registering of stimuli) is affected by biological changes and environmental influences. Perception occurs at the points of contact between persons and their internal and external environments. The first determinant of perception is the quality of sensory receptors. Changes in perception are of great significance because they influence actual behavior. Faulty perception of environmental specifics due to sensory receptor impairment may thus lead to seemingly inappropriate behavior that others might interpret as evidence of faulty thinking or reasoning. This often leads others to ignore or avoid elders who display such behavior.

In addition to perception, the processing of and response to stimuli depend upon cognition, which involves thinking and using information gained in present and past inputs, the latter being drawn from learning and memory; affective processes; and motor processes. With aging, there is a slowing of the central and peripheral nervous system. As a result, certain learning processes are slowed and there is an increased loss of short-term memory. This slowing of the nervous system also delays reaction time in the elderly. Perceiving fast-paced and content-loaded presentations becomes particularly difficult for elderly persons (Schmidt & McCroskey, 1981). Unfortunately, such performance on the part of the elderly is typically perceived by others as being due to a cognitive or personality defect, with avoidance as the consequence. While irreversible cognitive impairment may not be open to remediation, assessing for cognitive changes of the type described here and allowing older adults more time to think and express themselves can prevent the occurrence of social isolation.

That which appears on the surface to be cognitive impairment may also arise from depression. Depression and other mental health problems are important factors contributing to social isolation. Indeed, depression—especially that which occurs as reaction to loss—is the most common psychiatric disorder of later life. It is believed that older persons are particularly prone to depression because of the many losses that they often sustain in rapid succession (see Chapters 12 and 13). Depressed older persons may appear sad, unkempt, drab, underweight, and tired. Often they complain of lack of sleep even while they are seen to be sleeping most of the time. Such individuals become disinterested in their physical appearance and in keeping their immediate environment neat and clean. They lose confidence in their ability to manage financial and personal affairs. In general, they are afraid to do anything; everything becomes too much of a challenge.

Nurses also need to identify elderly persons who have been lifelong isolates. During young adulthood, it appears that some people develop a personality that tends to leave them as isolated persons for the remainder of their lives unless treatment reverses their absorption with self. In adulthood, the individual faces the developmental crisis of intimacy versus isolation (Erikson, 1968). During this period, the individual either learns how to reach out and use the self to form a commitment to a lasting relationship with another person, cause, or creative activity, or becomes absorbed with the self. In the latter case, one finds an inability to be intimate, spontaneous, or close with others, and a tendency to become withdrawn, lonely, and conceited. The person often experiences a long succession of unsuccessful relationships, overextending the self without any real interest or feeling, and then being unable to sustain close friendships.

Sociocultural Factors

Diminished economic resources, relocation, low educational level, loss of peer contact, and fear of crime are among the many sociocultural factors contributing to social isolation in the elderly. Low or decreased economic income and resources constrain social opportunities for some elderly persons, just as physical limitations do for others. A diminished income prevents some elders from participating in activities which might provide new roles and other meaningful occupation to replace roles lost through aging. Persons who particularly fall into this category are poorly educated and low-income women. In studies of the aged, when asked an open-ended question, such as "How do you spend your time?", people in this group tend to reply, "I do nothing. I sit around all day." These responses indicate social inactivity, and the lack of activity alternatives has serious implications for the health and self-esteem of such persons.

Relocation of elders occurs when neighborhoods change, when peers die or leave the area, and when adult children live at a distance. Usually, when elders relocate, it is simply not feasible to rebuild a social network of friends like the one they had before. In a brief period of time, one cannot develop the same closeness that took a lifetime to achieve. Also, the elderly no longer have certain natural mechanisms, such as school or the workplace, through which one initiates contacts with strangers.

Having peers is an important mechanism for adjusting to old age. An extensive association with friends becomes most important following either widowhood or retirement. Paradoxically, these events can themselves alter the formation and maintenance of friendships among older people. A change in marital or employment status which places the individual in a deviant position within an age or sex group interferes with opportunities to maintain old friendships. This is true both for elderly under 70 years of age where widowhood is not so prevalent (especially for males) and for elderly over 70 who are not retired.

Another outstanding sociocultural factor in the western world contributing to social isolation in the elderly is ageism. "Ageism" is a term coined by gerontologists to refer to the pejorative image of someone who is old simply because of his or her age (Butler, 1969). Like racism or sexism, it involves wholesale discrimination against all members of a category, though it usually appears in more covert form. For example, one comes across a belief that those in their sixties and beyond would not benefit from psychotherapy. Similarly, many helping professionals, including nurses, hold the belief that the elderly are dependent, asexual, meddlesome, and not valued by their families, and that elders have memory loss and limited interests (Solomon & Vicker, 1979). A fundamental if implicit element of ageism is that the elderly are somehow different from the rest of us.

Ageism probably became a national prejudice because of our society's emphasis on youth, productive capacity, and rapidly advancing technological expertise. In addition, early gerontological research which filtered into the public consciousness reinforced existing misconceptions of the elderly since it was based largely on institutionalized elderly who constitute only about 5% of the overall elderly population.

One result of ageism has been lowered self-esteem for a number of elderly persons and some closing of lines of communication between generations. As we know, communication is central to socialization throughout life. Through the linguistic process, humans share their needs, hopes, aspirations, reminiscences, and innermost thoughts. There is no reason to believe that communication becomes less important during the later years of life. Keeping lines of communication open for the elderly is crucial. Without viable interpersonal exchanges, like other human beings they will wither socially.

ASSESSMENT

Socialization is necessary for the elderly in making adaptations to the many changes they encounter in their lives. When their engagement in the socialization process has been so limited that they are socially isolated, this interferes with their adaptation to new settings, persons, and activities. Research in the area of sensory deprivation further demonstrates that lack of meaningful social interactions can lead to cognitive dysfunction in persons of any age (Zubek, 1969).

Therefore, it is essential for nurses caring for and working with the elderly to assess their socialization status and risk for or presence of social isolation in initial and ongoing diagnostic processes. Such assessments ought to be performed for healthy elders residing in the community, as well as for the sick, particularly those living alone. Assessment of the socialization status and presence of social isolation in elders who are newly-admitted to institutions (hospitals, nursing and rest homes, long-term and rehabilitation facilities, and segregated elderly housing) is crucial. Such assessments predict who of the newly-admitted might have adaptation problems. Interventions for resocialization can then be instituted early in the stay and before the older person is labelled as uncooperative by others. Such labelling can easily occur when an elder has become isolated in the community and enters a home for the aged or a similar setting. Misperceiving the norms because of loss of social skills, the elder makes blunders soon after his or her admission. Others then single the person out as a "troublemaker" and avoid the elder, which may lead to further isolation.

Often, as nurses begin to assess, they immediately focus on identifying problems. In some clinical situations, this may be appropriate. In others, this approach leads nurses to fail to assess each individual's strengths and abilities in the focused area of assessment. Assessing the elder's abilities in the area of socialization is particularly important for several reasons. First, it has been demonstrated that the majority of elderly persons maintain social ties with others, particularly family and friends. Second, focusing on strengths conveys to the older adult that he or she is maintaining a desired lifestyle, rather than implying that the life is full of problems. Third, most elders use functional ability to determine their health status.

The initial assessment of socialization status of the elderly person may be done as a part of the social history interview. Since language use is an integral part of socialization, assessment of an elder's basic communication skills is included in this initial assessment. Asking questions related to the following areas can elicit information needed to make inferences about the degree of socialization for the older adult.

Communication Skills

Observe the usual pattern of communication during the assessment interview: quality of speech (tone, pitch, pace, slurring, stuttering), content, verbosity, dialect, foreign language primarily spoken, presence of aphasia, non-verbal gestures, body movements, facial expressions. Note situational factors which affect communication and understanding. Is the person in pain which decreases the desire to communicate? Is there so much background noise that it is difficult for the person to attend to the conversation? Is the emotional state (anxiety, depression, grief) of the person limiting the ability to communicate? Observe the elder's comprehension. Does the person spontaneously respond in verbal interaction? Is there some slowness in responding (not unusual); great slowness? Does the person exhibit an understanding of the content of the conversation? Inquire about any difficulties with communication such as articulating words, forming ideas, memory losses, and understanding the dominant language spoken in the setting. Inquire if medications or other treatments affect communication patterns.

Social Status Information

Inquire about marital status, educational level, work history (current employment, past employment, retirement), place of residence (living arrangements and number of persons in the household, available transportation), economic status, and resources.

Social Network (socialization frequency and pattern)

Inquire about who the elder has seen in the past day or week. It is helpful to ask elders to reconstruct the previous day, since that gets at the elderly's categories of their relationships, not those of the interviewer. This approach often reveals those close friends the elderly have and think of as "fictive" family, for example, "she's like a sister to me." Asking the following types of questions provides information about who the elder confides in and who he or she perceives as sources of help in times of need: If you had a personal problem, with whom would you discuss it? If you became physically ill and could not care for yourself, who would you go to for help? If you needed money in a hurry, to whom would you turn?

Family Members

Ask the elderly person to name those family members living nearby, their ages, sex, and health status. How often is there some type of contact with these persons? What type of contact? Face-to-face? Telephone contact? Letter writing? Ask the same question about family members living afar. How well do family members get along with each other and make decisions? Would the client like family relationships to be different? Is there a family crisis or stressor with which members are now having to cope? How are they dealing with it?

Relocation

Inquire as to whether the elder has experienced relocation, either temporary or permanent. What impact has this relocation had upon usual social interaction activities?

Social Activities

Does the elder belong to church or community organizations, such as service groups, political groups, recreational groups, senior citizen's groups, or professional groups? Determine the elder's knowledge about and use of community services, such as health, social, and mental health services; senior citizen opportunities; or meal and transportation resources.

In addition to gathering information through an interview, nurses can obtain objective data on socialization through observation. For example, observing who is with the elder on first contact may be an important cue to who he or she can depend upon in time of need. Additionally, cues to identities of active members in the social network can be obtained by observing who becomes involved in the individual's problems and care. Note the frequency and pattern of interactions and the type of help provided (e.g., direct care, psychological support and visits, telephone calls, gifts, transportation, financial assistance). Observe how decision making occurs, if conflicts arise, and how they are handled.

As information on socialization is gathered through questioning and observations, analyze quality as well as quantity of interactions. Data for this analysis are obtained from sentiments and feelings projected by the elderly as they speak about their interrelationships. For example, does the verbal content and enthusiasm with which the individual describes interaction patterns convey satisfaction? Does the elder express a desire that things could be different? Or better? Does the elder seem overburdened with demands made by others?

During and at the completion of the foregoing assessment of socialization status, inferences or diagnostic hypotheses are generated from information collected about the individual elder's socialization pattern. An inference that the socialization pattern of the individual is inadequate raises the questions: What are the etiological factors associated with this decreased socialization pattern? Does the degree of inadequacy render the elder to be at risk for or actually to be socially isolated? Are critical defining signs and symptoms for social isolation present or absent?

Inferences made about the socialization pattern, along with questions they raise, provide a focus for a further search for cues critical to making a nursing diagnosis related to social isolation. For instance, nurses need to assess which factors contributing to social isolation exist for the elderly person judged to have inadequate socialization.

NURSING DIAGNOSIS

The purpose of a nursing assessment of an elder's socialization pattern is to determine if it is adequate or if there are problems amenable to intervention. Problems that are formulated during the diagnostic process are stated as nursing diagnoses which, in turn, provide a basis for nursing planning, intervention, and evaluation. The NANDA-approved nursing diagnostic category in the domain of socialization is *Social Isolation* (Duespohl, 1986). Its definition is: "Condition of aloneness experienced by the individual and perceived as imposed by others and as a negative or threatened state" (p. 292). Specific nursing diagnoses in this content area are based on identified etiologies and would be expressed as social isolation related to one or more of the following: delay in accomplishing developmental tasks; immature interests; alterations in physical appearance; alterations in mental state; unaccepted social behavior; unaccepted social values; altered state of wellness; inadequate personal resources; inability to engage in satisfying personal relationships. Note that in practical situations, a particular nursing diagnosis will likely include both the general diagnostic category and more than one etiology, since it is rare that social isolation would occur based solely on one antecedent factor. Thus, a nursing diagnosis in this area might be expressed as: Social isolation related to cognitive impairment and incontinence (Mundinger & Jauron, 1975). Finally, even when the actual presence of social isolation is ruled out, the existence of risk factors may suggest a potential problem which deserves attention.

PLANNING

Planning involves the establishment of goals and objectives for client behaviors, and is based upon several factors. The primary consideration when selecting outcome goals and objectives is that they are acceptable to clients and their families. Beliefs and values of clients and families, which are both individually and culturally determined, must be acknowledged.

A second consideration is to select goals and objectives that alter contributing factors associated with the diagnosis and enable clients to move toward one or more desired outcome behaviors. These expected outcomes should always be identified and stated during the planning phase in term of overall goals and specific, measurable objectives. For example, the overall goal may be for the client to reduce the sense of social isolation and enhance satisfying personal relationships, while specific objectives may state that the client will verbalize feelings of being part of a group or relationship; verbalize interest in activities and others; communicate with others; exhibit behavior acceptable to the dominant culture; and be seen in the company of others. These objectives must also identify a time frame within which they are to be accomplished.

A third consideration in planning is feasibility of the goals and objectives. Can they be achieved in a particular setting or community? Is the client capable of achieving them? Are family and other caregivers available to assist the client? If a community agency is required, is that resource available to the client? Finally, are the goals and objectives realistic and economically sound for the client?

INTERVENTION

A wide range of nursing interventions have been employed for three primary purposes: (1) to maintain socialization in the elderly; (2) to prevent social isolation for elders at risk; and (3) to resocialize elderly persons diagnosed as being socially isolated. For the sake of convenience, interventions are presented here in these three general groupings. However, this mode of presentation does not imply that interventions in different groupings are mutually exclusive. In fact, an intervention described under maintenance of socialization might also be appropriate in preventing social isolation. The success of any intervention depends upon careful matching of available treatments and therapies to the diagnosis and needs of the person in question.

Maintenance of Socialization

Strengthening Family Ties

As the elderly age, involvement with family becomes greater (Shanas, et al., 1968). In times of need, elders seek help first from family, then friends, and then bureaucratic agencies. Older adults expect the family to be their major source of help even when the assistance of outside agencies is undoubtedly necessary and useful. Research (e.g., Jacobsen, 1987) shows families do respond to these expectations.

The family is the natural, primary, and major resource of socialization, support, and assistance for the elderly. Therefore, nurses—

particularly those working with elders in long-term care facilities, retirement communities, and the community at large—would serve the socialization needs of the elderly best if they used strategies which encourage people to "connect" across family generations. Such strategies include active listening, information sharing, and family counseling. Since these intervention strategies are long-term processes, nurses in acute-care settings might not have opportunities to carry out such interventions. Nevertheless, all nurses can assess family interactions and refer families whose members have problems communicating with one another to community counselors, such as mental health clinical nurse specialists, social workers, clinical psychologists, and clergy.

Hall's research (1977) revealed that families in which the elderly have a personal, one-to-one relationship with various family members across the generations tend to be more effective in handling their lives and in coping with such stressors as retirement, illness, and death. By contrast, in families with symptomatic older people, members tended to be isolated from each other, and superficial and constrained in their contacts.

Community Senior Citizen's Programs and Centers

Under the Older American Act of 1965, which is periodically amended and renewed, federal, state, and local dollars are made available for programs and services for older adults. Depending on the funds available and the needs of the elderly in a particular community, a variety of recreational, vocational, and social activities is offered. These activities gather older persons together, enabling them to maintain social contacts with old friends and acquaintances, and to initiate new social contacts. Activities typically include congregate meals, field trips, educational offerings, and exercise, as well as legal counseling and health assessment. Programs of this sort are especially targeted for elders in the community who live alone. In large communities, there is usually a well-identified senior center building in which these activities take place. In smaller communities, senior activities occur in local churches and other buildings. Informing older persons and their families about such resources is a meaningful nursing intervention to maintain socialization and prevent social isolation.

Activities Programs

For various reasons, some older persons move to a retirement center, a nursing home, or some similar institution for the aged. There is great danger in such moves, as they can cause passivity and isolation. Maintaining socialization and preventing withdrawal can be accomplished through the implementation of an activities program. The key to such programs is that the activities, which might include promenades, excursions, study circles, bingo games, playing music, singing groups, and physical exercise, are chosen according to the elder residents' wishes. The activities themselves take place throughout the whole house or building—in the dining rooms, the day rooms, and the rooms of the elderly residents.

Prevention of Social Isolation

Communication

In addition to family members, friends, and grandchildren, the people who become important to the elderly in institutions are those with whom they come into daily contact, 24 hours a day, seven days a week—that is, the nursing staff. Communication and social interaction with the staff is probably the mainstay of institutionalized elders. However, communication between nursing staff and residents can have many difficulties because of sensory loss and/or speech impediments. Verbal communication can be enhanced if caregivers employ some of the following simple measures.

When speaking with an elderly person who is hard of hearing, speech should be directed to the ear which has not sustained a loss. For persons who use hearing aids, encourage them to wear the aid and be sure it is turned on when conversation is attempted. Many people who wear aids turn them off when there is a lot of background noise as it causes static, a most annoying sound. For all elders known to have a hearing loss, even those who wear a hearing device, stand or sit directly in front of them when speaking. Most hearing-impaired persons have adapted to their loss by lip reading.

Remember that older persons may need time to perceive, to respond, to learn, and to move and act. Use of self-pacing—which is defined as allowing the elder sufficient time to get started with a task, to integrate the information, and to respond before other verbal stimuli are given— reflects a respect for this general slowing as a natural aging process.

Problems of communication with elders of varying degrees of deafness can be met also by raising one's voice moderately, by enunciating clearly and slowly, and by written communication. Shouting at an older person is not a suitable remedy. Elders are sensitive to excessive strain, which embarrasses them, destroys their privacy, and is extremely tiring.

Support Groups

Use of groups as a means of providing support for persons with common problems or needs has a fairly long history. Recently, "artificial" social support and network interventions have been developed for use with the elderly. Some examples of these interventions implemented in urban settings are the organization of neighborhood networks for swapping services (Noberini & Berman, 1983) and the development of volunteer linking programs in which a helper who is trained, supervised, and organized by a formal agency provides help to an individual in need and living within the same community (Biegel, Shore, & Gordon, 1984). However, artificially-constructed support groups or networks are not a panacea for treating potential or actual social isolation or decreased social interactions. Evaluation research (Fennell, 1986) on some of these projects revealed a very low usage rate on the part of the elderly in the setting. One reason for this is that elderly persons hold dearly to the American cultural value of independence and do not wish to appear dependent.

Adult Day Care Centers

Adult day care programs serve those elderly who are at a dependency level in relation to physical or psychological needs. These programs are conducted in non-residential centers where an individual can obtain nursing, nutritional, and medical monitoring on a regular basis during the day while still residing in his or her own home. Adult day care facilities usually have activities to meet rehabilitative, recreational, and social needs of dependent elders. For example, an adult day care center might offer range-of-motion exercises, arts and crafts instruction, sing-a-long activities, one-on-one communication with staff or volunteers (usually elderly peers), medication administration, monitoring of vital signs, occasional excursions to local historic sites and fairs, and a warm, nutritious midday meal.

Resocialization

Role Models for Resocialization

Socialization is contingent upon effective role models, and especially upon models who undertake expressive and instrumental leadership. The expressive leader behaves and exhibits attitudes which reflect emotional and supportive relationships with others. The instrumental leader is one who sets rules and gives orders, directions, and suggestions. For the majority of persons, socialization begins in the nuclear family where parental models often differentiate along expressive and instrumental lines. In subsequent socialization in secondary social systems, such as schools and churches, similar patterns of leadership are evident.

On this basis, some nursing homes have utilized programs of "Leadership Role Models for Resocialization" to counteract the effects of pre-entry social isolation experienced by residents. That is, upon entering such a home an effort is made to resocialize the new resident. In these programs, volunteer senior citizens are assigned either expressive or instrumental roles, and are trained in the role prior to serving as leaders for group sessions with the residents. Group sessions are held for about one hour with a minimum of seven sessions, and leaders are guided on resocialization topics to introduce.

In homes where this intervention has been used, elderly persons in the instrumental leadership groups demonstrate increased socialization and integration behavior (Bennett, 1980). Elders belonging to expressive leadership groups showed increased morale. Elders belonging to groups in which there were two leaders, one expressing instrumental behavior and one demonstrating expressive behavior, showed increased socialization and conformity behaviors.

Reminiscence Therapy

Reminiscence is thinking about or relating past personally significant experiences. McMahon and Rhudick (1961) studied reminiscence in the elderly and found that it was positively correlated with adaptation to aging. Memories seem to help the aged work through losses and maintain their self-esteem. Reminiscence can be done orally, in writing, or through silent musing over the past, and is similar to what Butler (1963) has called "life review." As a nursing intervention, reminiscence is used to tap unspoken memories and encourage the elderly to verbalize them or put them into writing. The intervention is designed to increase ego integrity, decrease depression, and increase socialization.

Reminiscence therapy can be conducted with groups or individuals. The nurse's decision in this matter is guided by the nursing diagnosis, goals set with client(s), and the setting. Reminiscence sessions are held over a period of time, several weeks to a year, in order to permit the therapy to be effective. The sessions may be unfocused, free-flowing reflections on the past or subject-focused. For example, in working with slightly cognitively impaired elders, one might choose to focus the content of reminiscence therapy sessions on fall and winter holiday events during those particular seasons of the year. Introducing a specific topic usually stimulates memories and initiates interaction. Other topics might include early childhood memories, skills and hobbies, and past travels. Research on reminiscence therapy has suggested that it can decrease depression in the elderly (Hibel, 1971), decrease need for tranquilizers (Hala, 1975), and increase satisfaction with a new environment (Chennelly, 1979). Hamilton (1985) has offered a thorough review of this intervention and related research.

EVALUATION

Upon the implementation of interventions directed at maintaining or improving socialization and reducing social isolation, a continuous evaluation of client responses is instituted. Nurses collect information on responses by elderly persons relative to the behaviors stated in the goals and objectives for desired health outcomes, that is, relative to an elder's verbalizations, actions, abilities, etc.

Actual or observed responses by elderly clients provide evaluative information which, when compared with desired health outcomes, gives a clear indication of the success or failure of the prescribed interventions. The clients' responses provide the rationale for ruling out a problem as solved, for revising nursing interventions which are not effecting desired outcomes, or for continuing the same intervention approach.

The following case study illustrates how the ongoing evaluation of client responses supported the use of a reminiscence intervention for improving socialization in mildly cognitively impaired elderly.

CASE STUDY

Dr. A, an 89-year-old former surgeon, was a newly admitted resident to the intermediate care unit of an elderly retirement community when first encountered. In the year prior to his admission to the retirement community, Dr. A's wife of 50 years died. A depression accompanying his grieving interfered with his desire to renew old contacts and to initiate new ones. During this period, Dr. A's main companion was his dog, Maxwell. Having noted some cognitive and memory impairment on the part of Dr. A, his son—without consulting Dr. A—decided to place his father in a long-term care facility. Thus, Dr. A was relocated from the home in which he had spent a good many of his married years. He also became separated from his daily faithful companion, Maxwell.

Shortly after his admission, it was noted that Dr. A sat by himself in his room or in the chairs placed in the hallway. Other residents who went up to speak with him usually left quickly because all Dr. A would talk about was his wish to go home.

Since several other elders in this unit, as well as Dr. A, were assessed as drifting toward social isolation, it was decided to establish a reminiscence group. Six residents were identified by the staff as possible members. Each of these persons was approached and the group project was described. All agreed to participate and were individually assessed for cognitive impairment. The plan was to obtain a homogeneous group, either all with some cognitive impairment or all unimpaired. It has been observed in elderly group activities that if some members are cognitively impaired and others not, the non-cognitively impaired elderly tend to become impatient with those who are impaired. As a result, the cognitively-impaired elderly tend not to contribute and the unimpaired elderly become easily bored. In this case, all of the prospective members were assessed as having some mild to moderate cognitive impairment.

Group sessions were held twice a week on Tuesdays and Thursdays at the same hour of the day for a period of seven weeks. Topics discussed included fall and winter holidays and seasonal activities. To stimulate group reminiscence, objects such as fall leaves, a jack-o-lantern, and a football were brought to the group. Items such as apple cider and egg nog, which stimulate taste and smell senses, were also introduced at different sessions.

Prior to initiating this project, nursing staff who worked in the institution were asked to assess the members of the group as to initiating social contact with others, number of social contacts in a day, and attendance at planned unit activities.

The nurse leading the group sessions noted that for the first few weeks she had to initiate discussions, and that discussions generally occurred between herself and the different members of the group. Dr. A would respond when spoken to by the leader, but he did not initiate any discussion. Sometimes he would mention that he wanted to be taken home. By the fourth session, although discussions were still initiated by the nurse leader, once they were started members began turning to one another and sharing tales or asking questions. Dr. A no longer spoke of his desire to go home and he initiated conversation with members seated close to him in the group. By the last session, some members of the group were initiating the discussion and the nurse leader was able to sit back and observe.

At the conclusion of the project with this particular nurse leader, the nursing staff was again asked to evaluate the daily socialization patterns of the elderly group members. They reported that Dr. A was now going to the dining room by himself at mealtimes. Staff no longer had to find him and remind him. He now sat talking in the hallway with specific residents whom he seemed to select. Occasionally, he mentioned that he wanted to be taken home.

REFERENCES

Bennett, R. (Ed.) (1980). *Aging, isolation and resocialization.* New York: Van Nostrand.

Bennett, R., & Nahemow, L. (1961). Preadmission isolation as a factor in adjustment to an old age home. In P. Hoch & J. Zubin (Eds.), *Psychopathology of aging* (pp. 285–302). New York: Grune & Stratton.

Biegel, D., Shore, B., & Gordon, E. (1984). *Building support networks for the elderly.* Beverly Hills, CA: Sage.

Blau, Z. S. (1981). *Aging in a changing society* (2nd ed.). New York: Franklin Watts.

Brand, F. D., & Smith, R. T. (1974). Life adjustment and relocation of the elderly. *Journal of Gerontology, 29,* 336–340.

Butler, R. N. (1969). Age-ism: Another form of bigotry. *The Gerontologist, 9,* 243–246.

Butler, R. N. (1963). A life review. *Psychiatry 26,* 65–76.

Carpenito, L. (Ed.) (1987). *Nursing diagnosis: Application to clinical practice* (2nd ed.). Philadelphia: Lippincott.

Chennelly, S. (1979). *Reminiscing: A coping skill for the elderly.* Rochester, NY: University of Rochester, unpublished master's thesis.

Clausen, J. (1968). *Socialization and society.* Boston: Little, Brown.

Clausen, J., & Kohn, M. (1954). The ecological approach in social psychiatry. *American Journal of Sociology, 60,* 140–151.

Cohler, B. J., & Grunebaum, H. U. (1981). *Mothers, grandmothers and daughters.* New York: Wiley.

Cowgill, D., & Holmes, L. (Eds.) (1972). *Aging and modernization.* New York: Appleton-Century-Crofts

Duespohl, T. A. (1986). *Nursing diagnosis manual for the well and ill client.* Philadelphia: W. B. Saunders.

Erikson, E. H. (1968). *Identity: Youth and crisis.* New York: Norton.

Fennell, V. (1986). Exchange in an elders' highrise. Paper presented at Annual Meeting of the Southern Anthropological Society. Wrightsville Beach, NC.

Gordon, M. (1987). *Nursing diagnosis* (2nd ed.). New York: McGraw-Hill.

Hala, M. (1975). Reminiscence group therapy project. *Journal of Gerontological Nursing, 1*(3), 34–51.

Hall, M. (1977). Aging and family processes. In J. Lorio & L. McClenackan (Eds.), *Georgetown Family Symposia, Vol. II* (pp. 133–151). Washington, DC: Georgetown Family Center.

Hamilton, D. (1985). Reminiscence therapy. In G. Bulechek & J. McCloskey (Eds.), *Nursing interventions.* Philadelphia: W. B. Saunders.

Harbert, A. S., & Wilkinson, C. W. (1985). Growing old in rural America. In H. Cox (Ed.), *Aging* (4th ed.; pp. 113–117). Guilford, CT: Dushkin Publishing Co.

Heiss, J. (Ed.) (1976). *Family roles and interaction: An anthology* (2nd ed.). Chicago: Rand McNally.

Hibel, D. (1980). *The relationship between reminiscence and depression among institutionalized clients.* Iowa City, IA: University of Iowa, unpublished master's thesis.

Hyman, M. D. (1972). Social isolation and performance in rehabilitation. *Journal of Chronic Diseases, 25,* 85–97.

Jacobsen, D. (1987). The cultural context of social support and support networks. *Medical Anthropology Quarterly, 1,* 42–67.

Johnson, C. L., & Catalano, D. J. (1981). Childless elderly and their family supports. *The Gerontologist, 21,* 610–618.

Lawton, M. P. (1980). *Environment and aging.* Monterey, CA: Brooks Cole.

McMahon, A., & Rhudick, P. (1961). Reminiscing. *Archives of General Psychiatry, 10,* 292–298.

Mundiger, M. O., & Jauran, C. G. (1975). Developing a nursing diagnosis. *Nursing Outlook, 23,* 94–98.

Noberini, M. R., & Berman, R. (1983). Barter to beat inflation: Developing a neighborhood network for swapping services on behalf of the aged. *The Gerontologist, 23,* 467–470.

Parsons, T. (1955). Family structure and the socialization of the child. In T. Parsons & R. F. Bales (Eds.), *Family, socialization, and interaction process* (pp. 35–131). Glencoe, IL: Free Press.

Piaget, J. (1984). *The construction of reality in the child.* New York: Basic Books.

Rheingold, H. L. (1969). The social and socializing infant. In D. A. Goslin (Ed.), *Handbook of socialization theory and research* (pp. 779–790). Chicago: Rand McNally.

Rosnow, I. (1974). *Socialization to old age.* New York: Free Press.

Rudzites, G. (1984). Geographical research and gerontology: An overview. *The Gerontologist, 24,* 536–542.

Schmidt, J. F., & McCroskey, F. L. (1981). Sentence comprehension in elderly listeners: The factor of rate. *Journal of Gerontology, 36,* 441–445.

Shanas, E. P., Townsend, P., Wedderburn, D., Friis, M., Milhoj, P. & Stehouwer, J. (1968). *Old people in three industrial societies.* New York: Atherton Press.

Sokolovsky, J., & Cohen, C. (1978). Networks as adaptation. *Urban Anthropology, 7,* 323–342.

Solomon, K., & Vickers, R. (1979). Attitudes of health workers toward old people. *Journal of the American Geriatrics Society, 27,* 186–191.

Townsend, P. (1957). *The family life of old people: An inquiry in East London.* London: Routledge & Kegan Paul.

Uhlenberg, P. (1987). A demographic perspective on aging. In P. Silverman (Ed.), *The elderly as modern pioneers* (pp. 183–204). Bloomington, IN: Indiana University Press.

United States Bureau of the Census (1984). Demographic and socioeconomic aspects of aging in the U.S. Current Population Reports. P. 23, No. 138. Washington, DC: Government Printing Office.

Wentowksi, G. (1978). *Social networks and aging.* Chapel Hill, NC: University of North Carolina, unpublished doctoral dissertation.

Zubek, J. P. (Ed.) (1969). *Sensory deprivation: Fifteen years of research.* New York: Appleton-Century-Crofts.

Chapter 12

Effective Coping

Sharon M. Valente and Joan R. Sellers

INTRODUCTION

Coping is a process of interaction between individuals and their environment. Effective coping involves managing the demands of the environment and adapting to changes or loss such as those involved in aging or illness. It is inevitable that life will make demands upon human beings and generate stress. The question is how individuals will respond to those demands. Effective coping depends upon a balanced interaction between stressors and coping strategies. In this way, stress can result in growth.

As people grow older, they respond both to normal, age-related changes in their physical capacity, support network, and social roles, and to situations that are independent of the life-cycle pattern. These developmental and situational experiences may be positive or negative events. They may evoke a wide range of functional or dysfunctional responses as the person faces shifts in independence. For example, temporary anxiety, sadness, and loneliness are normal reactions and may improve coping, while defense mechanisms such as denial or sleep when overused may increase rather than reduce stress. People who cope effectively with one stressor may feel ill-prepared for the multiple stressors that often accompany aging.

To support coping, nurses must recognize the breadth of changes faced by elders and their rich history of strength and coping. Self-esteem grows out of relationships where individuals feel valued, nurtured, and respected. Thus, nurses may help restore feelings of hope, security, and self-respect in elderly persons. For example, nurses may enable elders to reconsider negative conclusions drawn from unmet goals by helping individuals to anticipate problems, modify goals, or rethink matters in a new way that reduces feelings of failure.

Nurses monitor responses and observe for signs that anxiety or sadness have become dysfunctional. This chapter focuses on effective coping and on specific threats to such coping which can arise for elderly persons. These threats may emerge in a variety of ways, but they typically include anxiety, powerlessness, depression, substance abuse, and suicide. Assessment guidelines and a case study help nurses identify risk factors, diagnose problems, develop an effective plan, and intervene constructively. Nurses also evaluate the effectiveness of efforts to ameliorate or remove such threats and to foster effective coping.

A subtle social prejudice and negative attitude may keep some nurses from seeing older persons realistically and from reinforcing their strengths. Increased awareness of feelings and biases can help nurses see elderly persons more realistically (Rice, 1988). Health care providers and advocates for the elderly, such as nurses and social workers, must collaborate, combine talents, and confront barriers which may restrict progress of elderly persons.

ASSESSMENT: THREATS TO EFFECTIVE COPING

Anxiety

Anxiety, an initial response to real or perceived threat, allows individuals to notice and react to danger. In the absence of anxiety or sadness, the person may deny smoking, substance abuse, and eating problems. Low anxiety often motivates hypertensive patients to modify diet, exercise, smoking, and caffeine or alcohol intake. High or chronic anxiety is linked to illness. Anxiety is functional when it matches the situation and does not disrupt activity, behavior, cultural values, and self-care.

Nurses evaluate anxiety, perceptions, resources, and coping strategies of elders, and reinforce their strengths. When high anxiety impairs memory, individuals need written instructions about appointments or treatments. Nurses observe indicators of anxiety including vital signs, perspiration, fidgeting, rapid speech or movements, and pupil dilation. Anxious elderly patients often complain of palpitations, tachycardia without organic etiology, nausea, insomnia, fears, dreams, worries, or a general apprehension. Historical data includes precipitants, onset, and duration of anxiety, and typical response patterns. People complain of nightmares and insomnia after a traumatic experience, such as a mugging or rape. How the person feels, interprets, and perceives the anxiety is important.

Elderly persons should receive a complete physical examination to evaluate medical causes of anxiety, such as drugs, hypoglycemia, hyperthyroidism, and pheochromocytoma, and to assess cardiac, renal, and autonomic systems before psychotropic medications are prescribed. Elders who interpret anxiety or bereavement reactions as "crazy behavior" are often afraid of reporting their anxiety.

The way in which nurses react to interactions with elderly persons during assessment is a useful diagnostic clue. If the nurse begins to feel sad with such a client, the person's sadness or depression should be explored. Anxious people typically evoke anxiety, limit setting, and structure. The key here is that the nurse must first *differentiate* his or her own feelings from feelings evoked by anxious clients. Hunches about the client's feelings should be validated by the client. It is imperative that the nurse be self-aware and identify personal feelings and biases when assessing elderly persons.

Powerlessness

Most people want to have an impact on others and some control over their own life. People with a sense of power believe they have some control over their feelings, interactions, responses, and environment. Powerlessness is the perception that one is a victim who has no control over the self, others, or events. Nurses need to assess perceived and actual powerlessness. Elderly persons may believe they are powerless when in fact they can learn simple strategies to ask for help or to change their behaviors. Nurses often intervene by helping patients ask for more information about their health, report side effects from treatments, or request a change in medications. Teaching elders how to be assertive with health care providers and family members can often reduce powerlessness. When they move into long-term care facilities or hospitals, patients report that their power to control events is actually reduced. In this case, nurses help patients identify strategies that may effectively impact things that can be realistically controlled.

Depression

Depression, America's most common mental health problem, affects between 20 to 50% of older Americans, twice as many men as women (Osgood, 1987). Depression can be endogenous or exogenous, that is, it can arise internally from biochemical or neurohormonal causes, or externally as a reaction to loss (e.g., loss of a bodily function or death of a loved one). Sadness, apathy, loss of pleasure, slowed behavior, and agitation signal unipolar depression. Bipolar depression occurs when sad, depressed moods alternate with elated, excited, hyperactive, euphoric periods.

Elderly persons with a major depression require thorough medical evaluation for physical illness that masquerades as or precipitates depression. It has been found (Sweer, et al., 1988) that 35% of 100 depressed elders had one of the following disorders: electrolyte abnormalities, renal disease, bacteriuria, medication reactions, thyroid dysfunction, Parkinson's disease, or chronic obstructive lung disease. History, physical examination, and laboratory tests detected these previously undiscovered diagnoses. A careful drug history should examine use of common prescribed, borrowed, or nonprescription drugs that cause depression.

History taking should include onset and course of sadness, apathy, euphoria, and difficulties with concentration, motivation, decision making, or relationships. Ask what has happened since the individual last enjoyed living. Inadequate control of pain, immobility, or symptoms may have reduced quality of life. Few elders take pain medication effectively or know how to use relaxation or other strategies to control pain. Anticipating and preventing symptom distress can lessen depression.

Assessment includes observation of speech, posture, eye contact, and walking. Posture and gestures can suggest feelings of guilt, worthlessness, and self blame. Depressed persons are typically alert to any clues in the nurse's voice, manner, or posture that they interpret as evidence that they are worthless.

History taking also includes typical daily and weekly activities. Isolation is a danger among the 29% of elders with impaired hearing and others with decreased vision, impaired speech, or vascular diseases. Watching television, sitting, or reading increase isolation and depression, while noncompetitive social activities relieve depression. For those who do not drive or engage in physical activity, letter writing, attending church socials, prayer meetings, or cooking are helpful. Other activities include needlework, woodworking, or recording family history. Recent events, losses, or broken relationships can trigger a depression.

A diagnosis of major depression requires four symptoms of depression for at least four weeks (see Table 12.1). Physical symptoms such as insomnia, anorexia, constipation, and fatigue are less accurate indicators of elderly depression than the cognitive (e.g., thoughts, memory, knowledge, concentration, judgment) or psychological signs. The Geriatric Depression Scale by Yesavage and Brink (1983), a self-administered 30-item test, effectively measures depression in elders.

TABLE 12.1 Information for Patients and Social Network

Warning signs of depression, substance abuse, and suicide in the elderly

Friends and family who observe patterns of any of the following symptoms in elders should consult with a mental health care provider.

Major Features of Depression
Four or more of the following symptoms for four weeks:

1. Disturbed mood, appetite, sleep, or activity level;
2. Social withdrawal;
3. Worthlessness;
4. Cognitive impairment;
5. Preoccupation with death or suicide thoughts.

General Signs of Substance Abuse

Physical: odor, slurred speech, poor coordination, unsteady gait, blackouts, nystagmus, gastritis, broken bones, burns, cirrhosis, hepatitis, disturbed sleep and sexual functioning.

Withdrawal: nausea, vomiting, anxiety, depressed or irritable mood, malaise, weakness, tachycardia, sweating, elevated blood pressure, coarse tremor, orthostatic hypotension, seizures.

Psychologic: history of rigid denial and multiple losses, mood swings, irritability, short attention span, decreased judgment, inhibitions, impaired memory, talks a lot and loudly.

Clues to Suicide

Verbal: suicide threats, messages that life isn't worth it.

Behavioral: saying goodbye, putting affairs in order, giving away prized possessions, suicide attempts.

Social: isolation, withdrawal.

Mood: helpless, hopeless, depressed, ambivalent

Depression must be differentiated from similar disorders, such as dementia, physical illness (e.g., pneumonia), drug abuse, and psychotic disorders with hallucinations, delusions, and distorted reality. Depressed older males are at *high risk* for suicide, so death wishes or suicide thoughts must be evaluated clearly and sensitively.

Substance Abuse

Although coping mechanisms are considered to be healthy, adaptive ways to deal with anxiety, sometimes these mechanisms prove to be ineffective and some elderly individuals rely on alcohol and/or drugs. This may result in unintentional or intentional substance abuse—it is not important to distinguish between these two alternatives. As in the general population, a substance problem is said to exist if the substance used impairs the elder's general functioning. This section, however, limits its focus to those who begin to abuse substances as senior citizens and those without severe psychiatric disorders; it does not address problems of illicit drug use.

Substance Abuse in the Elderly

It is estimated that at least 10% of Americans 65 years or older have an alcohol problem (Bienenfeld, 1987). There are at least three million alcoholics over the age of 55 (Brody, 1982). One-third of alcoholics over age 60 have "late" onset alcoholism which is discussed in this chapter (Bloom, 1983).

Although those 60 and older represent at least 12% of the United States population, the elderly take 25% of all prescription drugs. This represents between four and five million elderly individuals (Caroselli-Karinja, 1985). Documentation is limited with regard to medically addicted elderly. Researchers agree, however, that because the elderly will be increasing proportionately in the population, the problems of the elderly prescription drug addict require increased attention.

Developmental Issues and Risk Factors

Nurses in acute medical settings spend much time with elderly persons. This is not surprising because the elderly patient population experiences tremendous physical and psychological changes as part of the normal aging process. The need of elderly persons to visit many physicians for disparate problems often results in the acquisition of multiple prescriptions which may go undocumented by the general practitioner.

Practitioners often forget that the normal aging process results in heightened sensitivity to the toxic effects of both alcohol and drugs; also, that the mixing of alcohol and medications alters the effects of both. The risk of the misuse of alcohol and drugs increases because of lowered self-esteem associated with job and/or income loss, relocation, a loss of significant others, and a decrease of physical or intellectual capacity that often accompanies the aging process.

Although helping professionals care for many elderly persons, it may be difficult to identify alcohol and drug problems. Impairment in functioning or losses in general are not easily evident in elders as they may be in younger persons. The loss of a job, for example, of a driver's license, of a significant other, or of motor coordination may not stand out as a clue in the elderly person. Similarly, sleep and/or sexual dysfunction may not appear related to a substance problem. Finally, cognitive impairment may be mistaken for a normal aging problem whereas the same symptom in a younger person may signal the need for further assessment (Abrams & Alexopoulos, 1987).

Challenges in the Assessment of Substance Abuse

There are many clues which alert nurses to the possibility of a substance problem (see Table 12.1). Still, it is tempting to consider these clues to be merely the result of aging. Denial, the most common response by abusers when questioned, also confounds assessment. Abstinence, or the decreased use of alcohol and/or medications, is the best means of determining whether the substance is a primary or secondary problem, or perhaps not a problem at all.

Descriptions of the clinical presentation of the elderly alcoholic are numerous. Often, one finds self-neglect, confusion, off-hand questions or jokes about alcohol intake, mood swings, depression, marital and social problems, complaints about loss of libido, insomnia, and loneliness. Malnutrition, vitamin deficiencies, or anorexia may be present since "empty calories" are provided by alcohol and appetite decreases. Injuries from falls may be apparent, along with incontinence, diarrhea, myopathy, hypothermia, neuritis, cirrhosis, hepatitis, and a history of blackouts or delirium tremens.

History taking should include physical, social, and psychological features. These data should be gathered from the patient, friends, family, and especially other physicians treating the patient. Useful questions include asking for specifics (e.g., time, place, and amount of last alcohol or drug use). Feelings about use of alcohol and drugs should be explored. Alcohol or drug preferences, early drinking history, and periods of abstinence should be considered. Ask if there are particular times or places where the individual seems to use more alcohol or medications. Determine what kind of effects the person believes the substances have had in his or her life. Often the aging person has religious beliefs which are relevant. It is important to share observations about substance abuse in a patient, nonjudgmental manner.

Bloom (1983) identified late-onset alcoholism as a form of "learned helplessness" or a type of coping mechanism. The series of losses the elder often faces teaches that life events cannot be predicted, prevented, or controlled. Substance consumption limits the anxiety and, at least initially, provides peace of mind.

There is less documentation on methods of assessing prescription drug abusers. Often, the presenting problems include pain, headaches, insomnia, anxiety, depression, and/or obesity. Typically, how the person describes these problems is more revealing than the symptoms themselves.

The prescription addict may complain in a particularly vigorous way or be unusually manipulative or pressuring in order to meet his or her needs. The individual may be intolerant of interviews or exhibit inconsistent anxiety. Some persons may threaten to leave against medical advice if hospitalized. Others may be particularly "respectful" of the physician; the physician represents more than the resource that most patients expect. Weiss and Greenfield (1986) describe seven clues that identify the elderly prescription addict. According to these researchers, nurses should suspect addiction when the patient reports a history of trauma (fractures or burns not explained by occupation), bizarre infections (e.g., malaria or tetanus), hepatitis, heart valve infection, seizures, pulmonary disorders, and general debilitation.

As individuals age, tolerance to alcohol and medications decreases. The elderly are more vulnerable to toxicity, and the intermixing of alcohol with drugs or drugs with drugs may be lethal. Problems with multiple drugs are common (Streltzer, 1980). Alcohol interacts with more than 150 commonly prescribed medications (Bienenfeld, 1987). Factors which increase the danger include the tendency in some elderly persons to save or share medications, and to alter their schedules of substance use.

Elderly widows and widowers living alone are particularly vulnerable to alcohol abuse and suicide. Alcoholism can arise among the elderly at any age as an attempt to cope with stress, depression, loneliness, and growing old (Osgood, 1987). Acting as a depressant that dulls the senses, alcohol provides brief escape from loss, pain, stress, problems, and alienation, but then evokes depression and broken relationships. Osgood (1987) recommended reducing the risk of alcoholism by planning for retirement and leisure as a way of preparing for aging, bereavement, and role changes.

Nurses need to know agency policies for reporting substance abuse problems to a client's employer or family. Nurses must balance their respect for the autonomy of elderly persons who are competent but refuse to accept help with the principle of beneficence, or doing good. Beneficence can lead to attitudes of paternalism where health-care professionals intervene coercively or deceptively to protect individuals from themselves or "for their own good." The aged and mentally ill are particularly vulnerable to paternalistic attitudes and policies (Bromberg & Cassell, 1983).

Suicide

Suicide in the Elderly: Patterns and Risk Factors

People over age 60 have the highest rate of completed suicide (McIntosh, 1985; Osgood & McIntosh, 1986). They compose 12% of the U.S. population, but commit 17 to 25% of all suicides (Osgood, 1987). Although not all depression, substance abuse, or suicide can be prevented, nurses who identify clues to suicide can recommend treatment, begin crisis intervention, and often reduce serious risk (Hatton & Valente, 1984; see Table 12.1).

The first national survey of suicide in long-term care facilities (LTC) in the United States (Osgood, Brant, & Lipman, 1988) reported overt suicidal behavior, such as shooting, hanging, or jumping; and intentional life-threatening behavior, such as refusing food, fluids, or medications. Of 30,269 total residents, 294 (1%) engaged in some form of suicidal behavior during 1984–1985. Researchers found that 15.8 per 100,000 were overt completed suicides; 94.9 per 100,000 demonstrated life-threatening behavior. In contrast, the suicide rate for the general United States population is about 12 per 100,000. Males, caucasians, and the old-old (age 75+) had highest rates of completed suicides. These high-risk groups should be monitored for overt suicidal and intentional life-threatening behavior.

To detect suicide, nurses assess risk factors, suicide signals, and behaviors indicating that an individual is considering suicide (see Table 12.1). Effective assessment includes specific questions, such as (1) how each person has coped with the toughest times of life; and (2) whether the elder has ever been so discouraged that suicide was an option (see Table 12.2). Elders may be reluctant to share their suicide thoughts directly unless asked.

Nurses determine a person's lethality by reviewing the suicide plan, method, means, and the likelihood death will result. A person with a precise plan in the next three days, a lethal method (e.g., gun, hanging, knife, lethal overdose, or jumping), available means, and no rescue plan is high risk (Hatton & Valente, 1984). The individual is likely to die unless placed in a safe environment with suicide precautions. Elders often die on the first suicide attempt. Those with vague, imprecise plans, or nonlethal methods (e.g., cutting wrists) often respond to a no-suicide contract and allow more time for intervention.

Safety is the first priority. Fearing their impulses, many suicidal elders are willing to enter the hospital. For example, one man finally decided to be hospitalized after friends had stayed with him constantly for three days to monitor suicidal impulses. Individuals may be involuntarily hospitalized when they demonstrate a present danger to themselves or others. Most states require evidence of a patient's danger and a professional's signature before involuntary hospitalization.

Individual resources, supportive others, and hope that can lower suicide risk should be evaluated. Indicators of increased risk include depression, exhausted family resources, a state of intolerable stress, and living alone (Richman, 1986). Religion, humor, relationships, work, or activities are strengths that may reduce suicide risk.

Challenges in Suicide Assessment

Older persons challenge nurses to look behind a "polite" facade that can disguise discouragement, depression, suicide. For survivors of the eco-

TABLE 12.2 Assessment Questions

Do you think your needs are being met?

How do you deal with stress? (Do you drink? Keep it inside?)

Are you currently functioning as well as usual?

How are you taking care of yourself?

Whom do you talk with about your concerns?

Have you felt so distressed that you are thinking of killing yourself or others? Tell me about it.

If you felt that way, what would you do? How? When?

What would you expect to happen after your attempt? (E.g., Rescue? Death?)

Could you promise me that you would not accidentally or on purpose harm yourself until (specify date)?

Under what circumstances would you think that suicide was the only acceptable way out?

If you have thought of suicide, how did you avoid suicide? How did you cope?

I wonder if any of your habits or behaviors endanger your life? (E.g., seatbelts, safe sex practices, take diabetic or heart medications or treatments, combine alcohol and sleeping pills?) Please tell me about these.

nomic depression of the 1930s, mental health is among the "taboo" topics that include sex, finances, and political persuasion. The person who says, "Things aren't so bad; I manage pretty well," may also have a lethal suicide plan, just in case things get worse. Nurses need to reinforce strengths while exploring how the individual copes when illness, hospitalization, or fatigue overwhelm coping.

A second challenge is differentiating thoughts of death that typically accompany aging from suicidal ideas. Conducting a life review, achieving a sense of accomplishment, making funeral plans, disbursing important belongings, and preparing for death are among the developmental tasks facing elderly people. Elders people their world with short-term relationships as long-standing friends die or become unable to converse intelligently. One 73-year-old, recently-bereaved widow, Ms. B, said, "Having dentures or implants won't matter since I won't be around much longer." The nurse asked if Ms. B was planning to die soon. "Oh no," she said, "but I'm not paying a fortune and waiting forever to have implants if I'll only have a short time to enjoy them. I want new teeth to use now!"

A third challenge lies in determining whether suicidal ideas function as a way of controlling fears of reduced quality of life, as a reminder of existing choices, or as a way to plan how to manage the worst possible scenario. Often when elderly persons have strategies for managing the worst situations, then they can cope with the present. Suicide ideas emerge when elders find their quality of life unacceptable.

A fourth challenge concerns identifying the hidden wishes behind suicide threats. Some who threaten suicide are actually pleading for "reassurance" that they are loved, valued, and needed.

Rational Suicide and Ethical Conflicts

People with Huntington's chorea, AIDS (Acquired Immune Deficiency Syndrome), or early Alzheimer's disease may choose death before the indignities of terminal illness destroy self respect. Many nurses who understand such wishes for suicide do not know how to assess rational suicide.

Suicidologists debate whether or not a person of sound mind can plan suicide (Maris, 1983). Many believe that the decision to suicide is, in itself, evidence of confusion or distorted thought processes. Some suicidologists believe that suicidal plans usually evolve from a temporary crisis. But when a person has AIDS or a terminal illness, the problem is not simply a "temporary" crisis. Proponents of rational suicide advise evaluation of the following criteria for terminally-ill persons with suicide plans: (1) a mental status examination showing clear mental processes without depression; (2) understandable motivation for suicide; (3) society would understand motives for suicide; and (4) evidence that all other options have been thoroughly explored before suicide is selected (Siegel, 1986). It would be a *mistake* to conclude that a suicide plan was rational before depression was treated or symptom distress was fully explored and reduced.

The nurse's duty is to document a comprehensive mental status assessment, assess each criteria of rational suicide (Siegel, 1986), and recommend a psychiatric consultation. When a patient with Huntington's chorea told a clinical nurse specialist about his suicide plan, the nurse responded, "I can understand your wish to avoid undue suffering, however at present you *only* have a slight hand tremor. I will *not* help you suicide. I will help you improve the quality of your life and control over your symptoms." The man mistakenly thought symptom control was impossible; the nurse explained that a long time remained before early symptoms progressed. Finally, the nurse asked the man to discuss suicide ideas with loved ones and a therapist. She invited the therapist and staff to meet and discuss this issue (Saunders & Valente, 1988).

A professional nurse-client relationship implies a legal and professional duty to refrain from assisting a suicide. Nurses may not knowingly give a lethal dose of medication or help the client plan a lethal dose. Nurses who have a suffering, terminally-ill loved one may have a conflict between their personal views about the right to die and their professional duties toward clients. It is imperative that nurses make use of appropriate consultation in order to remain objective and sort out personal reactions.

CASE STUDY

The intertwining of threats to effective coping can be illustrated in the following case study. Accompanied by her husband, Mrs. R, a 60-year-old caucasian, came to a small hospital complaining of groin pain for the past year. Mrs. R sat quietly; Mr. R answered questions and completed the admission and history forms. Mr. R explained that his wife used Tylenol® and Valium® to relieve the groin pain and had delayed seeking treatment despite the fact that the pain had continued for more than a year.

Mrs. R was an accommodating, relatively nonverbal patient. She was a "good" patient who followed instructions and participated minimally in her care, but exhibited somewhat flattened affect. For example, she had little reaction to the fact that the extensive tests and laboratory work had not uncovered any cause for her pain.

The nurse earned the patient's trust and learned that Mrs. R had a son who had suicided about two years ago. The nurse suspected that Mrs. R's flattened affect and withdrawal might be related to her grief over her son's death. The nurse requested a consultation with the psychiatric nurse specialist and the licensed clinical social worker. Together this team planned the assessment and encouraged Mrs. R to talk about important life events and problems, including the suicide of her 35-year-old son. The son had experienced a career reversal with financial losses and had returned home to live with his parents. One Saturday evening, Mr. R expected to go to the movies with his wife as usual. Mrs. R expressed her reluctance to leave the house becasue of her "mother's intuition" that something was wrong. Mr. R convinced her to leave the house by insisting that his evening would be ruined, and she could "babysit" their son all day Sunday. Upon returning home, they found the son hanging from the stairwell.

As the nurse asked specific questions, Mrs. R described her inability to sleep, enjoy food, concentrate, or feel happy. She also reported ongoing fatigue, tearfulness, and apathy. She doubted she could go on with life. She had felt lazy and had "not been out of the house much." Thus, Mrs. R spent most of her time in the location of her son's suicide. She admitted that her husband was "fed up" with her reluctance to go out, so he was spending increased time away from home. She was now drinking one to three glasses of wine at dinner.

Later, Mr. R agreed that his wife was drinking more because he found that bottles were empty soon after they were opened. With this increased information, the social worker assessed that Mrs. R had a sense of powerlessness and internalized anger directed toward her husband and herself. Using a coping mechanism called conversion, Mrs. R had expressed this anger not in words but in physical symptoms, such as groin pain. Unconsciously, she punished her husband because the groin pain made sexual relations impossible. Mrs. R medicated herself by using alcohol and more than 10 mg Valium® to help her forget. She acknowledged her increased alcohol intake but felt she could abstain at will. Mrs. R felt guilty that she did not prevent her son's suicide and imagined other people might think she was a weak person and a terrible mother.

Mrs. R had moderately good ego strength before her son's suicide. Her intelligence, judgment, reality testing, and even her "intuition" had been accurate. Now, she maintained low self-esteem and commented that her coping strategies had failed her in the grieving process. She said, "A son should not die before the mother," and that his death had made her lose faith in herself. Mrs. R said that, "Nothing I've ever been through in my life has prepared me for coping with my son's death." She agreed that her responses to the suicide and her weak support system were ineffective. The resulting depression and drug use in response to bereavement was evident. The nurse evaluated Mrs. R's suicide risk as low because there was no plan or thoughts of suicide.

After a thorough psychosocial assessment, Mrs. R was discharged with a team recommendation that she start individual psychotherapy for her depression, grief work, and self-esteem, and then family psychotherapy. As the therapy progressed, the physical signs disappeared within one month.

NURSING DIAGNOSES

There are four main nursing diagnostic categories approved by NANDA (Duespohl, 1986) that relate to the topics of this chapter. These categories and their definitions are:

1. Anxiety: A vague, uneasy feeling, the source of which is often nonspecific or unknown to the individual.
   The NANDA-approved identified etiologies that lead to a nursing diagnosis of "*Anxiety, Related to*" are: unconscious conflict about essential values/goals of life; threat to self-concept; threat of death; threat to or change in health status; threat to or change in socioeconomic status; threat to or change in role functioning; threat to or change in environment; threat to or change in interaction patterns; situational/maturational crisis; interpersonal transmission/contagion; unmet needs.

2. Ineffective Individual Coping: Ineffective coping is the impairment of adaptive behaviors and problem-solving abilities.
   The NANDA-approved identified etiologies that lead to a nursing diagnosis of *"Ineffective Individual Coping, Related to"* are: situational crises; maturational crises; personal vulnerability; multiple life changes; no vacations; inadequate relaxation; inadequate support systems; little or no exercise; poor nutrition; unmet expectations; work overload; too many deadlines; unrealistic perceptions; inadequate coping method.

3. Powerlessness: The perception of the individual that one's own action will not significantly affect an outcome. Powerlessness is the perceived or actual lack of control over a current situation or immediate happening.
   The NANDA-approved identified etiologies that lead to a nursing diagnosis of *"Powerlessness, Related to"* are: health care environment; interpersonal interaction; illness-related regimen; life style of helplessness.

4. Violence, Potential for, Self-Directed or Directed at others: A condition in which the individual exhibits behaviors indicative of an impending violent action.
   According to NANDA, the nursing diagnosis of *"Potential for Violence"* should be specified in terms of etiology to include violence that is self-directed or directed at others.

Taking as an example the case study presented above, an individualized nursing care plan for Mrs. R might at least include a nursing diagnosis of ineffective individual coping, related to: the situational crisis arising from the suicidal death of her son (incorporating symptoms of chronic depression, fatigue, lack of appetite, and anger directed at herself and her husband); inadequate coping methods arising from the use of alcohol and Valium®; and unmet expectations arising from her poor self-esteem, feelings of powerlessness, and failed role expectations. Other nursing diagnoses, such as anxiety and powerlessness, might also be included in a comprehensive nursing care plan for this individual, along with additional etiological factors underlying her ineffective individual coping, such as her interactions with her husband.

PLANNING

The planning step of the nursing process establishes goals that describe the desired health state to be achieved by the individual who is receiving nursing care. This step also specifies objectives and time frames which are measurable indicators that are important in evaluating the degree to which the client has or has not achieved the desired health state.

In the case of Mrs. R, planned goals and objectives might include:

| *Goals* | *Objectives* |
The patient will:	The patient will:
1. Discuss feelings and reactions to son's death.	1. State she is aware of specific feelings about son's death within one week and differentiate feelings related to son's death from other feelings within 10 days.
2. Identify positive attributes.	2. Discuss positive attributes with nurse within four days.
3. Notice and reduce two negative thinking patterns.	3. Identify two negative thinking patterns and discuss other more positive ways to evaluate events within one week.
4. Reduce powerlessness by describing strengths and relationships.	4. Explain strengths, discuss two supportive relationships, and practice asking for support within three days.
5. Recognize dangers of increased drinking. Find alternative ways to manage stress.	5. Learn relaxation strategies to use, such as progressive relaxation or imagery, instead of drinking, starting today.

INTERVENTION

Nursing interventions are those actions which assist the elderly person in moving toward stated goals. Interventions that are selected must be individualized and are determined by the nursing assessment, diagnosis, and plan. Nurses must continually assess to determine whether or not interventions are effective. In the case of Mrs. R, the following nursing interventions (based on stated goals) are suggested, together with their rationale.

Nursing Actions	*Rationale*
1. Use active listening and empathy; explore feelings; reassure Mrs. R she is not atypical.	1. Most bereaved and depressed people feel sad, alone, helpless, or guilty. Expressing feelings lessens alienation. Knowing typical feelings of bereavement reduces hopelessness.
2. Use cognitive strategies to reduce the negative thoughts accompanying depression (Ronsman, 1987). a) Encourage daily log of pleasure/mastery activities; b) Praise small steps of activities; c) Encourage activities where she can help others. d) Teach positive affirmations (positive statements about the ability to master a task or feel better, e.g., I will tell the nurse how I feel; this will help me feel less guilty).	2. Depression lifts as negative thinking declines. Awareness and active participation in therapy facilitates change. Daily log helps patients recognize the pleasure and mastery experiences they have. Without reinforcement, patients discount small steps and achievements. Helping others raises self esteem.

EVALUATION

In the week before her discharge, Mrs. R met her goals and objectives. Although initially hesitant to talk about her son's death, she related the facts in a monotone. With the nurse's support, Mrs. R began to share feelings of sadness, shock, and numbness. Feeling shy and embarrassed to share feelings, she needed reminders that this was important to recovery.

Despite fearing it was bold, impolite, and rude, Mrs. R made a list of positive attributes, strengths, and relationships. As a child, she had been punished for talking or bragging about herself so boldly.

Mrs. R began to identify several patterns as she formed a negative conclusion or personalized events. She could laugh at her own tendency to create a gloomy picture and she impatiently wanted to change all these patterns immediately. The nurse reminded her that awareness was the first step and change takes longer.

CONCLUSION: HEALTH PROMOTION AND WELLNESS

Nurse researchers agree that older adults are treatable for anxiety, powerlessness, depression, substance abuse, and suicidal behavior (Osgood, 1987). Helping professionals, patients, family, and significant others need access to current research through education and community resources. Professionals should also examine their own attitudes and biases which may affect patient care, and make use of team approaches.

Optimally, nurses will be able to allow elderly persons to lean temporarily on their ego strengths until the older adults are able to select healthy coping tools or secure new means of dealing with stress. In addition, nurses promote wellness by educating elderly persons. Elders may explain that they have never been told of the dangers or side effects of self-medicating. Written directions for how to take medications safely or carefully chosen articles about depression may help.

Support groups in institutional settings composed of patients with similar concerns are often beneficial. Such groups show elders they are not alone and do have choices (control). Groups such as Alcoholics Anonymous or Emotional Health Anonymous provide similar supports in the community. One-third of members in these groups are over age 50. Community groups such as Al-Anon or Narc-Anon are for family members or close friends of the identified person. These groups encourage awareness of the ways loved ones may offer support or unwittingly sabotage a person's progress.

Sensitive nurses who know current issues confronting elderly persons and who are imaginative with regard to interventions can make a huge impact as advocates and caregivers for the elderly. Families may not appear to require assistance, but often do benefit from nursing intervention. Families have often felt frustrated and do not know how to help their elderly loved one. It is important to alert them to watch for evidence of regression.

Community resources are available for the long-term promotion of wellness. Agencies catering to an elder population maintain up-to-date resource information. They offer a social environment where elderly persons can alleviate depression, engage in activities, and thus decrease aloneness. Senior citizen centers offer perfect settings for elderly persons to rebuild self-esteem through small or large accomplishments and social interactions. Finally, community resources such as Meals on Wheels, home health agencies, or Visiting Nurse Associations may assist in monitoring the elder's continued well being.

REFERENCES

Abrams, R. C., & Alexopoulos, G. S. (1987). Substance abuse in the elderly: Alcohol and prescription drugs. *Hospital and Community Psychiatry, 38,* 1285–1289.

Bienenfeld, D. (1987). Alcoholism in the elderly. *American Family Practice, 36,* 163–169.

Bloom, P. J. (1983). Alcoholism after sixty. *American Family Practice, 28,* 111–113.

Brody, J. A. (1982). Aging and alcohol abuse. *Journal of the American Geriatrics Society, 30,* 123–126.

Bromberg, S., & Cassell, C. K. (1983). Suicide in the elderly: The limits of paternalism. *Journal of American Geriatrics Society, 31,* 698–703.

Caroselli-Karinja, M. (1985). Drug abuse and the elderly. *Journal of Psychosocial Nursing, 23,* 25–30.

Duespohl, T. A. (1986). *Nursing diagnosis manual for the well and ill client.* Philadelphia: W. B. Saunders.

Hatton, C. L., & Valente, S. M. (1984). *Suicide: Assessment and intervention* (2nd ed.). Norwalk, CT: Appleton-Century-Crofts.

Maris, R. (1983). Suicide: Rights and rationality. *Suicide and Life Threatening Behavior, 13,* 223–231.

McIntosh, J. L. (1985). Suicide among the elderly: Levels and trends. *American Journal of Orthopsychiatry, 55,* 288–293.

Osgood, N. J. (1987). The alcohol-suicide connection in late life. *Postgraduate medicine, 81,* 379–384.

Osgood, N. J., Brant, B. A., & Lipman, A. A. (1988). Patterns of suicidal behavior in long-term care facilities: A preliminary report on an ongoing study. *Omega, 19,* 69–77.

Osgood, N. J., & McIntosh, J. L. (1986). *Suicide and the elderly: An annotated bibliography and review.* New York: Greenwood Press.

Rice, B. (1988). Attitudes toward aging. *Nursing '88, 18,* 45.

Richman, J. (1986). *Family therapy for suicidal people.* New York: Springer.

Ronsman, K. (1987). Therapy for depression. *Journal of Gerontological Nursing, 13*(12), 18–25.

Saunders, J. M., & Valente, S. M. (1988). Cancer and suicide. *Oncology Nursing Forum, 15,* 575–581.

Siegel, K. (1986). Psychosocial aspects of rational suicide. *American Journal of Psychotherapy, 40,* 405–418.

Streltzer, J. (1980). Treatment of iatrogenic drug dependence in the general hospital. *General Hospital Psychiatry, 2,* 262–266.

Sweer, L., Martin, D. C. Ladd, R. A., Miller, J. K., & Karpf, M. (1988). The medical evaluation of elderly patients with major depression. *Journal of Gerontology, 43,* 53–58.

Weiss, K. J., & Greenfield, D. P. (1986). Prescription drug abuse. *Psychiatric Clinics of North America, 9,* 475–490.

Yesavage, J. A., & Brink, T. L. (1983). Development and validation of a geriatric depression screening scale. *Journal of Psychiatry Resident, 17,* 37–49.

Chapter **13**

Loss, Grief, and Hope

Sister Karin Dufault

INTRODUCTION

The maturing and aging processes bring with them multiple circumstances that call for saying goodbye to significant people, places, objects, status, goals, and feelings of well being. Experiencing losses is commonplace in the process of development, but is accelerated during the last decades of a full life. Some losses call forth a response of grief; others are easily adjusted to with minimal pain. Accommodation and integration of significant losses, being able to feel the pain of the loss and yet hope, can lead to discovering opportunities for hellos never fully expected. Mourning is a time for healing, adaptation, and growth.

This chapter will explore the phenomena of grief and mourning as a response to loss, and will focus on some common *significant* losses associated with aging. It will also describe hope as a resource in coping with loss that has enabled grieving persons to travel the journey toward healing.

GRIEF AND MOURNING

Human responses to significant losses suffered in later life are varied. They reflect the individuality of bereaved persons and of the losses that they experience. The term used to describe the feelings or emotions evoked by loss, and the behaviors in which they are often manifested, is "grief." Perhaps the most important thing to emphasize is that grieving is a natural and healthy emotional response to the suffering caused by important losses. Rather than being an abnormal or unhealthy reaction, grief is the ultimate price of loving, of attachment, of meaningful relationships (Dufault & Martocchio, 1982; Shneidman, 1983).

Mourning or "grief work" is the process of working through the grief in order to come to terms with a loss and achieve an outcome that has been variously characterized as resolution, completion, adaptation, or integration. The mourning process with all its thoughts, feelings, and behaviors evolves and fluctuates in a dynamic fashion. Mourning has both social or public aspects (evident, e.g., in funeral practices and ritual), and private or intrapersonal dimensions. It is the latter that most concern us here. In some instances, the grieving person is unable to mourn in a manner that allows for coming to terms with the grief and reinvesting in life—which may result in dysfunctional or pathological grief, a phenomenon that will be described in greater detail later in this chapter.

Grief and the defining characteristics of mourning can be understood through a description of general patterns within the mourning process. Among researchers and students of grief, there is agreement that the uncomplicated mourning process follows a more or less predictable course with distinctive manifestations (Bowlby, 1961; Engel, 1964; Lindemann, 1944; Parkes, 1987; Switzer, 1970). This course includes: a period of shock and somatic distress; feelings of hostility, guilt, and preoccupation with thoughts of the loss; confusion and withdrawal; and, finally, work toward a healthy integration.

This pattern does not suggest a single timetable or one, exclusive way that individuals grieve and mourn; rather, elderly people, like every other age group, experience high variability and fluctuation in their thoughts and feelings. Speaking of phases of mourning is intended to provide a framework for understanding, for guiding observations and assessments, and for making nursing judgments. These phases are not intended to be mutually exclusive, sequential, or additive. The framework was developed in relationship to the death of a loved one as the central loss; however, many elements are transferable to other types of significant loss (Dufault & Martocchio, 1982).

Shock and Disbelief

The most immediate response to news of a loss is shock and disbelief which can often last for several weeks. Reported physiological manifestations include muscular weakness, tremors, tearfulness, dry mouth, hypotension or hypertension, tachycardia, arrhythmias, tightness in the throat, rapid, shallow or gasping breaths, diaphoresis, flushed skin, cold clammy sensations, dysphagia, diarrhea or constipation, indigestion or anorexia, and an overwhelming feeling of discomfort and exhaustion. The frail elderly are especially at risk for medical complications from these physiological responses.

Extremes of behavior may be present, ranging from being unable to move, think, or feel (hypoactivity) to being unable to sit quietly and a compulsion to be busy making arrangements, cooking, cleaning, etc. (hyperactivity). A sense of numbness and unreality may protect against the full realization of the loss, allowing for an automatic approach to routine activities. Even though there may be an intellectual comprehension of the loss, doubt remains that it is true. "There must be a mistake."

Yearning and Protest

For several weeks to several months, the bereaved may be preoccupied with thoughts of the loss, yearning for a return of the way things used to be and searching for answers to many troubling questions. Anger is often expressed or at least felt toward any causal agent—the significant loss (person or object), God, caregivers, family, friends. Those who try to comfort may be the object of striking out. Guilt and regret may take the form of questioning what one could or should have done to make things different. "If only I had . . . ."; "why didn't I . . . ?" Negative thoughts toward others can contribute to feelings of alienation, of being evil, of mental instability, and of adjusting poorly. "Why do I think this way? I must be losing my mind." Fear may prevent sharing such thoughts with others.

Common during this phase are sleep disturbances, nightmares, dreams related to the loss, anorexia, weight loss, fatigue, chest pain, motor restlessness, changes in sexual patterns, sadness, emptiness, fear and irritability, and preoccupation with images of the loss, especially loss of a loved one.

Anguish, Disorganization, and Despair

The reality and finality of the loss penetrate consciousness when the numbness and anger are exhausted. Often what follows is a sense of confusion, loss of motivation and enthusiasm, indecision, aimlessness, and lack of confidence. Loneliness, apathy, depression, and meaninglessness can plague the bereaved as they withdraw from social contacts and usual activities. Previous friendships, hobbies, and spiritual, recreational, or work activities may seem irrelevant and meaningless when not shared with the loved one.

Difficulty concentrating and lapses in memory may increase anguish and fears that emotional control and mental faculties are in danger of being lost. As a defense against the fear of losing more, a self-centered-ness can be mistaken by the bereaved and by others as selfishness. The fragility of life becomes vivid and fear develops about injury to other loved ones or self. At the same time, health-compromising behaviors may be present, such as excessive smoking or drinking, especially if the bereaved tended to use such means to cope before the loss. The wish and need to cry is strong during this time; it fulfills an important function in acknowledging the loss and in receiving support from others.

Sadness and disorientation may occur as the survivor lives through the "first times," special events without the loved one. Specific reminders of the loss, such as a picture or song may precipitate a flood of renewed grieving that is overwhelming and catches the person by surprise. A reluctance to share the experience can be present, particularly if the person believes that he or she "shouldn't be feeling like this by now."

Selective memory may be operative during this time as the bereaved bring up, think about, and talk about memories of the loss, framing mental images devoid of any negative characteristics. With this process of idealization, renewed feelings of guilt, remorse, fear, or regret may resurface.

Identification in Bereavement

The bereaved may adopt behaviors, admired qualities, goals, ideals, and mannerisms of their loved one. Some take on the symptoms of illnesses that were present or may have caused the death. One prospective, exploratory study of the phenomena of identification in bereaved persons found that 14% of the sample reported feeling physically ill since the loss, 15% felt "just like the person who died," 8% reported acquiring habits of the deceased, 12% believed they had the same illness, and nine percent had pains in the same parts of their body as the dead person (Zisook, Devand, & Click, 1982).

Reorganization and Restitution

Usually during the second six months the phase of reorganization and restitution occurs, and may continue for a few years. During this time, periods of depression are interspersed with periods of well being as life takes on meaning once again. New information is integrated into the lives of the bereaved. Slowly, sadness decreases and aspects of ordinary life are resumed. The bereaved once again begin to take notice of the beauty around them. Life stabilizes, though some of the pain of the loss may remain for a lifetime.

HOPE

Throughout the mourning process, dimensions of hope can and do coexist in the bereaved. Hope is characterized by the confident yet uncertain anticipation of a future significant good (Dufault, 1981; Dufault & Martocchio, 1985). It is not necessarily limited to a single focus, but may focus on different goods, and adjust to changing circumstances. Hope enables the bereaved to believe in a tomorrow that holds a rainbow after the shower of sorrow. Hope provides the general sense that the future is possible and will bring with it positive elements even though the how and what and when are unknown, thus protecting the hoping person against despair when deprived of the love of the deceased. With this spirit of hope, no matter how weak or vague, there is an overall motivation to carry on with life's responsibilities and to be open to mysteries yet unknown.

In addition to the general sense of hope, bereaved people often describe very specific hopes, that is, particularly valued outcomes, goods, goals, or states of being (hope objects), some of which are very concrete and others quite abstract. Articulation of hopes helps clarify, prioritize, and affirm what the bereaved person perceives as most important in life, and can restore lost meaning in life. Hopes can encourage investment in and commitment to something specific which extends beyond the present painful moment. In this way, hope can provide an object toward which the person's own energies and those of others can be positively directed. In the processes of hoping for a particularly hope, other potential hopes can be identified that aid in gradually relinquishing hopes which have become unrealistic and in substituting new hopes that have relevance to the present and future.

Recognizing the factors that give rise to hope or influence the bereaved person to hope, such as a particular belief system or precious people, can support, reinforce, and facilitate hoping processes. These sources of hope, whether external or internal to the person, strengthen the sense of confidence that there is a way out of the bondage of grief. In contrast, threats to hope bring occasions of worry, fear, guilt, and discouragement.

For some bereaved elderly, a future without the loved one is hard to envision. Reality is clouded by the pain of separation and much that once seemed important loses its luster. Nevertheless, patience, courage, faith, imagination, and the ability to connect with others provide strength that make hope and healing possible. Nursing attention to a careful assessment of the grief and mourning processes in elderly persons, as well as the process of hoping, will provide an important basis for helping behavior.

ASSESSMENT

Before describing the components of the nursing assessment of the bereaved older adult, it may be helpful to explore personal qualities of caregivers who are most likely to provide effective bereavement care. Lattanzi (1982) suggested that nurses who possess the following characteristics are most likely to offer effective bereavement care: (1) communication skills and empathy; (2) personal knowledge and understanding of grief and loss; (3) sensitivity and compassion; (4) personal presence, for instance, the ability to "be" with people; and (5) awareness of personal limitations. Another important characteristic is security in one's own fundamental convictions so as not to be threatened in personal values and faith commitments by the bereaved's doubts (Corr, Martinson, & Dyer, 1985).

Nursing assessment seeks first to determine what the older adult considers to be a significant loss, and then to understand the meaning of the particular loss for the individual. Most frequently, when asked about significant losses, elders will describe the death of loved ones. The loss of a spouse, siblings, parents, friends, or children through death or other separation can be profound. The response to the loss of a loved one varies in intensity, duration, and manner of expression, and is influenced by numerous factors that can be included in an assessment. These factors include: (1) the survivor's relationship with and degree of attachment to the lost person; (2) circumstances surrounding the death; (3) personal characteristics of the survivor, previous grief experiences, and manner of coping with loss; (4) the social and cultural milieu influencing expression of grief; and (5) the nature of the support network (Barton, 1977; Broden, 1970; Dufault & Martocchio, 1982; Engel, 1964; Littlefield & Rushton, 1986; & Martocchio, 1985).

The death of a pet can also have a great impact. Pet death is particularly difficult for elderly persons who have directed their attachment needs toward an unconditionally receptive pet as a source and object of caring following the loss of a significant person. The pet's companionship, trust, acceptance, and displays of affection contribute in a positive way to the self-worth, comfort, security, and pride of the owner (Bustad, 1980; Mugford, 1979; Stewart, et al., 1985).

Separation from or loss of a pet can elicit enduring reactions of grief when the owner's need for emotional fulfillment leads to psychological investment in the pet. This may be compounded when the owner had difficulty reaching a decision on euthanasia for the animal (Quackenbush & Glickman, 1984). Usual behavior patterns are as altered as when human loss is experienced. Unfortunately, the same sympathy and support is often not offered and the significance of the loss not recognized, nor are rituals available to help with expression of grief. One study indicated that the older the person, the greater the difficulty of adjustment at the loss or death of a pet, partly because there is a reduced likelihood that elderly owners will replace their lost animal companions (Stewart, et al., 1985).

Loss of meaningful possessions because of relocation, theft, or disaster can also be extremely difficult. Loss or change in possessions can contribute to loss of continuity with life history and loss of a sense of self or identity (Sherman & Neuman, 1977). One study concluded that, "If the elderly see their possessions as extensions of themselves or as a personal record of their memories and experiences, then depriving older people of objects they care about may be equivalent of destroying their identity" (Csikszentimalyi & Rochberg-Halton, 1981, p. 82). McCracken (1987) found that possession loss by elderly women in the course of relocation to a nursing home was difficult and threatening. For some individuals, the loss of possessions, such as items given by a loved one (spouse, parent, grandparent), contributed to loss of continuity with life history. Loss of other possessions emphasized role changes, such as a missed second bedroom (hospitality role) and dining table (hostess and presider).

Loss of employment, financial stability, and certain social contacts through retirement, as well as loss of function (particularly mobility and physical capacity) through illness, accident, or the aging process, can lead to much grief. Often there are multiple losses for the elderly occurring concomitantly with little time to grieve them separately, leading to an experience of "bereavement overload" well described by Kastenbaum (1969). In some instances, the person has had time to prepare for losses through anticipatory grief (Rando, 1986); at other times, the losses are sudden and unanticipated. Some studies indicate that expected death does little to lessen psychological distress experienced after the death; others support the adaptation value of anticipatory grief (Gerber, et al., 1975; Lundin, 1984; Norris & Murrell, 1987). These conflicting findings support the need to evaluate carefully each individual's pre- and post-bereavement responses.

Some instruments have been developed to identify individuals at risk for difficulty in the grieving process or to identify the problems of individuals who experience prolonged bereavement-related distress with widowhood. For example, the Grief Resolution Index (Remondet & Hansson, 1987), includes four measures of short-term adjustment (survival expectation, fear, preparation, and desperation indexes) and four measures of long-term adjustment (depression inventory, anxiety, adjustment to widowhood, and health indexes). Parkes and Weiss (1983) have developed an eight-item Bereavement Risk Assessment instrument that has been refined through research and is used at

St. Christopher's Hospice in England. Factors include the survivor's age, length of preparation for the person's death, pining or clinging behavior, anger, guilt, perceived family support, and occupation of the principal wage earner. Additionally, nurses assess the potential coping ability of the bereaved.

Hospice programs have provided leadership in the development of initial assessment guides used during bereavement care, particularly following the funeral by a week or two (Bohnet, 1986). The initial assessment during this period provides a baseline for measuring progress, as well as data for planning appropriate interventions.

Nurses caring for bereaved older adults are well advised to be generous in both initial and ongoing risk assessments in order to allow broad latitude for individual variability in grieving. It is equally important to grant ample time for the hard work of mourning a significant loss.

NURSING DIAGNOSIS

Grieving

The principal nursing diagnostic category for this chapter is *grieving*, which may be related to an actual or perceived loss, or to an anticipated loss (Carpenito, 1987). In this framework, a particular nursing diagnosis would specify the nature of the loss, and would indicate whether it is currently present or anticipated. Because grieving is a normal and healthy response to loss, it is an appropriate diagnostic category for nurses who seek to promote wellness and to facilitate the healing that is found in constructive grief and mourning. At the same time, it can be noted that normal grieving may be associated with dysfunctional or distorted behaviors that can be recognized in a variety of secondary nursing diagnoses, such as ineffective individual coping related to depression in response to the loss; hopelessness; self-care deficits; sleep pattern disturbance; social isolation; spiritual distress; disturbance in self concept; and alterations in thought processes.

Dysfunctional grieving itself is defined as "a condition in which the individual experiences delayed or exaggerated response to a perceived, actual, or potential loss" (Duespohl, 1986, p. 191). This sort of distorted grieving or unresolved mourning may be related to an actual or perceived object loss; a thwarted grieving response to loss; absence of anticipatory grieving; a chronic fatal illness; loss of significant others; loss of physiological or psychosocial well being; or loss of personal possessions. In view of the implications for nursing care of dysfunctional or pathological grieving, it will be helpful to discuss this phenomenon at greater length.

Dysfunctional or Pathological Grieving

For some individuals, the grieving process becomes extended or excessively intense, making reorganization and restitution improbable or impossible (Parkes & Weiss, 1983). These are the bereaved who are sometimes described as "dying of a broken heart." Anger, guilt, depression, and self-blame are more pronounced and do not ease with time. Dysfunctional grief of this sort has also been called unresolved grief and has been defined as a "pathological response of prolonged denial of the loss or a profound psychotic response" (Carpenito, 1987, p. 271).

Because the range of normality differs in each case of grief, it is difficult to describe pathological grief. Parkes (1970) and Volkan (1970) identified the following characteristics that require psychiatric intervention: (1) an extreme depressive reaction manifested by persistent sadness with no shifts to a normal state, an unresponsiveness to warmth, extreme expressions of guilt and of identification symptoms; (2) psychotic break with reality (neurotic anxiety; obsessions; phobic, hysteric, or schizophrenic reactions; acting and speaking as though the loss was still present); (3) suicidal tendencies (the use of self-punitive acts often to expiate guilt); and (4) excessive drinking, substance abuse, or promiscuity (as substitutes for the deceased).

Ramsay's research (1979) indicated that those who experience pathological grief reactions are those who, prior to their loss, tended to avoid confrontation and attempted to escape from difficult situations. Windholz, Marmar, and Horowitz (1985) concluded that about 20% of widows and widowers possessed risk factors that placed them in a high-risk group for difficulty in grieving. The factors included high initial symptomatic response to the loss; lack of perceived social supports; unanticipated loss without time for assimilation; and the presence of multiple concurrent life events.

Absent or delayed grief reactions are also reported. Bowlby (1980) described survivors who respond with absent grief as taking pride in carrying on as though nothing has happened. They are active, involved, and appear on the surface to be managing well, making no reference to the loss, and accepting no support. They usually are tense and often short-tempered, and seem to fight off threatening emotions too painful to bear. The price for the refusal to grieve may be depression marked by significant physical symptoms. Delayed grief reactions are ones that may appear days, months, or years after absent grief, and resemble heightened symptoms of the normal grieving process.

Raphael (1977) described risk predictors of high distress during the grieving process that can be identified in the nursing assessment. The predictors include: (1) high level of perceived lack of support in a social network; (2) previous highly ambivalent relationship with the deceased; and (3) the presence of at least three concurrent stressful events. Lindstrom (1983) added other variables that identified high-risk families in need of more intense bereavement follow-up. Included among them were: (1) dysfunctional family relationships in which either one spouse is completely passive and dependent, or exerts a controlling influence on the family; (2) geographic and emotional distance from family and friends; (3) a personal style of the survivor related to isolation, anger, self-reproach, and hostility during the anticipatory phase; (4) extreme denial manifested by withdrawal from the dying person, avoidance of staff, and refusal to discuss dying or death with them; and (5) multiple concomitant losses.

Much research remains to be done in order to provide clarity about the expected duration of uncomplicated grief, the phenomenology of dysfunctional grieving, valid and reliable methods of assessing grief, and appropriate interventions based on prospective, controlled studies (Middleton & Raphael, 1987).

PLANNING

The desired outcome or goal associated with grief and the work that is entailed in the mourning process has been described well by Nichols and Nichols (1975): to remember the loved one without emotional pain and to reinvest emotional energy in life so that the capacity to love is not lost. Cantor (1978) speaks of the same outcome as "enriched remembrance" that may not preclude sadness. In order to achieve these important goals, several objectives or "tasks" of mourning (grief work) must be satisfied (Jackson, 1974; Worden, 1982). In the following list, the first two tasks relate to the earliest phases of grieving, while the last four are most associated with the reorganization/restitution phase.

To face the pain. In facing the often excruciating pain, the bereaved person recognizes the full reality of what is happening as a normal part of life. Not only the facts, but the meaning of those facts are faced, overwhelming as they may seem.

To permit the emotional expression of the full range of feeling. The tendency is to suppress or avoid the intense emotions associated with grieving because they are frightening. Avoiding the pain and the expression of related feelings is perhaps the major obstacle to successful outcomes of grieving.

To achieve emancipation from bondage. The bereaved person works through unfinished business with the deceased and establishes a new or renewed identity that focuses on recognition of internal and external strengths and resources independent of the loved one. New needed skills are learned that were previously possessed by the deceased, such as managing the finances, cooking, or cleaning. This task may include the ability to dispose of items no longer needed by the bereaved.

To adjust to an altered environment. Living in the space previously shared with another calls for a readjustment. It means participating in activities that were once shared and enjoyed with the loved one and now can be enjoyed alone or with others. It means filling the time previously spent with the deceased by traveling, working, volunteering, or other meaningful activities. It can also mean sitting comfortably in the loved one's favorite chair.

To renew or form new relationships. Meeting this objective calls for emotional investment in others and developing new interests. For older people this may call for a substantial amount of effort. Often it is made possible by others reaching out to the bereaved. Sometimes the renewed concern may be directed toward others who are suffering, other mourners or individuals in crisis. It may include an ability to renew one's faith in life and to integrate the loss into a religious belief system even when some abandonment from God had been experienced.

To be able to live with memories. To live with the memories requires that the bereaved let go of the relationship and realize that it is now a part of the past, "fixed in history but no longer actual as it once was in our present" (Corr, Martinson, & Dyer, 1985, p. 224). It means saying goodbye to the loved one with the full resources of the self, with sadness, grace, and equanimity, treasuring memories but not living in memories. The bereaved person is able to remember pleasures, yet not forget disappointments. This task calls for learning to live with the hurts, sufferings, joys, and happinesses associated with the deceased loved one in a more or less comfortable fashion.

INTERVENTION

Understanding grief and the mourning process as a normal part of loving provides the basis for effective nursing interventions. Nursing actions in response to the bereaved call for a delicate blending of being present, listening, expressing honest feelings, and inviting the bereaved to share their experiences and emotions. To understand specific interventions appropriate to the time continuum of grief and mourning as the bereaved may be experiencing them, attention will be focused on supportive actions prior to the death of the loved one, at the time of the death, and after the death.

Before Death

Norris and Murrell's findings (1987) support the notion that nursing interventions directed at supporting caregivers and alleviating their stress while caring for the needs of ill relatives may enhance or promote the bereaved person's health following the death. As more and more older persons find themselves caring for elderly parents, spouses, and children, they may find themselves having difficulty maintaining their own health and high family stress. The results of the National Hospice Study bereavement interview data (Mor, McHorney, & Sherwood, 1986) also revealed that health problems in the bereaved before the loved one's death were the key determinant of health care use and morbidity after the death. Home health and hospice nurses have a special expertise to offer in this situation, though the referral may best be made through the intervention of office or hospital nurses.

In addition to assessing health of the caregiver prior to the death, nurses can learn about other existing resources and reinforce those resources both before and after the death. These resources include interpersonal support (provision of information, material goods and services, emotional support), religious-spiritual beliefs, and intrapersonal coping (cognitive and behavioral strategies) (Richter, 1987).

The trusting relationship that is established by nurses with family members during the dying of their loved one provides an important base for a continued relationship following the death. The family values and needs are viewed within a context by nurses over time which later helps to assess more accurately which interventions might be most appropriate during the bereavement period. Verbal and nonverbal communication is more likely to be understood in the light of the grieving processes.

By enabling the family to participate in care and assisting them in understanding the dying process, nurses play a role in providing for family members' comfort in fulfilling the wishes of the dying person and in knowing that family have contributed to the safety, security, belonging, and symptom management of their loved one. Time is often available to begin the planning of the funeral and burial so that multiple decisions do not become necessary at the time when people feel least able to make the best decisions, that is, immediately following the loss, when shock and disbelief seem overwhelming.

At the Time of Death

Nursing interventions can be especially important for the bereaved immediately following the death itself, particularly for those who experience death for the first time. Survivors may be unfamiliar with what to do or with how to respond to all the sudden thoughts and feelings that accompany the death.

In some instances, family members may wish to prepare the body for the mortuary and may appreciate the assistance or presence of a nurse. By encouraging family to express themselves in word and loving gesture to the deceased before the body is taken to the mortuary, an opportunity is given for positive memory and a step toward the healing process. Nurses are also involved in care and disposal of items that had been used in the sick room, both in the home and hospital. The manner and timing of doing so is tailored to the needs of the family after consultation with them.

After Death

Nurses have not traditionally been involved with families after death, aside perhaps from attendance at the funeral and an initial contact or two by the concerned nurse who last cared for the deceased either at home or in the hospital. Over the course of the last several years, however, nurses have become increasingly active in longer term follow-up through involvement with the hospice movement and specific bereavement programs.

By virtue of their relationship with survivors, nurses can provide an environment where the bereaved can relive the dying and death experience and where reassurance can be offered that the family did well in supporting their loved one. Nurses can assist the bereaved to understand their grief responses and to accept them as normal and healing, thus promoting the mourning process. They can also help bereaved older adults to identify coping strategies that have been useful to them in managing previous losses and to draw upon such strategies in the new situation. Further, nurses can provide information regarding strategies that have been useful to others who have struggled with loss so that bereaved individuals might broaden their options. And nurses can help structure opportunities for the use of such strategies. Bereavement groups (e.g., Widowed Person's Services, 1982) and research (Garrett, 1987; Rigdon, Clayton, & Dimond, 1987) have identified the following coping strategies that older bereaved people cite as having been helpful:

1. helping others
2. making new friends
3. joining groups
4. setting goals
5. maintaining independence

6. adopting a pet
7. maintaining a sense of humor
8. sustaining family ties
9. avoiding isolation and self-pity
10. realizing that grief is different for each person
11. having faith
12. giving yourself time
13. making your own decisions
14. grieving in your own way

Specific behaviors of others have also been identified that bereaved elders perceive as helpful (Rigdon, Clayton, & Dimond, 1987). These include being there and doing something as indicated by the following categories: (1) being available; (2) expressing concern; (3) keeping in touch; (4) extending social invitations; (5) providing physical labor; (6) providing transportation or financial and legal assistance; and (7) giving "care packages." Nurses' awareness of these behaviors can help them structure their own interventions and provide guidance to family, friends, and acquaintances of the bereaved.

Availability was most confirmed when people offered to help. The offers of help came immediately after the death and were rare after the first six months, perhaps supporting the notion that grief is considered by many to be a short-term crisis rather than a period of longer term transition. *Expressed personalized concern* for the bereaved as individuals gave the bereaved a sense of well being and the opportunity to talk about themselves and their feelings. Telephone calls, visits in their home, letters, and cards from others helped the bereaved to *keep in touch* and continue communications.

Social invitations were appreciated as opportunities to get out and do something with others, to be involved and to keep busy. Bereaved persons recognized that others were not letting them stay home and pine away at a time when the bereaved might feel like doing so. *Manual labor* in the form of yardwork, car maintenance, homemaking, and house maintenance provided helpful strongarm help by some that was needed and much appreciated. Others assisted the bereaved with estate settlements and *business affairs,* as well as in completion of benefit forms and payment of medical and funeral expenses.

Transportation assistance is needed by many bereaved elders who find themselves with no access to a car, fear of traveling alone at night, poor eyesight, reluctance to impose on others, and few friends or relatives. Going to the physician's office, grocery store, church, or other outings can be a difficult task without access. Another significant mode of help was the giving of food gifts and *"care packages,"* symbols of concern.

In all of these ways, nurses can assist bereaved persons by "being there and doing something." Perhaps more importantly, nurses can encourage the bereaved, their families, and their friends to support the bereaved in giving help as well as in receiving it.

Nurses can also direct bereaved persons to self-help groups which have become an effective intervention in our society in recent years for widows and parents, particularly for those at risk for high distress or who have actual characteristics of high distress. Vachon, Lyall, and Rogers (1980) demonstrated that widows in a "high distress" group who participated in a self-help group reported better physical health, less anticipation of further difficulty in adjusting to their loss, less contact with old friends, and more investment in new relationships than did a high-stress control group.

Self-help groups are defined as groups in which people with a common problem come together for the mutual support and constructive action that leads to the achievement of shared goals. Guides for conducting such groups have been provided by Lieberman and Borman (1979), Silverman (1978; 1986), Silverman and Morrow (1976), and Vachon, Lyall, and Rogers (1980).

Post-bereavement self-help groups include two general categories: (1) those that assist the bereaved to deal with personal grief, the practical problems resulting from loss, and reorganization of life around changed roles (e.g., THEOS—"They Help Each Other Spiritually," Widow-to-Widow, Widowed Persons' Service, and other widow/widower programs); and (2) those that assist survivors to cope with grief made particularly difficult because of the circumstances, such as suicide, homicide, or sudden death of a child (e.g., Seasons, Compassionate Friends, Mothers Against Drunk Drivers [MADD], and Military Widows). One-to-one outreach, group meetings, peer counseling, and periodic presentations and discussion for members and professionals are common to all (Osterweis, Solomon, & Green, 1984). When such groups are not available in a community, nurses can provide guidance and direction to bereaved persons in establishing self-help groups.

As a part of hospice services, many hospice programs have developed bereavement support groups. Initially, these are intended to provide both education and emotional support primarily to survivors of individuals who have died in the program, but they are often then made available to other bereaved persons in the community. Such groups may vary from being limited to a specific number of sessions or a particular time period, to being relatively open-ended.

Finally, nursing interventions can help elderly persons draw on the past comfort of hope in its most general sense that has helped these elders to keep going even when tempted to give up. Open communication surfaces more specific hopes that provide a direction and reason for rising each morning. An environment is created that helps identify new objects and sources of hope, and provides energy for actualizing the hope. Threats to hope are realistically faced and actions taken to reduce them or deal effectively with them. The fundamental belief that a new day will dawn and that hope will heal the broken heart imparts strength and courage.

EVALUATION

A measure of the successfulness of nursing interventions directed toward assisting the elderly in their grieving process is their ability to love again. Positive features accrue out of loss and grief that are identifiable. Middleton and Raphael (1987) summarized this by saying, "Those that have fulfilled their potential to have mature, giving relationships with as many people as practicable and who, in terms of the quality of relationships, have the most to lose when someone near to them dies, are seemingly paradoxically those best able to cope."

Other measures indicating that the nursing interventions have been effective during the grieving process would be evidence that the bereaved person has been able to express grief, has shared the meaning of the loss, has interacted with significant others, and is able to verbalize plans and actions to rebuild meaningful, hopeful life.

CONCLUSION

This chapter has reflected upon the complex human experiences of loss and grief, and upon the role of nursing in assisting elderly persons to experience mourning as a time for healing, adaptation, and growth. The nursing process served as a framework for examining loss, the human responses to loss, and nursing actions that can influence elderly persons to complete the healing journey with hope as a beacon. Listening and teaching are primary nursing roles with the bereaved. Helping bereaved persons and their families and friends to understand and journey through the valley to new life and awareness is challenging and rewarding.

REFERENCES

Barton, D. (1977). The process of grief. In D. Barton (Ed.), *Dying and death: A clinical guide for caregivers* (pp. 107–122). Baltimore: Williams and Wilkins.

Bohnet, N. L. (1986). Bereavement care. In M. Amenta & N. L. Bohnet, *Nursing care of the terminally ill* (pp. 247–262). Boston: Little, Brown.

Bowlby, J. (1961). Processes of mourning. *International Journal of Psychoanalysis, 42,* 317–340.

Bowlby, J. (1980). *Loss: Sadness and depression*. Vol. 3 in *Attachment and loss*. New York: Basic Books.

Broden, A. R. (1970). Reaction to loss in the aged. In B. Schoenberg, A. C. Carr, D. Peretz, & A. H. Kutscher (Eds.), *Loss and grief: Psychological management in medical practice* (pp. 199–217). New York: Columbia University Press.

Bustad, L. K. (1980). *Animals, aging and the aged*. Minneapolis: University of Minnesota Press.

Cantor, R. C. (1978). *And a time to live: Toward emotional well being during the crisis of cancer*. New York: Harper & Row.

Carpenito, L. J. (Ed.). (1987). *Nursing diagnosis: Application to clinical practice* (2nd ed.). Philadelphia: Lippincott.

Corr, C. A., Martinson, I. M., & Dyer, K. L. (1985). Parental bereavement. In C. A. Corr & D. M. Corr (Eds.), *Hospice approaches to pediatric care* (pp. 219–240). New York: Springer Publishing Co.

Csikszentimalyi, M., & Rochberg-Halton, E. (1981). Object lessons. *Psychology Today, 15*(12), 79–85.

Duespohl, T. A. (1986). *Nursing diagnosis manual for the well and ill client*. Philadelphia: W. A. Saunders.

Dufault, K. (1981). *Hope of elderly persons with cancer*. Cleveland, OH: Case Western Reserve University, unpublished doctoral dissertation.

Dufault, K., & Martocchio, B. C. (1985). Hope: Its spheres and dimensions. *Nursing Clinics of North America, 20*, 379–391.

Dufault, K., & Martocchio, B. C. (1982). Bereavement: The price of loving. *Advances in Geriatric-Long Term Care Nursing, 1*(8), 1–7.

Engel, G. L. (1964). Grief and grieving. *American Journal of Nursing, 64*, 93–98.

Garrett, J. E. (1987). Multiple losses in older adults. *Journal of Gerontological Nursing, 13*(8), 8–13.

Gerber, I., Rusalem, R., Hannon, N., Battin, D., & Arkin, A. (1975). Anticipatory grief with aged widows and widowers. *Journal of Gerontology, 30*, 225–229.

Jackson, E. N. (1974). Grief. In E. Grollman (Ed.), *Concerning death: A practical guide for the living* (pp. 1–12). Boston: Beacon Press.

Kastenbaum, R. (1969). Death and bereavement in later life. In A. H. Kutscher (Ed.), *Death and bereavement* (pp. 28–54). Springfield, IL: Charles C Thomas.

Lattanzi, M. E. (1982). Hospice bereavement services: Creating networks of support. *Death Education, 8*, 54–63.

Lieberman, M. A., Borman, L. D., & Associates (1979). *Self-help groups for coping with crisis: Origins, members, processes and impact*. San Francisco: Jossey-Bass.

Lindemann, E. (1944). Symptomatology and management of acute grief. *American Journal of Psychiatry, 101*, 141–148.

Lindstrom, B. (1983). Operating a hospice bereavement program. In C. A. Corr & D. M. Corr (Eds.), *Hospice care: Principles and practice* (pp. 266–277). New York: Springer Publishing Co.

Littlefield, C. H., & Rushton, J. P. (1986). When a child dies: The psychology of bereavement. *Journal of Personality and Social Psychology, 51*, 797–802.

Lundin, T. (1984). Morbidity following sudden and unexpected bereavement. *British Journal of Psychiatry, 144*, 84–88.

Martocchio, B. C. (1985). Grief and bereavement. *Nursing Clinics of North America, 20*, 327–340.

McCracken, A. (1987). Emotional impact of possession loss. *Journal of Gerontologi-cal Nursing, 13*(2), 14–19.

Middleton, W., & Raphael, B. (1987). Bereavement: State of the art and state of the science. *Psychiatric Clinics of North America, 10*, 329–343.

Mor, V., McHorney, C., & Sherwood, S. (1986). Secondary morbidity among the recently bereaved. *American Journal of Psychiatry, 143*, 158–163.

Mugford, R. (1979). The social significance of pet ownership. In S. A. Corson & E. O. Corson (Eds.), *Ethology and non-verbal communication in mental health* (pp. 111–122). London: Pergamon.

Nichols, R., & Nichols, J. (1975). Funerals: A time for grief and growth. In E. Kubler-Ross (Ed.), *Death: The final stage of growth* (pp. 87–96). Englewood Cliffs, NJ: Prentice-Hall.

Norris, F. H., & Murrell, S. A. (1987). Older adult family stress and adaptation before and after bereavement. *Journal of Gerontology, 42*, 606–612.

Osterweis, M., Solomon, F., & Green, M. (Eds.) (1984). *Bereavement: Reactions, consequences, and care.* Washington, DC: National Academy Press.

Parkes, C. M. (1987). *Bereavement: Studies of grief in adult life* (2nd ed.). Madison, CT: International Universities Press.

Parkes, C. M. (1970). The first year of bereavement: A longitudinal study of the reaction of London widows to the death of their husbands. *Psychiatry, 33*, 444–467.

Parkes, C. M., & Weiss, R. S. (1983). *Recovery from bereavement.* New York: Basic Books.

Quackenbush, J. E., & Glickman, L. (1984). Helping people adjust to the death of a pet. *Health and Social Work, 4*, 42–48.

Rando, T. A. (Ed.) (1986). *Loss and anticipatory grief.* Lexington, MA: D. C. Heath.

Raphael, B. (1977). Preventive intervention with the recently bereaved. *Archives of General Psychiatry, 34*, 1450–1454.

Ramsay, R. W. (1979). Behavioral approaches to bereavement. In P. Sjoden & S. Bates (Eds.), *Trends in behavior therapy* (pp. 211–247). Orlando, FL: Academic Press.

Remondet, J. H., & Hansson, R. O. (1987). Assessing a widow's grief: A short index. *Journal of Gerontological Nursing, 13*(4), 30–34.

Richter, J. M. (1987). Support: A resource during crisis of mate loss. *Journal of Gerontological Nursing, 13*(11), 18–22.

Rigdon, I. S., Clayton, B. C., & Dimond, M. (1987). Toward a theory of helpfulness for the elderly bereaved: An invitation to a new life. *Advances in Nursing Science, 9*(2), 32–43.

Sherman, E., & Newman, E. S. (1977). The meaning of cherished personal possessions for the elderly. *International Journal of Aging and Human Develop-ment, 8*, 181–192.

Shneidman, E. S. (1983). Reflections on contemporary death. In C. A. Corr, J. M. Stillion, & M. C. Ribar (Eds.), *Creativity in death education and counseling* (pp. 27–34). Lakewood, OH: Forum for Death Education and Counseling.

Silverman, P. R. (1978). *Mutual help groups: A guide for mental health workers* (NIMH, DHEW Publication No. ADM 78-646). Washington, DC: U. S. Government Printing Office.

Silverman, P. R. (1986). *Widow to widow.* New York: Springer Publishing Co.

Silverman, P. R., & Morrow, H. (1976). Mutual help during critical role transitions. *Journal of Applied Behavioral Science, 12,* 410–418.

Stewart, C. S., Thrush, J. C., Paulus, G. S., & Hafner, P. (1985). The elderly's adjustment to the loss of a companion animal: People-pet dependency. *Death Studies, 9,* 383–393.

Switzer, D. K. (1970). *The dynamics of grief.* New York: Abington.

Vachon, M. L. S., Lyall, W. A. L., & Rogers, J. (1980). A controlled study of self-help interventions for widows. *American Journal of Psychiatry, 137,* 1380–1384.

Volkan, V. D. (1970). Typical findings in pathological grief. *Psychiatric Quarterly, 44,* 231–250.

Widowed Person's Services (1982). *Training program.* Austin, TX: Author.

Windholz, M. J., Marmar, C. R., & Horowitz, M. J. (1985). A review of the research on conjugal bereavement: Impact on health and efficacy of intervention. *Comprehensive Psychiatry, 26,* 433–447.

Worden, J. W. (1982). *Grief counseling and grief therapy: A handbook for the mental health practitioner.* New York: Springer Publishing Co.

Zisook, S., Devand, R. A., & Click, M. A. (1982). Measuring symptoms of grief and bereavement. *American Journal of Psychiatry, 139,* 1590–1593.

Part **IV**

Delivering Nursing Care Within an Aging Society

The implementation of gerontological nursing care faces a variety of challenges. In the three chapters that follow, those challenges are addressed both at the organizational or systemic level and at the level of the individual nurse. More importantly, each of the challenges considered is shown to have potential as an opportunity to improve the delivery of nursing care within an aging society.

In Chapter 14, Lorna Guse and Lesley Degner demonstrate ways in which nurses can work not only as advocates for individual elderly persons and members of their families, but also as social agents who can affect policies bearing upon client populations. Similarly, in Chapter 15, Stephanie Zeman notes how nurses can work with family systems both to assess and to enhance the potential for family caregiving. Finally, in Chapter 16 Kay Weiler, Kathleen Buckwalter, and James Curry identify sources of work-related stress and the nature of ethical dilemmas which typically affect gerontological nurses. Exposing work-related stress and ethical dilemmas in this way enables nurses to see how they can draw upon professional guidelines and develop their own personal philosophy of practice to improve care of older adults. In short, these three chapters taken together are intended to indicate how gerontological nursing can be enhanced and to empower individual nurses to exercise their professional autonomy in constructive ways.

Chapter 14

Nurses as Advocates and Social Agents

Lorna W. Guse and Lesley F. Degner

INTRODUCTION

In this chapter we examine the role of nurses as advocates and social agents within an aging society. First, we look at the advocacy role of nurses at the level of individual and family care. Later, we consider the role of nurses as social agents in stimulating, developing, and participating in social change at a broader level. To move from the role of nurses as advocates to the role of nurses as social agents, we examine professional autonomy and the interdisciplinary team. We also review important developments within the nursing profession, such as educational specialization in gerontological nursing and the state of the art of nursing research in aging and care of the aged.

The structure and function of any institution or system are key forces in social changes. What are the hallmarks of the present system of health care, and is such a system in step with the needs of an aging population? It is clear that our population is aging and that this is an ongoing and cumulative process. It is less clear what the response to these changes should be, and the ways in which nursing practice can be enhanced given such changes. What are the challenges to nursing care of the aged and to nurses as advocates and social agents? These issues facing nursing today have important implications for the future.

NURSES AS ADVOCATES

What is an advocate? An advocate is ". . . one who attempts to influence the persons or groups who have control over the situation with which the client group is dissatisfied in order to make the decision makers more responsive to client needs" (Berger, 1976, p. 2). While Berger's definition is acceptable, it refers to the "client group," and as such seems more applicable to the role of nurses as social agents rather than to the role of nurses as advocates. Furthermore, for this definition, the client group is portrayed as relatively passive. But unless client groups are involved in some way in the "attempt to influence," they will not develop skills in this process and their relative dependence on the advocate may become an issue in itself.

As a group, older adults are sometimes perceived as being less self-directive than younger persons because of their decreasing physical energy or because of cohort-based norms that place value on the eminence of "experts" like the physician (Kerschner, 1976). In the institution and in the community, nurses may be called upon to represent the views of individuals and families, a traditional role that nursing continues to assume.

This type of advocacy does not usually promote change beyond the level of individual or family. The goal is to make those changes that are pertinent and tailored to the client. In general, the aim is not to simulate change in policy and planning on a larger scale. This is not a criticism. Our aging population is not a homogeneous group, and nurses at a primary level of caregiving respond to individual needs. The role of advocate for the individual and the family is different from the role of social agent where the goals are relatively global and population-based. This is an important distinction for nursing action.

Nurses have accepted the role of advocate, and issues related to advocacy have been reported and discussed in the literature (e.g., Abrams, 1978; Robinson, 1985). Unlike Berger's definition which involves client groups, nurse advocacy has been defined more often at the level of the individual and family. The definition given by Kohnke (1980) often is quoted. She stated that advocacy is ". . . the act of informing and supporting a person so that he can make the best decisions possible for himself" (p. 2038). After the client has made the decision, the role of advocate is ". . . to support clients in the decisions they made" (p. 2039).

The role of advocate may be uncomfortable for some nurses and advocacy is not without hazards. Acting on the client's behalf may lead nurses into direct conflict with other workers and this has led some nursing authors to promote the skills of advocacy in negotiation and compromise (Robinson, 1985). Becker (1986) suggested that nurses assess the risks in the advocacy role and provided a checklist of questions that nurses should answer in this assessment (see Table 14.1). Special attention should be paid to the clarity with which the health-care team understands the role of nurses in the nurse-patient relationship.

The advocacy role of nurses often occurs within the context of a health-care team. The concept of the team and the team approach has been widely embraced within the health-care system. Provision of care in the institution and in the community often is shared by an interdisciplinary team of health workers. Certainly, this is true when the recipients of care are elderly and, in fact, the field of gerontology grew out of converging interests in a number of independent disciplines. Central to the development of the team and interdisciplinary care is the assumption that each discipline has knowledge and skills that are diverse but basically compatible for achieving the goals of client care. Whether or not the team approach works or is the best approach with a client group is still to be persuasively demonstrated (Ducanis & Golin, 1979). This gap in the literature indicates a need for research on the structure, process, and outcome of interdisciplinary team work.

TABLE 14.1 Assessing the Risks in the Advocate Role

1. Are channels of communication between health care professionals open and clear regarding client needs and choices?
2. Once channels of communication are open and clear, are these channels being maintained?
3. Are members of the health care team clear regarding the obligations and responsibilities of the nurse in the nurse-patient relationship?
4. Has trust been established and maintained in the nurse patient relationship?
5. What role in the decision-making process does the patient have (i.e., degree of autonomy)?
6. What influence do significant others have in health care decisions regarding the patient?
7. What role expectations do the patient and family have of the nurse and other members of the health care team?
8. What information and knowledge must the nurse have to support and teach the patient?
9. What are the legal and ethical implications involved in assuming the advocate role in this situation?

Source: P. H. Becker (1986). Advocacy in nursing: Perils and possibilities. Reprinted from *Holistic Nursing Practice*, Vol. 1, No. 1, p. 60, with permission of Aspen Publishers, Inc., © November 1986.

AUTONOMY AND INTERDISCIPLINARY TEAMWORK

Care of the aged is a field where the interdisciplinary approach seldom has been questioned. The value of the team approach for this population has been based on the complexity of the aging process and on heterogeneity among the elderly. However, it has been argued that the elderly themselves may have difficulty dealing with a "team" or group of caregivers. Thus, it may be the nurse's role and responsibility to introduce and interpret the interdisciplinary team concept and services to the geriatric client (Pesznecker & Paquin, 1982). The concept of "team" is relatively new to the layperson, and the elderly in particular may be more comfortable dealing with one health worker whose role is familiar, such as the nurse. For these reasons, the nurse may be in a good position to become a client advocate within the health-care team and to promote the advocacy function of the team itself.

Some nurses have difficulty with the team approach and sense a loss of autonomy within such a structure. McKay (1983) pointed out that the traditional definition of autonomy has emphasized independent decision making in accordance with one's training. She suggested that this must be broadened to encompass both independent *and* interdependent decision making. Interdependence is a key defining property of an organized group as opposed to a collection of individuals, and what one member of the group does will have effects beyond that member and for other individuals. At times, nurses will be autonomous and make independent decisions within their sphere of professional expertise. However, because the interdisciplinary health team is considered essential to health care, nurses will also be highly involved in interdependent decision making.

In order to function effectively as team members, nurses must develop and use skills related to the group process. Using work originally carried out by R. F. Bales, Sampson and Marthas (1981) suggested that the group process involves both task-based and group maintenance functions. *Task-based functions* refer to the activities related to achieving the substantive goals of the group (in this case, client care goals), while *group maintenance functions* refer to activities aimed at promoting effective working relations within the group. Task-based functions include proposing and evaluating ideas, and representing the client's preferences. Group maintenance functions consist of offering encouragement to other members of the group and promoting harmony within the group through open communication and compromise. In team work, the group maintenance function is crucial to the success of the task-based function.

As members of the health-care team, nurses must develop skills to perform both of these functions. Task-based functions may be more comfortable for nurses whose education and experience focus on client care and the direct application of the nursing process to meet client needs. Group maintenance functions, while intuitively obvious once they have been explicitly identified for attention, may not otherwise or always be extensively or formally examined by nurses working in groups. Sampson and Marthas (1981) suggested that in order to understand group effectiveness, health-team members should examine the group norms, that is, the shared standards of behavior, attitudes, and perception within the group. Similarly, Ducanis and Golin (1979) emphasized that the team must have a "sense of shared direction" in order to operate effectively.

In providing care to the elderly, a number of health workers and professional disciplines are represented on the team: nursing, medicine, social work, psychology, physical and occupational therapy, nutrition, and other specialties and sub-specialties. Group norms must be identified and developed concerning team leadership, role definition and role function of the various specialties, and communication (Pesznecker & Paquin, 1982). It is common for the physician to be perceived as the leader of the team, but group leadership should be based primarily on criteria of suitability and not solely on professional background.

Nurses are primary, ongoing providers of care. Compared with other health workers, nurses have relatively sustained contact with the client and family. Nurses often coordinate community and institutional care. As a result, they are likely candidates for leadership. Designating a leader is dependent on a number of factors, including factors outside of the group and involving agency and institutional directives. However, given the opportunity, nurses by virtue of their client contact and coordination role can fulfill the leadership role. Furthermore, the elderly client may feel more comfortable with the nurse compared with other specialty and sub-specialty health-care workers whose roles are not as familiar.

Role definition and role function for each team member must be determined in order for the group to work together effectively. Similarities, differences, and areas of overlap among health workers may be a source of strength or a source of contention and misunderstanding. For the elderly, the assumption has been that the physical and social changes associated with the later years of life require the expertise of a number of health workers. As a result, the team approach has been advocated, although there is often difficulty in defining who does what. These are issues that must be worked out within the team, and norms must be developed when the division of labor within the team is unclear. Effective communication is critical for this process to occur.

Ducanis and Golin (1979) argued that if interdisciplinary teams are to function at an optimal level, health workers need to be educated to function as part of a team. Within nursing education and practice, more work needs to be done to assist nurses in learning about group maintenance functions. Naturally, the task-based functions require that members of the team be competent within their respective areas of expertise. Nursing competence in care of the elderly has been based on both general and specialized education.

EDUCATION IN GERONTOLOGICAL NURSING

The specialty area of nursing care for the elderly has been recognized by the profession as a separate field of practice and specialized educational programs have been developed. The American Nurses' Association established a national practice division, Geriatric Nursing, in 1966. Later the division's name was changed to Gerontological Nursing Practice, reflecting the broader context of nursing care. In Canada, the Canadian Gerontological Nursing Association was established formally in 1985 and a national conference is sponsored by this organization every two years in Canada in order to bring together expert nurses and others interested in the field of gerontological nursing.

Gerontological nursing has been described as a young and often little-understood specialty in nursing (Wells, 1979). In fact, there is debate as to how gerontological nursing should be handled in basic nursing preparation. Some argue that it should be integrated within the basic program and that students should be educated in the rudiments of caring for the elderly as part of adult care. Others believe it should be set apart as a specialized area, with separate theory in courses and with clinical experiences in gerontological nursing offered at the undergraduate level. One of the complicating factors in this argument is the lack of nurse educators who are qualified to teach in the area of gerontological nursing. Thus if specialized education is viewed as the preferred approach, another question follows: Where do the instructors and leaders in gerontological nursing come from? This is also a problem for practicing nurses who want continuing education or inservice programs in this field.

There is a pressing need for personnel prepared in gerontology. This need will be even greater in the future as the elderly segment of the population increases. At this time, the rate of population aging is slower in Canada, but by the year 2000 the overall age structure of the American and Canadian population will be quite similar with nearly 12% of the population over age 65 (Kane & Kane, 1985). There is a demand for nursing graduate and post-graduate expertise. Master's specialization in gerontological nursing has been available in the United States since the early 1970s. In Canada, such specialization is not currently available. Nurses prepared in gerontological nursing at the doctoral level are required for education and research activities (Martinson, 1984).

The educational preparation and role of the gerontological nurse specialist has been described in the literature (Steffi, 1984). This clinical specialty is relatively new, but a number of roles have been identified for the gerontological nurse specialist to assume in the institution and in the community. Eliopoulos (1979) described the roles of implementor, educator, advocate, and innovator. As implementor, the gerontological nurse specialist facilitates the integration of gerontological knowledge into nursing practice. This knowledge is communicated to other nurses through the role of nurse educator. The gerontological nurse specialist has an in-depth and a scientifically-based knowledge of the aging process and the needs of the elderly. This broad body of knowledge can be used in providing individual care and in representing the client as an advocate. The advocacy role pertains to the needs of the elderly, and the nurse can also act as an advocate for gerontological nursing itself as a needed specialization. As an innovator, the gerontological nurse specialist searches for new ways to apply knowledge and ultimately to improve client care.

In the community and institution, the clinical nurse specialist in gerontology is an important resource for staff members. Indeed, the educator role of the gerontological nurse specialist within an organization will likely be in even greater demand for the future. The elderly present complex nursing care needs. The gerontological nursing specialist is knowledgeable about the processes of normal aging, as well as the common disease and illness patterns that occur in the later years. Such a background ensures that health concerns presented by elderly persons are not dismissed as "part of growing old," but are assessed according to the current state of knowledge in the fields of nursing and gerontology.

The growth of information on aging and health problems associated with aging has been increasing, particularly in the past 10 years. Some information is population-based. For example, social demographers have described our present cohort of elderly and have provided projections of future cohorts. There are increasing numbers and proportions of elderly persons in the population. The most rapid growth is with the "oldest old," that is, those age 85 and over (Manton & Soldo, 1985). More is known about these demographic changes than is known about the health changes that are associated with an increase in life expectancy (particularly at advanced age).

Caution is warranted when making generalizations concerning the future based on the present elderly population because of cohort differences and historical and environmental influences. Furthermore, population trends are not transferable directly to the level of the individual and the family. The gerontological nurse specialist in the community and institution will continue to need information and research applicable to individual client care. Such knowledge is essential for implementing the advocacy function.

RESEARCH IN GERONTOLOGICAL NURSING

Research in gerontological nursing has been almost nonexistent until very recently and a variety of textbooks are just beginning to appear (Steffi, 1984). Research that focuses on nursing care of the aging individual is limited. In particular, there is a lack of clinical studies (Wolanin, 1983). A great deal of research has been carried out in gerontology by social scientists and other health professionals. Nursing can make use of this work as it is deemed appropriate. For example, while there have been few studies of social support among the elderly carried out by nurses (Adams, 1986), this is a relatively well-researched area in social science. Nurses can use this established literature from the social sciences to answer nursing questions, guide nursing actions, and point the way to future nursing research work.

Kayser-Jones (1981) defined two goals for gerontological nursing research: (1) to provide a sound basis for the practice of gerontological nursing; and (2) to improve the quality of care for the aged. Indeed, the first goal should go a long way toward meeting the second one. Nursing research should assist the nurse in providing the best possible care. Kayser-Jones (1981) also noted that the conduct of nursing research studies on aging depends on the number of nurses who have the preparation to do this work. The quantity and quality of these studies will reflect the post-graduate education of nurses who have specialized in aging and health care. More master's and doctorally-prepared gerontological nurses are needed.

A number of problems and gaps in gerontological nursing research have been identified (Cormack, 1985; Steffi, 1984; Wolanin, 1983). New research and more research is needed in virtually every area of care of the elderly. More work is needed to evaluate nursing interventions for elderly clients. Fewer studies are being carried out with elderly persons in the community by comparison with studies on elderly hospital patients and the institutionalized elderly. This stands in contrast to the fact that in the United States, only six percent of persons over 65 live in nursing homes or other institutions (Zopf, 1986). In Canada, the percentage is slightly higher. There is also a lack of emphasis in gerontological nursing research on health promotion and maintenance, and on restoration of health.

Some of the problems identified in gerontological nursing research are not unique to nursing. The same problems have been identified in the social science research on aging. For example, studies of elderly persons have not always discriminated between younger and older subgroups, yet clearly there are important differences in terms of health status and sociodemographic characteristics. Sample size is an issue; in most studies small numbers predominate. There is a need for replication in order to validate findings in areas of research where beginning work is being done. The most frequent criticism is based on the limitations of cross-sectional research and the overwhelming response is a call for more longitudinal studies.

Foster and Archbold (1981) recommended that future research in gerontological nursing include the following: theory-generating (inductive) studies; nursing intervention studies; development of additional measurement instruments for research in this area; and research on the ethics of research on the elderly. These researchers suggested that other disciplines have developed theory and produced empirical findings that may be of use to nursing. Moreover, they indicated that collaborative research with other disciplines is needed. Indeed, the team approach in research is based on similar assumptions to those underlying the formation of the interdisciplinary team in practice. In the research team, individuals with varied knowledge and expertise pool their resources to study a research question that is of mutual interest.

Foster and Archbold (1981) also emphasized policy research. They wrote that ". . . research into social policies *per se* and their impact on the lives of the elderly must be a major thrust of gerontological nursing research" (p. 293). This type of research is not based on individual and family care, but it has implications for nursing care in a broad sense. Social policy research could indicate deficits or problems in policy that affect nursing care of the elderly. Such findings provide impetus for innovation. Research on social policy is an important area and will require a competent cadre of nurses both to carry out the research and to implement the findings.

NURSES AS SOCIAL AGENTS

What is social agency? How can nurses engage in social action to bring about needed change? These are important questions for nursing and for gerontological nurses. Nurses acting as social agents generate ideas, introduce innovations, develop a climate for planned change, and implement and evaluate the changes (Lancaster, 1982). As social agents, nurses do not act directly for any particular client, but act for a client group as a whole. In this context, the client group is the elderly, and the area for ideas and potential change is health care.

There are some differences between nurses as advocates and nurses as social agents. Social agents take a large-scale or macro-approach to health care and the client group. Population-based data is critical information to social agents, while practicing gerontological nurses likely will find that this information is not meaningful at an individual or family level. Social agents look for trends and patterns in the client population and examine population needs compared with health-care services. Social agents work with individuals and organized bodies representing the client group so that the plan for action is grounded in the reality of their needs. Defining these needs is a separate and critical task that must precede direct action at the level of the institution, the community, or the society.

Nurses acting as social agents must be knowledgeable and competent in gerontological nursing. Furthermore, additional knowledge and skill in how to plan and implement social policy change is necessary. Nurses are often skilled in identifying gaps and deficits in the health-care system, but the difficulty lies in determining the steps that follow such an identification. In addition, a major issue facing gerontological nurses is whether or not they can agree on priorities for social action and act as a coordinated unit in taking action. Organization and teamwork is crucial for gerontological nurses to go beyond providing care within a structural context and begin planning for change of that very structural context itself.

The circumstances within which nurses can assume the role of social agent differ somewhat in the two major countries in North America. In Canada, the national association of professional nurses, the Canadian Nurses' Association (CNA) has published a document indicating that social policy change is a concern of that association and listing the steps for achieving such change (Canadian Nurses' Association, 1985). In recent years, the CNA has lobbied and supported the federal government in introducing legislation that would curtail the erosion of principles of availability and accessibility of health services (Labelle, 1986). Although nurses have identified some shortcomings in the Canadian health-care system in terms of health care for an aging population, concerted effort for change has not been staged at this time. It seems likely that the impetus will have to be initiated by the national nursing interest group, the Canadian Gerontological Nursing Association. This organization is relatively young, but it would appear to be the most appropriate body to begin to develop innovative ideas and plans for social policy change aimed at benefitting the aging population in Canada. At the community and institutional level, similar interest groups and committees are potential leadership bodies.

While the Canadian and American health-care systems are different in many ways, these systems also share some common features, particularly in terms of services to the elderly (Kane & Kane, 1985). In the United States, the major health insurer of the elderly is Medicare, a federally-funded and administered health insurance program for eligible persons over the age of 65 and for the permanently disabled. In

Canada, the elderly receive health care as part of a universal system of health care. Both systems are based on a biomedical model with emphasis on short-term acute care. The dominant professional group is the medical profession and the hospital is a key structure in this system.

It has been cogently argued that the most appropriate types of formal care for an aging population are not the ones most readily available in Canadian and American society (Chappell, Strain, & Blandford, 1986). The health concerns typically experienced by the elderly are related to chronic conditions and problems of disability and mobility. These are not well addressed by a health-care system that focuses on acute and institutional care. The health concerns of the elderly are not typically amenable to medical intervention. Canadian research indicates that only a small portion of the elderly live in nursing homes. Further, for those who reside in the community, it is a minority that are heavy utilizers of hospital services. One study reported that 5% consume almost two-thirds of total hospital days used by elderly persons (Roos, Shapiro, & Roos, 1984). As a result of this research, there is increasing interest in developing and expanding home care services for the elderly as a more appropriate future direction for our society and its health-care systems.

There are a number of issues and areas for change for nurses acting as social agents and working on behalf of the elderly. One such area involves institutionalization and the development of programs to facilitate community living. The trend toward home care services is consistent with the prevailing view in the gerontological and nursing literature that long-term institutionalization is undesirable except for the minority who require such total care. While many favor the trend toward increasing the diversity of community supports for elderly persons, there is by no means consensus. Some policy makers fear that community programs will destroy family responsibility for aged members, although there is no empirical evidence to support this claim. In fact, American and Canadian research has provided evidence of a complementary relationship between formal care and informal or family caregiving (Chappell, 1985; Hooyman, Gonyea, & Montgomery, 1985). This is an area of debate that will have strong implications for the future care of the elderly. It is an area of debate that should concern gerontological nurses and, in fact, all nurses who are interested in care of the aged.

Gerontological nurses are in key positions to identify the critical issues for nursing care of the elderly now and in the future. In order to have an impact on policy at any level, be it the institution, the community, or the society, nurses will have to work together and agree among themselves on the major issues and the appropriate steps in promoting change when it is clearly required. Again, the impetus for such work would seem to rest with gerontological nursing interest groups—local, regional, and national—with each addressing issues at an appropriate and manageable level. Nurses must become well-versed in the available information and pertinent research in order to present persuasive arguments for change. In addition, they must become knowledgeable about the dynamics and processes for bringing about change. Political involvement and lobbying efforts are important strategies for the future.

CHALLENGES FOR GERONTOLOGICAL NURSING

Many challenges face gerontological nursing today and the future likely will involve even more demands for those concerned with nursing care in an aging society. Within gerontological nursing, there are concerns related to educational preparation and the state of the art of gerontological nursing research. The personnel shortage at all levels of education and practice is a major issue. The enhancement of nursing practice depends on the quality and quantity of practitioners and on the growth of nursing research. Nurses have looked to schools of nursing to take a leadership role in care of the elderly (Brower, 1984; Rankin & Burggraf, 1983). Similarly, nurses have looked to their professional associations (ANA or CNA) and gerontological interest groups for guidance on education and practice issues.

We have examined the role of nurses as advocates at the level of the individual and family, and the role of nurses as social agents for client groups. The success of both these roles depends not only upon nursing competence, but also on the ability of nurses to work among themselves, with other health workers, and with clients. Nurses function within structures such as the institution and the community, and even more broadly within larger health-care systems. Nurses can bring about change as advocates and as social agents working on behalf of the elderly. The challenge rests with nurses to make this a reality.

REFERENCES

Abrams, N. (1978). A contrary view of the nurse as patient advocate. *Nursing Forum, 17*, 258–267.

Adams, M. (1986). Aging: Gerontological nursing research. In H. H. Werley, J. J. Fitzpatrick, & R. L. Taunton (Eds.), *Annual Review of Nursing Research, 4*, 77–103. New York: Springer Publishing Co.

Becker, P. H. (1986). Advocacy in nursing: Perils and possibilities. *Holistic Nursing Practice, 1*(1), 54–63.

Berger, M. (1976). An orienting perspective on advocacy. In P. A. Kerschner (Ed.), *Advocacy and age* (pp. 1–16). Los Angeles, University of Southern California Press.

Brower, H. T. (1984). Gerontological nursing needs. *Journal of Gerontological Nursing, 10*(2), 6.

Canadian Nurses' Association (1985). *Social policy function.* Ottawa, Canada: Author.

Chappell, N. L. (1985). Social support and the receipt of home care services. *The Gerontologist, 25,* 47–54.

Chappell, N. L., Strain, L. A., & Blandford, A. A. (1986). *Aging and health care: A social perspective.* Toronto: Holt, Rinehart & Winston of Canada.

Cormack, D. F. S. (1985). *Geriatric nursing: A conceptual approach.* Oxford: Blackwell.

Ducanis, A. J., & Golin, A. K. (1979). *The interdisciplinary health care team.* Germantown, MD: Aspen.

Eliopoulos, C. (1979). The gerontological nurse specialist. In A. M. Reinhardt & M. D. Quinn (Eds.), *Current practice in gerontological nursing* (pp. 197–203). St. Louis: C. V. Mosby.

Foster, S. B., & Archbold, P. G. (1981). Past and future directions in gerontological nursing research. In C. Eisdorfer (Ed.), *Annual Review of Gerontology and Geriatrics, 2,* 285–295. New York: Springer Publishing Co.

Hoovman, N., Gonyea, J., & Montgomery, R. (1985). The impact of in-home services termination on family caregivers. *The Gerontologist, 25,* 141–145.

Kane, R. L., & Kane, R. A. (1985). *A will and a way: What the United States can learn from Canada about caring for the elderly.* New York: Columbia University Press.

Kayser-Jones, J. (1981). Doctoral preparation for gerontological nurses. *Journal of Gerontological Nursing, 12*(3), 19–23.

Kerschner, P. A. (1976). Power, pluralism and the aged. In P. A. Kerschner (Ed.), *Advocacy and age* (pp. 17–22). Los Angeles: University of Southern California Press.

Kohnke, M. (1980). The nurse as advocate. *American Journal of Nursing, 80,* 2038–2040.

Labelle, J. (1986). Nurses as a social force. *Journal of Advanced Nursing, 11,* 247–253.

Lancaster, J. (1982). Change theory: An essential aspect of nursing practice. In J. Lancaster & W. Lancaster (Eds.), *The nurse as change agent* (pp. 5 23). St. Louis: C. V. Mosby.

Manton, K. G., & Soldo, R. J. (1985). Dynamics of health changes in the oldest old: New perspectives and evidence. *Millbank Memorial Fund Quarterly—Health and Society, 63,* 206–285.

Martinson, I. (1984). Gerontology comes of age. *Journal of Gerontological Nursing, 10*(7), 8–17.

McKay, P. S. (1983). Interdependent decision making: Redefining professional autonomy. *Nursing Administration Quarterly, 7*(4), 21–30.

Pesznecker, B. L., & Paquin, R. (1982). Implementing interdisciplinary team practice in home care of geriatric clients. *Journal of Gerontological Nursing, 8*(9), 504–508.

Rankin, N. M., & Burggraf, V. (1983). Aging in the '80s. *Journal of Gerontological Nursing, 9*(5), 270–275.

Robinson, M. B. (1985). Patient advocacy and the nurse: Is there a conflict of interest? *Nursing Forum, 22,* 58–63.

Roos, N. L., Shapiro, E., & Roos, L. L. (1984). Aging and the demand for health services: Whose aged and whose demand? *The Gerontologist, 24,* 31–36.

Sampson, E. E., & Marthas, M. (1981). *Group process for health professions.* New York: Wiley.

Steffi, B. M. (1984). Why gerontological nursing? In B. M. Steffi (Ed.), *Handbook of gerontological nursing* (pp. 3–7), New York: Van Nostrand Reinhold.

Wells, T. J. (1979). Nursing committed to the elderly. In A. M. Reinhardt & M. D. Quinn (Eds.), *Current practice in gerontological nursing* (pp. 187–195). St. Louis: C. V. Mosby.

Wolanin, M. O. (1983). Clinical geriatric nursing research. In H. Werley (Ed.), *Annual Review of Nursing Research, 1,* 75–99. New York: Springer Publishing Co.

Zopf, P. (1986). *America's older population.* Houston, TX: Cap and Gown Press.

Chapter 15

Nurses and Family Systems

Stephanie Zeman

INTRODUCTION

Many of today's elderly are healthier, better educated, and more financially stable than their parents and grandparents were. They are also living much longer. In 1900, average life expectancy in the United States was in the mid-40s, but today people in North America can expect on average to live well into their seventies (National Center for Health Statistics [NCHS], 1984). Longevity, however, is a mixed blessing, bringing with it a higher incidence of physical and mental impairments. Statistics show that most people over 65 have one or more chronic conditions—which increase in number as they age (NCHS, 1981).

Although the chronic care needs of our elderly are among the nation's major health concerns, episodes of acute illness with a need for provision of home care after discharge are not uncommon. According to the 1987 "Profile of Older Americans" published by the American Association of Retired Persons (AARP, 1987), "hospital expenses accounted for the largest share of health expenditures for older persons in 1984, followed by physicians and nursing home care (21% each)." Discharge planning and the appropriate management of home care are the key to helping older adults enjoy the highest level of wellness and quality of life attainable in their later years. This is especially true for those who become disabled enough to require long-term assistance with their care. In the over-65 age group living at home in 1987, 23%

required help with one or more personal care activities, while 27% needed assistance with some aspect of home management. However, despite a variety of available resources, research indicates that the bulk (about 80%) of elder care is provided by family members (AARP, 1987). In 1986, the National Association for Home Care estimated that as many as eight million people were in need of home care services. The overwhelming majority were over 65 years of age (Select Committee on Aging, 1987).

Nurses working with the elderly and their families in hospitals or in the community can make the difference between a successful home care situation and one in which caregiver burnout and the unmet physical or psychosocial needs of the patient and family bring about a crisis. In many instances, nurses function as discharge planners or as part of a multidisciplinary discharge planning team. However, it is most often the bedside nurse who knows the patient and his or her family best, and who can offer a detailed assessment of the patient's needs and the caregiver's ability to meet those needs.

WHO ARE THE CAREGIVERS?

Aging is often referred to as a woman's issue for good reason. Women are not only seen as the more caring, nurturing sex, but since women on the average also live longer than men, they are more likely to be caregivers for their spouses or other family members. A recent report published by the House of Representatives Select Committee on Aging (1987) stated that 72% of all caregivers were female, had an average age of 57 years, and were living in the same household as the care recipient. Daughters (29%) and wives (23%) are usually designated as the "prime caregivers," and have the bulk of the responsibility for the actual care given. Husbands (representing 13% of caregivers), sons (9% of caregivers), and significant others are less likely to be found in this role.

Statistics show that the majority of caregiving is from the young-old (65–75 years of age) to the old-old (85 years and older) (AARP, 1987). The length of long-term illnesses, the high cost of institutional care, and the cost of professional home care are seen as major reasons for families providing the care themselves.

The following three case studies illustrate the complex problems associated with providing long-term care at home.

Independence and Self Care: Joan

The older person's need for self care and independence has long been recognized as a major concern in caregiving situations. Joan is 73 and despite being wheelchair bound since a crushing injury brought about amputation of both her legs over 20 years ago, she has been able to manage all of her personal care, cook, clean, and keep house with a minimum of help from her husband, Peter. Two weeks ago, Peter died suddenly and Joan has realized that without the help he gave her, she is unable to live alone. Joan's only son, Tom, lives near and has asked her to come and live with him so he can take care of her. Joan, however, refused, asking to be placed in a nursing home and explaining that she never wants to be a burden to her son. A public health nurse, working as an advocate with Joan and her son, was able to provide a solution by showing them that the situation could be mutually beneficial if Tom would allow Joan to contribute to caring for his house in return for the help he would be giving her. After some modification to Tom's house and the rental of an emergency response system for Joan, she was able to perform her own self-care and felt that she was still contributing to her family by doing light housework and providing Tom with hot meals at night. Joan and Tom have the added benefit of being able to support each other during their period of mourning for Peter.

Aging as a Woman's Issue: Anne

Anne, at 77 years of age, was seen outside the intensive care unit where her husband, John, was dying of cardiac and circulatory disease. John, 93, was not expected to survive the night. The gerontological nurse specialist offered support and hoped to find resources to help Anne cope with his death. Anne spoke of caring for her husband at home for the last 15 years "since his mind became confused." Concerned about her grief and the possibility of isolation at a time when she needed support, the nurse was about to suggest some community resources when Anne interrupted her. "You don't need to worry about me," she said, "I'll be fine. I have plenty to do. You see, I still have my 96-year-old mother living with me."

The "Sandwich Generation": Jim and Gail

It is not unusual for the middle-aged generation to find themselves caught between the needs of their children and aging parents. Part of the "Sandwich Generation," Jim and Gail are in their mid-40s and have two teenaged children. Over a four-year period, both of Gail's parents died of cancer. Although they lived over 200 miles away, Gail, an only child, spent weeks away from home helping her father when her mother became ill. A year and a half later, when her father developed terminal cancer, Gail brought him home with her. With the help of a local hospice, Jim and Gail cared for her father until he died. The two illnesses meant time away from the children and a total disruption of their personal and social life, but both Gail and Jim felt love and a sense of responsibility toward Gail's parents and wished that there was more that they could have done to help. Gail was able to keep her job during this difficult time by asking for a leave of absence and using her vacation time. However, the family suffered financially. When Gail's father died, they were unable to take a vacation despite the fact that all of them felt physically and emotionally exhausted. The following spring the family made plans for an extended vacation, hoping for some "quality time" together, but the vacation plans had to be put on hold again. Three weeks before they were to leave, Jim's father broke his hip and the attending doctors found that he had advanced bone cancer. A family obviously torn between their needs and the needs of their dying father, they once again prepared to accept the caregiver's role.

The caregivers in each of these case studies were able and willing to provide the care required by their older relatives despite the long-term commitment and disruption to their life styles. Nurses working with families providing care have an opportunity to improve the quality of life for both the patient and caregiver by careful assessment of needs, physical and psychosocial intervention, education, and referral to community resources.

ROLES FOR NURSES

Caregiving can be an overwhelming task in the care of the elderly. Without the use of appropriate resources, it can quickly take its physical and emotional toll on those providing the care. Whether nurses find themselves in the role of hospital discharge planners or are working in the community with the elderly and their families, they are able to assess the patient and caregivers with a holistic and nonjudgmental view, taking into account all of the factors which will determine the level of care needed and the caregiver's ability to provide it.

In acute-care settings, every bedside nurse becomes a discharge planner. Consequently, patient assessments should begin on the day of admission or as soon as possible thereafter. Shorter lengths of stay in recent years mean that most patients are hospitalized only through the acute phase of their illnesses. The recuperative period for most patients will take place at home. For this reason, extra care must be taken to help the family provide for the patient's physical and psychosocial needs, safety, and comfort until the elderly person is able to resume self care. Short-term home care is usually easier to manage than long-term chronic care for the following reasons: Medicare or Medicaid may pay for professional care in the home for a few weeks after an acute illness if skilled care is required, and caregiver burnout is less of a problem when there is "an end in sight." However, when an acute episode brings about the need for long-term chronic care, the life styles of the patient and the caregivers will be affected, and for the majority of patients chronic care at home will not be covered by insurance. In either case, the information provided by physicians, nurses, social workers, and other professionals will be used to develop the discharge plan. No discharge plan should be completed, however, without input from the patient and the family caregiver(s).

Community health nurses (public health nurses, visiting nurses, nurses working in outpatient clinics, etc.) are more likely to be involved with families who "grew into" the caregiving role as its older member(s) became frail and more dependent over a period of time. For this reason, long-term care situations should be evaluated periodically to reassess for any changes in the patient's condition and need for care. Caregivers should also be observed at these times for signs of fatigue, illness, or emotional stress. While nurses in critical care units are often the ones to detect severe abuse, nurses working in the community will be more aware of self neglect, isolation, and other forms of abuse (Fulmer, 1984; Hickey & Douglas, 1981). Some communities provide multidisciplinary teams to evaluate the elderly in their homes and give support to the families working with them (Morishita & Hansen, 1986; Tynan & Cardea, 1987).

ASSESSING THE CAREGIVING POTENTIAL: PHYSICAL NEEDS

Since caregivers include the elderly who practice self-care, the assessment of caregiving potential begins with the patient. Although a major illness may have brought about the need for hospitalization or caused a decline in the patient's health status, the majority of older persons will also have several chronic conditions requiring additional care. Data reported by the U.S. Department of Health and Human Services in 1986 (AARP, 1987) showed that the most frequently occurring chronic conditions in the elderly were: arthritis (48%), hypertension (39%), heart disease (30%), and hearing loss (29%). Orthopedic impairments, cataracts, diabetes, and visual impairments were also reported frequently by the elderly. For this reason, patients and their families should be taught to avoid the "tunnel vision" which sometimes occurs when the overwhelming nature of diseases like cancer or Alzheimer's disease causes caregivers to forget there may be other conditions which merit attention. Although all of the patient's health care needs should be met, steps must be taken to avoid exacerbation of one disease from the use of medications or treatments for another.

Patients and their families should also have some idea of the prognosis or course of the illness. How much recovery can be expected after a stroke? Can the Alzheimer's victim with overlying depression be expected to function more effectively when the depression has been treated? Will recovery from a total hip replacement bring the patient back to the level at which he or she functioned before a fall?

Once health status and the patient's level of functioning are determined, they will form the basis for the home care plan. The patient's ability to perform self-care is of major importance in determining how much help will be needed. Since the overall goal of the home care plan will be for the patient to reach the highest achievable level of wellness and functioning, self-care abilities and potential should be assessed carefully. Even terminally ill patients will benefit from measures to improve comfort and quality of life, as the hospice movement has demonstrated. Thus self-care, depending on the patient's abilities, should be part of the care plan, as it has the potential to improve self-image and to help patients feel less dependent.

In order to prevent physical complications, provide mental stimulation, and help increase a sense of self-worth, it is particularly important for the elderly to understand the need for self-care and for increasing activity within their capacities. Unfortunately, bedside nurses sometimes inadvertently contribute to a patient's sense of dependency by meeting every need and failing to encourage self-care. Home health nurses occasionally see elderly persons whose decline after discharge is directly related to lack of encouragement for self-care by families "determined to do all they can" for their frail older members. Less frequently, families misinterpret the abilities of elderly persons and expect them to do more than they are able. For these reasons, care plans must reflect expected progress or decline in the individual's condition within a specified time frame and with provision for additional reassessment and evaluation.

Since successful caregiving depends on many factors, nurses should offer assistance to help the family decide on a primary caregiver, someone who will have the bulk of the responsibility for the patient's care. While statistics show that this person will probably be a spouse or daughter, most families will make the decisions based on such things as: Which child lives closest to the parent or has provided care in the past? Who feels the most comfortable with the patient and is most willing to provide care? What is the health status of potential caregivers? Which of the adult children are employed, and who has children to look after? Which family member has enough space in his or her home, and how long will caregiving last?

Nurses can be most helpful during this process by discussing the levels of care needed and the physical strength and stamina required of the caregiver, especially if professional help will not be utilized. When the caregiver has been identified, nurses can assess the primary caregiver's need for information on normal aging, the patient's care needs, medication use, and safety in the home. Since the need for care is not limited by education or culture, nurses must also consider the possibility of illiteracy or language barriers, and be prepared to arrange appropriate resources to assist elders and their families with these problems (Seabrooks, Kahn, & Gail, 1987).

Of major importance to patients and caregivers monitoring their progress, is an understanding of normal aging. Education on age changes helps elderly persons and their caregivers improve their ability to distinguish between normal age changes and symptoms requiring medical attention. Nurses can and should use the time spent at the client's bedside to teach the elderly and their families about normal aging and how to cope with the changes it brings. During this time nurses can also suggest alterations that can be made within the home to accommodate the sensory changes associated with aging and provide a safer environment for the elderly client. The following list of modifications were suggested to Tom and Joan (Case Study #1) to provide for Joan's safety in her son's home.

Normal Age Changes	*Modification Required*
The eyes react more slowly to sudden changes in light.	Lamps or light switches should be available at the entry to every room.
Older adults need two to three times the amount of light adequate for younger eyes.	Use brighter lights (150–200 watts) in halls, stairwells, and reading lamps. Use night lights in bedrooms and bath.
Color perception is altered due to yellowing of the lens of the eye. Glare can be a problem, especially if cataracts are present.	Use contrasting colors on rugs, stairs, walls, and furniture. Reduce glare on reflective surfaces, such as waxed floors and counter tops.
Normal aging can cause some hearing loss, especially high tones.	Door bells and fire alarms may need to be modified. An amplifier can be placed on the telephone. Use headphones for radio and television to block out background noises.

Normal Age Changes	*Modification Required*
The sense of smell may decrease with age.	Odors of smoke or gas may not be detected. Use fire alarms and check gas stoves for pilot light dysfunction or leakage problems.
Aging brings on a reduction of the perception of heat and cold.	Reduce tap water temperatures to avoid burns. Use bath thermometer; keep heating pads on low. Observe skin frequently when using heat or cold packs.
Circulatory changes lessen the body's ability to maintain body temperature.	Keep thermostats over 70 degrees at all times. Arrange for emergency response system and make sure it is on the patient at night in case of a fall.

In addition to modifications to accommodate normal age changes, special consideration must be given to the needs brought on by physical disabilities. Joan also required other modifications appropriate for the wheelchair bound.

Other lists might include:

Balance may be altered and reflexes slowed with age.	Remove electrical and telephone cords from traffic areas; use slip-resistant mats under rugs. Remove clutter and rearrange furniture to avoid falls. Secure hand rails on stairs; use railings if needed. Use grab bars and non-skid mats in bath and shower.

Caregivers may have to be willing to convert a living room or dining area into a bedroom if necessary or provide room for extra equipment as needed (commode, walkers, wheelchairs, hospital bed, etc.). This arrangement usually results in a loss of privacy and space for both the elder and the caregiving family, and should be planned for in advance.

In order to avoid potential problems with dehydration, constipation, malnutrition, urinary infections, and other complications, the elderly and their caregivers should be encouraged to attend classes on aging or make use of the many publications available on normal aging and preventative health for the elderly (e.g., Stoppard, 1984).

ASSESSING THE CAREGIVING POTENTIAL:
PSYCHOSOCIAL NEEDS

Caregiving requires flexibility and sacrifices on the part of the family or significant other providing care. If the experience is to be managed successfully, the psychosocial needs of both the elderly person and the caregiver(s) have to be considered. Since caregivers often underestimate the level of assistance required, a conference is useful to evaluate their understanding of the elder's needs. If major changes in life style are necessary, there should be a frank discussion of the priorities of everyone involved. Caregivers who plan ahead to meet their own needs, as well as those of the older adult, will find that they are more supportive of each other and better able to cope with problems when they occur.

During the conference, the nurse can help caregivers to recognize and acknowledge losses associated with aging and multiple chronic illnesses. Older adults resist dependence as long as they can, but when physical decline brings about loss of status, power, privacy, financial security, and independence, depression may occur. Support from family and friends has the potential of preventing or lessening the depression while making the grief more bearable. This is especially true if the older adult can accept the reality of illness and the family's offer of care.

Adult children may find it painful to realize that their parent is no longer capable of making decisions alone, and role reversal can be a major problem for both the aging parent and the adult child (Zarit, 1985). When long-standing patterns of responsibility suddenly shift from the elder parent to a daughter or son, the parent may resent being dependent on the child. Problems occur when the balance of power is upset and conflicting opinions exist about decisions affecting the way care is provided. Family issues may also cause arguments when, for example, grandparents feel they have a right to discipline grandchildren who, in fact, may be participating in their care. Most elderly patients state that they "do not want to be a burden" to their families. Often they can be helped to feel like contributing family members if they are given opportunities to participate in family activities and are allowed to perform minor chores (sorting laundry, peeling vegetables, etc.) to the extent that they are able (Rogers, 1985).

When permitted, elderly persons have the potential to enrich the lives of others. They are usually excellent family historians and can bring a sense of continuity to the family. But adult children should not expect aging parents to change annoying habits or alter the way they relate to other family members. It is said that although the elderly may mellow with age, they also become more like themselves (Stoppard, 1984). Aggressive or demanding people become more so as they try to deal with the anxiety created by old age, illness, and dependency. Anger directed at family members is often a reflection of the frustration brought on by loss of control. Recognition of this fact can help caregivers cope with occasional unexplained displays of temper. Some older adults appear to be more accepting of their situation and prefer seclusion and tranquility. Whether or not they are verbal about their needs, the values of the elderly must not be ignored.

Older adults have the right to expect care that not only provides for their physical needs, but also assures them freedom from mental distress and the security of a safe environment supportive of their self-care efforts. The ability to maintain an effective perception of reality is also important to older adults since loss of one's sense of time and place contributes to depression, disorientation, and confusion. Older people also need love and physical affection. Everyone benefits from an occasional tender touch or hug; such moments can help older adults to feel more secure and can enhance their sense of safety and well being. In the busy process of meeting physical needs, caregivers should also remember to provide for the patient's spiritual needs.

Aging parents often ask their children to help them plan for their death. Whether the request is simply to advise relatives of their wishes, to make legal arrangements for a will, living will, or power of attorney, or to ask for help in distributing personal belongings, caregivers are likely to find these the most difficult of tasks. Many adult children prefer to deny that elderly parents are declining, yet it is important to help these older adults express their wishes. Most communities have hot lines and support groups for relatives and friends in need of help in dealing with the impending death of a loved one (Katterhagen, 1987). Nurses should be aware of these resources and anticipate the family's need for referral.

The psychosocial needs of caregiving families are similar in many ways to those of the elderly client. The right to pursue a high quality of life includes freedom from physical and emotional distress, respite from caregiving responsibilities, time to pursue personal interests, and a right to avoid financial stress when providing for an aging parent. Families also have a need to feel that their efforts are appreciated, but above all, they will strive for a sense of normalcy and preservation of family values. Those who have confidence in their ability to provide care will also be better able to maintain their sense of control.

The importance of respite from the responsibilities of caregiving cannot be overemphasized. Time for relaxation is essential if physical and emotional fatigue, illness, and burnout are to be avoided. This is especially true when families find themselves in the midst of a cacophony of emotions. Love, hate, anger, frustration, helplessness, guilt, and other emotions often coexist for most caregivers. Those suffering from physical and emotional fatigue may be forced to consider nursing home placement as an option to home care. The point at which caregivers can no longer provide care varies for each situation. Frequently, incontinence, confusion, or combativeness are beyond the tolerance level of the family (Knight, 1985). Other reasons for families to consider alternate care arrangements include decline in the physical health of the caregiver, unrealistic expectations on the part of the patient or caregiver, financial burdens, and caregiver burnout.

One of the best tools to help the elderly client and caregiver plan for the provision of care while taking into account the psychosocial needs of both is a contract for care. Using the home care plan as a foundation, the contract should state how each of the client's care needs will be met, who will be responsible for the care, and how the psychosocial needs of the elderly client and caregiver will be dealt with. To do this, the client and family will need to list and prioritize the things that are important to them. Items should include such things as privacy, social obligations, or even sleeping late on Saturdays. Anything considered important to a family member and threatened by the caregiving process should go on the list. A comparison of care needs and family priorities gives everyone a chance to divide the responsibilities fairly, keeping priorities intact to the extent possible. Where concessions have to be made, there is an opportunity for other family members to help out. Frequently, community resources can be used to give caregivers time to attend to their own needs.

The contract is also useful to clarify responsibilities. Who will take over if the caregiver becomes sick? If the family is depending on the use of adult day-care services, will the older adult agree to go? Can adult children living in other areas provide financial assistance if needed?

When using a contract, families should be urged to "assume nothing and anticipate everything." Obviously, no contract can cover every possibility, but putting expectations in writing gives everyone involved a clearer picture of the patient's needs and how the responsibilities for care are to be met.

ELDER ABUSE

Research (e.g., Block & Sinnat, 1979; O'Malley, et al., 1983) has shown that the stress involved in caring for older relatives at home increases the potential for elder abuse. Caregivers unable to secure adequate respite from their duties often report feeling trapped, especially if the provision of care has continued over a period of years. This is particularly true if older adults refuse to accept outside help or limit the type of help they will accept from other family members. Caregivers may find the personal habits of the older adult have deteriorated to an unacceptable level and become a source of daily disagreements. Short-term memory problems and personality changes can also make it difficult for families to cope with elderly persons who endanger themselves by trying to perform tasks without assistance.

Caregivers experience many conflicting emotions, often simultaneously. However, when faced with constant feelings of anger, frustration, and resentment, the caregiver may develop abusive behavior. Elder abuse takes many forms, but while physical abuse is the most obvious, psychological abuse is believed to be the most frequent (Douglas & Pearson, 1987). Often occurring because of a lack of understanding about the needs of the older adult, neglect can range from such things as failure to provide enough mental stimulation to the purposeful withholding of basic needs, such as food, water, shelter, and medical care. Other forms of abuse include misuse of money or property and psychological abuse (verbal threats or assaults). Whatever the form of abuse, fear of greater harm, abandonment, institutionalization, even feelings of responsibility toward adult children (financial or emotional), may keep an older adult from admitting that he or she is being abused.

The law now mandates that physicians, nurses, and other professionals report any suspected incident of elder abuse (Ambrogi & London, 1985). A careful assessment of the older person and the caregiver is essential to evaluate for possible abuse. If possible, nurses should observe the elder's living quarters to check for cleanliness and any equipment required for care. Is the elder progressing as expected? Are there any unexplained bruises or injuries? Is there a comfortable relationship between the elder and caregiver? Has the elder suddenly become quiet or begun to show signs of depression? Is the elder's weight stable? If any observations lead a nurse to suspect abuse, he or she is mandated to inform Adult Protective Services who will intervene to provide protection for the older adult (Ambrogi & London, 1985). Adult Protective Services workers can also assist families to work out care problems or find alternate care arrangements, if necessary.

Nurses have the opportunity to help prevent elder abuse through provision of education on aging and information on community resources. They can suggest the use of support groups to give families a way of venting emotions without jeopardizing the welfare of their older relatives while learning how other families cope with many of the same problems they are experiencing.

NURSING HOME PLACEMENT

About 5% of the elderly in the United States are in nursing homes at any given time. The need to pursue nursing home care should *never* be construed as a failure by the family trying to provide care. At times, adult children promise their parents: "I will never put you in a nursing home." This is a promise that some will have to break. If this promise is made, and often even if it is not, adult children experience high levels of guilt when nursing home placement is required. Nurses working with family members can help by asking them to discuss what they really meant. Most families will agree that the promise was really to provide the best care possible in the most comfortable place possible. When home care is no longer an option, that place may have to be a nursing home. To help the elderly person and family get through the placement and adjustment period, nurses can teach the family how to support the older adult and be an advocate for his or her care. It should be mentioned here that competent adults of any age cannot be forced into nursing homes against their will. Even confused and incompetent persons have the right to be informed of decisions made on their behalf and to be given an opportunity to adjust to the impending move (Coons, et al., 1986).

Once a nursing home has been chosen, the family should help the older adult select personal belongings to take along. Some nursing homes also allow small pieces of furniture (perhaps a chair or chest of drawers) and a television set. The family will also want to bring the elderly person's own bedclothes for comfort and familiarity. All items should be marked with the elder's name and brought on the day of admission. A family member can help the older adult to place belongings about his or her new room, and can remain present for most of the day. Families can also help orient new residents to their room, the unit, the nursing staff, meal times, and activities. At day's end, departure without tears, along with a promise to return the next day, will help the older adult adjust a little more easily. However, it is especially important for promises to be kept and essential for the family to return at the time they specified to avoid having the elder feel abandoned.

Problems will most certainly arise, especially during the adjustment period. Families who are taught how to assess situations can function as advocates for their older relatives. Depending on the severity of the situation, a good rule of thumb is to start by discussing the problem with the direct caregiver, usually a nursing assistant. Often, small problems can be resolved simply by pointing them out. More serious problems should be discussed with the charge nurse, social worker, director of nurses, or administrator, as needed. Families also have the option of seeking assistance from the area Long Term Care Ombudsman, whose job is to function as a patient advocate and mediator between patients, families, and the nursing home (Coons, et al., 1986).

Nurses in long-term care facilities can help families realize that even the mentally impaired elderly can live out their lives in dignity with some measure of comfort and independence. It has been pointed out that "as the impaired person becomes less able to communicate verbally, families need to focus on shared activities to help their relatives stay involved in the world around her or him" (Coons, et al., 1986, p. 6). Since impaired elderly usually lose their recent memory first, it is essential for families to learn how to reminisce and share treasured memories. Family photos, music, and personal belongings can be used to trigger memories, and families should be encouraged to use them. When verbal communication fails completely, families can be taught to use verbal tones, body language, and touch to convey their love and caring.

Many families need extra help and support to cope with changes and declines in the condition of an elderly relative. This is especially true if the elder has developed combative or undesirable behaviors. It is helpful for families to understand the progress of the disease and the fact that it brings about these behavioral changes. Referral to other resources, such as family support groups, clergy, or social workers, should also be considered at this time.

Family members may wish to participate in hands-on care for their older relative. This often happens as the elder becomes terminal and the family feels the need to "do more." In these circumstances, nurses can provide physical help and emotional support. With that assistance, this final time together can have special meaning for both the elderly person and the family.

CAREGIVER PROBLEMS IN UNIQUE SITUATIONS

Providing home care for the elderly is always complex, but when they have problems which set them apart from their peers, specialized resources must be created to meet their needs.

Older Refugees: Song

Song, a 62-year-old, Vietnamese refugee, was discovered to be hypertensive at the Public Health Clinic in her community. With the aid of an interpreter, the nurse was able to determine that Song also slept poorly, had nightmares, and was suffering from symptoms suggestive of depression. The nurse asked Song to bring a relative with her to the next appointment. Two weeks later, Cory, Song's daughter-in-law, explained that since coming to the United States five years ago, Song had kept to herself, refusing to learn English and spending the day in their apartment waiting for the family to come home from work and school. Cory stated that Song came to this country reluctantly with her family, fearing that if she stayed behind, no one would care for her in her old age. Song expected that even in this "new" country, she would have the respect and honor accorded to the elderly "at home," and she eagerly tried to help her grandchildren learn the customs and language of their original culture. However, Song's family was anxious to become Americanized and her grandchildren had little time to spend with her. Song became more and more isolated, refusing to give in to the "new ways," saying that at her age she was much too old to learn. Cory also noted that Song recently seemed to be losing interest in maintaining her personal care.

Providing care for older refugees presents special problems for caregiving families. In many cultures, old age begins at a much earlier time of life, often in the mid-forties. Refugees in this age range may perceive themselves as being old and have the expectation that they will be treated with the dignity and respect accorded to the elderly in their country of origin. Additionally, many refugees came to the United States because of war, poverty, or mistreatment. As a result, the physical state of most of these refugees reflects their previous poor quality of life. At 40 or 50 years of age, many of them suffer from chronic conditions usually seen only in the elderly in North America. Health insurance for this population is a major problem. Also, many illegal aliens do not seek care, either because they cannot pay for it or they fear deportation.

The psychosocial needs of older refugees are not well understood and appropriate resources for their care are slow to develop. Some of the barriers to providing care for this group include their mistrust of the American health care system, dependency on cultural supports and folk medicine, and the difficulties of providing health education materials in different languages.

Stress is believed to be a major problem for many elderly refugees for a number of reasons. In a study recently completed by the Refugee Policy Group (Gozdziak, 1988), it was found that many of the elderly refugees interviewed complained of persistent headaches, stomach aches, and other ailments frequently attributed to "stress and survivor's grief." Cambodians were found to have the most difficulty adjusting to a new culture and reported persistent nightmares probably related to their experiences in the Cambodian War. However, many older refugees feel it is shameful to discuss psychological problems and might not accept help even if bilingual counselors were available.

Adult children of aging refugees, already burdened by the struggles of adapting to a new country, have a much more difficult time trying to meet the additional needs of their older parents. As a result, many older refugees feel rejected and may fear that their families will not be able to provide for them. Intervention on their behalf requires an understanding of the problems of refugee families and the importance of cultural values, especially to the elderly. Refugee assistance programs, such as Women's Association for Hmong and Lao, Inc. (1544 Timberlake Road,

St. Paul, MN 55117; tel. 612-488-0243 or 487-3972), and the United Polish American Services (308 Walnut, Philadelphia, PA 19106; tel. 215-923-1900) are just beginning to recognize and understand the needs of older refugees. Local Area Offices on Aging can be contracted for information on programs available in the community.

Significant Others: Jan and Mary

Caregiving is almost always a highly stressful situation. Taking on the responsibility for the welfare of another often requires additional support (physical, emotional, financial, and legal) from friends, relatives, and the community. There are, however, some caregiving situations in which participants are unwilling or unable to ask for assistance when it is needed.

Jan and Mary lived together for over 18 years. For the past two years, Jan, who is 68, has cared for Mary, 72, who is suffering from Alzheimer's disease. Mary was recently hospitalized with pneumonia and malnutrition, and it became clear that Jan would need some additional help with her caregiving efforts. However, while Mary was in the hospital, her physician contacted her only living relative, a distant niece living in another state, and advised her to place Mary in a nursing home. Despite Jan's insistence that Mary would be better off at home with her, the family made plans to have Mary transferred to a nursing home near them. Jan is heartbroken and fears that she may never see Mary again, but Jan will not disclose the fact that they have had a lesbian relationship for almost 20 years. When Mary leaves, Jan will be grief stricken, but unable to share the depth of her feelings with friends since none of them are aware of the relationship she had with Mary. Jan knows that even if she were to disclose their secret, nothing would change since the law does not consider the rights of gay couples to be equal to the rights of family members.

Mary's problem is compounded by the fact that while today's society is more accepting of gay and lesbian relationships, many older homosexuals are not comfortable being open about their lifestyles. Many have been together for a good number of years, and when one member of the couple dies, the other grieves in much the same way a widow or widower would grieve. Support systems for this group are hard to find, but a good example of resources for older gays is a group called Senior Action in a Gay Environment (SAGE, 208 West 13th Street, New York, NY 10011; tel. 212-741-2247). Based in New York, SAGE has been in existence for ten years providing social services, legal assistance, senior centers, and regular activities for older homosexuals in the New York area.

COMMUNITY RESOURCES

Information on national organizations and federal, state, and local resources can be obtained by contacting local Area Offices on Aging (AOA). Each AOA provides an updated directory of community resources including information on:

- Counseling services (Alcoholics Anonymous, Alzheimer's Disease and related disorders, mental health services, family counseling, widowed persons services, adult protective services, and emergency and TTY [Tele-Type] emergency numbers).
- Health-related services for education and support (cancer, diabetes, heart, and lung diseases, arthritis, dental care, preventative health programs, home health services, respite care, loan closets, hospice services, and visiting nurse services).

Directories also include information on consumer protection, employment, financial assistance and counseling, legal assistance, discount programs, transportation, and volunteer services. The most visible of the programs for elderly persons in the community are the "drop in centers," where seniors may come to share activities and the noonday meal with their peers. Elders who are not independent enough to attend the senior centers may be enrolled in Adult Day Care, an option which provides activities and a meal under more closely supervised conditions while families can enjoy a short respite from caregiving responsibilities. Seniors who do not attend these programs may benefit from telephone reassurance, Meals on Wheels, or friendly visitor programs in their own homes.

Area Offices on Aging can also supply the elderly with information on senior housing options. In most areas, independent housing, communal living, life-care communities, and nursing homes will be available. Information is also available on home maintenance, weatherization, energy assistance, and programs developed to match seniors in need of a place to live with others who have extra room.

Additional educational information on a large number of topics related to aging and caregiving is available from:

The American Association of
  Retired Persons
  1909 K Street, N.W.
  Washington, DC 20049
  tel. 202-872-4700

American Association of Homes
  for the Aging
  1129 20th Street, N.W., Suit 400
  Washington, DC 20036
  tel. 202-296-5960

National Council on The Aging   National Institute on Aging
   600 Maryland Avenue, S.W.   Information Center, Box 87
   West Wing 100   2209 Distribution Circle
   Washington, DC 20024   Silver Spring, MD 20910
   tel. 202-479-1200   tel. 301-496-1752

CONCLUSION

Nurses who assist with the development of plans for home care have a
responsibility to extend their assessment beyond the needs of the
elderly client to include an evaluation of caregivers and their ability to
provide long-term care. Elder care, safety, and self-care abilities can be
used as a foundation upon which the care plan is built. Family consulta-
tions are a good way for nurses to assess caregiver abilities. Input to
and approval of the care plan by the elderly person and caregiver(s)
supplies nurses with additional information and provides an opportunity to suggest community resources for additional education and support. A contract between the elderly person and his or her caregiver(s)
is an effective means of clarifying everyone's understanding of the
requirements for care and how they will be met. Contracts can also
include a recognition of the psychosocial needs of both the elderly
person and caregiver(s), allowing those involved to plan for ways in
which everyone's needs can be satisfied.

Nurses work with the elderly and their caregivers in a variety of
settings. The ability of nurses to view the caregiving situation holisti-
cally enables them to assist families to develop effective home care
plans with the potential of reducing the occurrence of complications,
accidents, medication reactions, abuse, and caregiver burnout. Elder
advocacy is the key role for nurses in working with family systems and
the elderly person.

REFERENCES

Ambrogi, D., & London, C. (1985). Elder abuse laws—Their implications for
    caregivers. *Generations 10*(1), 37–39.
American Association of Retired Persons (1987). Profile of older Americans
    (Pamphlet #PF3049 1187 *D996). Washington, DC: Author.
Block, M. R., & Sinnat, J. D. (1979). *The battered elder syndrome: An exploratory study.*
    College Park, MD: Center on Aging, University of Maryland.
Coons, D., Metzelaar, M., Robinson, A., & Spencer, B. (1986). *A better life.*
    Columbus, OH: The Source for Nursing Home Literature.
Douglas, R., & Pearson, L. (1987). *Domestic mistreatment of the elderly: Toward preven-
    tion.* Washington, DC: American Association of Retired Persons.

Fulmer, T. (1984). Elder abuse, assessment tool. *Dimensions of Critical Care Nursing, 3*, 216–220.

Gozdziak, E. (1988). Older refugees in the United States: From dignity to despair. Paper presented at the National Symposium on Older Refugees in America, June 1988, Washington, DC.

Hickey, T., & Douglas, R. (1981). Neglect and abuse of older family members: Professional perspectives and case experiences. *The Gerontologist, 21*, 171–176.

Katterhagen, A. (1987). Care for families: Expanding hospice bereavement programs. *Generations, 21*(2), 39–41.

Knight, B. (1985). The decision to institutionalize. *Generations, 10*(1), 42–44.

Morishita, L., & Hansen, J. (1986). GNP and LTC team. *Journal of Gerontological Nursing, 16*(6), 15–20.

National Center for Health Statistics [NCHS] (1984). *Advance report of final mortality.* Washington, DC: Government Printing Office.

National Center for Health Statistics [NCHS] (1981). *Health characteristics of persons with chronic activity limitations* (Series 10 #137). Washington, DC: Government Printing Office.

O'Malley, T., Everett, D., O'Malley, H., & Campion, E. (1983). Identifying and preventing family-mediated abuse and neglect of elderly persons. *Annals of Internal Medicine, 98*, 998–1005.

Rogers, J. (1985). Low technology devices. *Generations, 10*(1), 59–61.

Seabrooks, P., Kahn, R., & Gail, G. (1987). Cross cultural observations. *Journal of Gerontological Nursing, 13*(1), 18–21.

Select Committee on Aging, House of Representatives, Subcommittee on Human Services (1987). Exploding the myths: Caregiving in America (Comm. Pub. #99-611).

Stoppard, M. (1984). *The best years of your life.* New York: Villard Books.

Tynan, C., & Cardea, J. (1987). Home health hazard assessment. *Journal of Gerontological Nursing, 13*(10), 18–20.

Zarit, S. (1985). New directions. *Generations, 10*(1), 6–8.

FOR ADDITIONAL READING

Gelman, D., Hager, M., Gonzalez, D., Morris, H., McCormick, J., Jackson, T. A., & Karagianis, E. (1985). Who's taking care of our parents? *Newsweek*, May 6, 1985, pp. 61–68.

Johnson, S. (1982). The dilemma of the dutiful daughter. *Working Woman*, August, 65–69.

Rempasheski, V., & Phillips, L. (1988). Elders versus caregivers: Games they play. *Geriatric Nursing, 9*(1), 30–34.

Wood, J. (1987). Labors of love. *Modern Maturity, 30*, 29–34, 90–91. United States Department of health and Human Services (1985). Home safety checklist for older consumers. Washington, DC: Government Printing Office.

Chapter 16

Nurses, Work-Related Stress, and Ethical Dilemmas

Kay Weiler, Kathleen Coen Buckwalter, and James P. Curry

INTRODUCTION

Nurses working with the elderly encounter many complex and potentially stressful care situations. This chapter identifies some of the more common sources and outcomes of work-related stress for gerontological nurses, and then sets forth some useful strategies for managing stress and developing systems of support to enable nurses to function as ethical agents.

The conceptual model upon which this chapter is based is depicted in Figure 16.1. The model derives from research on work stress and morale among nursing home employees (Curry, 1987; Curry, et al., 1985). For purposes of this chapter, ethical dilemmas and philosophies of care have been added to the model as antecedent conditions. In the following sections, the antecedents and outcomes of work stress highlighted in this model are briefly reviewed, with special attention to ethical dilemmas faced by gerontological nurses.

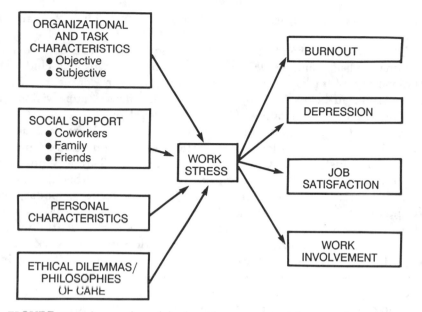

FIGURE 16.1 A causal model of work stress antecedents and outcomes.

SOURCES OF WORK-RELATED STRESS

In an Institute of Medicine report (1986), the quality of care in nursing homes was linked to the nature of staff-resident interactions. Clearly, those interactions can be affected by the stresses experienced by nurses working with the elderly. And yet, very little research has examined the causes and consequences of work-related stress (defined as the cumulative impact of events occurring during the performance of job-related duties which require substantial behavioral adjustment) in this population. Those studies that have been done are largely anecdotal, prescriptive, and cross-sectional in design. There are indications in the literature, however, that a high degree of stess is inherent in the role of caregiver. For nuses caring for elderly clients, this stress can result in role conflict and ambiguity, poor self-esteem, and burnout (Goldin, 1985; Heine, 1986; Klus & Thoreson, 1980; Morrow-Winn, 1985). The most frequently cited causes of stress for nurses include: continual exposure to physical and emotional pathology and death; and conflict with families of elderly persons, co-workers, supervisors, and representatives from other departments (Goldin, 1985; Klus & Thoreson, 1980). Many studies, primarily focused on nurses in hospital settings, have concluded that workload, absence of positive reinforcements, and low autonomy and task variety also contribute to stress-producing situations (Constable & Russell, 1986; Jacobson, 1982; Pines & Kanner, 1982).

The antecedent conditions noted in Figure 16.1 are defined and summarized as follows. *Objective organizational characteristics* include: (1) the variety of tasks in nursing positions; (2) the degree to which supervisory authority is delegated; (3) the closeness of supervision; (4) the degree of specialization; (5) the skill level of the work; (6) the quantity of the work; and (7) the pace of the work. *Subjective organizational characteristics* include: (1) task routinization; (2) communication; and (3) distributive justice (cf., Curry, et al., 1985; Gray-Toft & Anderson, 1985; and House, 1981). *Social support*, for purposes of this discussion, includes perceived support from supervisors, co-workers, spouse, and friends or relatives (Constable, 1983; House & Kahn, 1985). *Personal characteristics* refer to variables such as age, sex, educational attainment, length of nursing service, occupational position or title, work status (e.g., full or part-time), marital status, and number of relatives living nearby. These last two factors can also be viewed as crude indices of social support. Finally, an *ethical dilemma* is defined as a situation in which no choice is clearly correct and the alternatives are all equally unsatisfactory, while a *philosophy of care* incorporates both the American Nurses' Association (ANA) standards of care (e.g., *Code for Nurses*, 1985; *Standards and Scope of Gerontological Nursing Practice*, 1987) and the nurse's personal beliefs regarding the client's right of autonomy, the client's role in the decision-making process, and the client's right to respectful treatment (Lueckenotte, 1987). These last two elements, ethical dilemmas and a philosophy of care, are discussed in greater detail in the following section.

ETHICAL DILEMMAS AND A PHILOSOPHY OF CARE

The ethical principles of autonomy, beneficence, distributive justice, and non-maleficence as applied to client care (see Table 16.1) form the basis for ethical decision making in the clinical setting (Beauchamp & Childress, 1983; Kapp, 1987; Mappes & Zembaty, 1986; Veatch & Fry, 1987). These principles are involved in ethical decisions which nurses must make in the care of elderly clients, and their application may be a potential source of stress and conflict for the nurse in the care of elderly clients.

The principles identified in Table 16.1 appear to present readily acceptable ethical standards for nursing practice. However, gerontological nurses face complex real-life situations evolving from difficult circumstances which do not have readily identifiable solutions. Factors which contribute to the complexity of the ethical decisions which ger-

TABLE 16.1 Ethical Principles

Autonomy: the right to self determination; the individual makes the decisions and acts on the basis of those decisions.

Beneficence: the goal of helping or doing good for others.

Distributive Justice: equal treatment for all; a fair distribution of resources and benefits.

Non-maleficence: to do no harm; may be described as a part of beneficence.

Paternalism: is the interference with a person's liberty of action justified by reasons referring exclusively to the welfare, good, happiness, needs, interests, or values of the person being coerced.

ontological nurses make include: the elderly client's level of decision-making ability; the stability of the client's decision-making ability; the physician's suggested course of action; the opinions and concerns of family members; the client's stated wishes regarding treatment or the presence of a legally appointed substitute decision maker for health care decisions; the seriousness of the decision to be made; and the professional and individual nurse's philosophy of care.

Each of these factors will be explored in relation to the ethical dilemmas which gerontological nurses may confront on a daily basis. Ethical problems do not have prescribed answers; however, discussion of their critical elements and a summary of potential processes for problem resolution are helpful in analyzing such problems.

Capacity or Incapacity

The starting point of each ethical problem regarding an elderly client is the determination of whether or not the client is competent. If asked, few nurses would acknowledge that they have considered the client's competency. However, each nurse has assessed the ability of clients to distinguish: their personal identity, their relationship to significant others, the problem which exists, the decision which is being considered, and the potential outcomes which could result from the selection of the available alternatives (Thompson, Pender, & Hoffman-Schmitt, 1987). This assessment provides information regarding the client's neurological status and also contributes to the nurse's decision regarding the client's capacity to make decisions. If the elderly client demonstrates an understanding of the problem, acknowledges the potential risks and benefits of the proposed treatment, and appreciates that the information has personal relevance, the nurse should conclude that the person has the capacity to make the decision (Haddad, 1988; Nelson, 1986).

If the client does not demonstrate this level of understanding, the person is incapable of making treatment decisions and may be labeled as incompetent. The terms "incapable" and "incompetent" may be perceived by health care professionals as synonymous. In fact, these terms are distinctly different. Under United States law, each adult is presumed to be competent; the strict label of incompetency is only appropriate for an individual who has been adjudicated to be incompetent (Nelson, 1986; Northrop, 1988). However, gerontological nurses frequently encounter competent elderly clients who do not have the capacity to make a specific health care treatment decision. Because of the frequent confusion between the two terms, a recent congressional report (U.S. Congress, Office of Technology Assessment, 1987) has suggested that the term "incompetent" should be reserved for clients who have been adjudicated incompetent. Individuals who are unable to make a specific treatment decision should be described as "incapable."

This distinction between the elderly client's capacity or incapacity is relevant in ethical problem resolution because of the deference which is given to the client's proclaimed decision. If the elderly client is capable, the principle of autonomy asserts that he or she has the right to self-determination, the right to accept or reject treatment, and the right to have those decisions respected by caregivers. If the client is incapable of making treatment decisions, the principles of beneficence and paternalism influence nurses and other health care professionals to protect the client from harm and to structure decisions which they believe will benefit the client (Nelson, 1986).

Stability of Capacity

Once the decision regarding capacity or incapacity has been established, the next issue which arises is whether that status appears to be stable. If the individual demonstrates decision-making capacity and that capacity appears to be stable, the principle of autonomy again indicates that the wishes of the client should be honored.

If the client has capacity, but of a limited duration, the direction of the decision will determine whether the decision is questioned. If the client's decision is consistent with the proposed medical treatment, there is generally little discussion regarding the ethical basis for the decision (Brennan, 1986). If the client's decision is contrary to the suggested medical treatment, controversy may ensue; however, the right to self-determination should prevail. If the client's decision is in conflict with the proposed medical treatment and has substantial consequences for the person's welfare, an ethical dilemma may arise. This conflict may precipitate re-examination of the client's initial categorization of capacity (Haddad, 1988; President's Commission, 1982).

Physician's Suggested Course of Action

Because physicians are responsible for the diagnosis and medical plan of care for clients, they are placed in a role of authority and responsibility. Some physicians believe that decisions in life-threatening situations should be medical decisions and that the client or surrogate decision maker should merely give consent to the treatment. Others believe that they should educate and advise the client while the client maintains the right to form the final decision. Increasingly, physicians are seeking collaborative decision making with client, family, colleagues, and other health care providers (U.S. Congress, Office of Technology Assessment, 1987).

Regardless of the decision-making framework which the physician has chosen, if the physician's decision is congruent with the decision of client, family, and nurse, it is unlikely that an ethical dilemma will arise. However, if the physician's plan of care differs from the client's or family's wishes, or from the nurse's assessment of the situation, an ethical dilemma may arise for the nurse (Brennan, 1986; Wilson-Barnett, 1986).

This conflict emerges from the nurse's dual responsibilities as a patient advocate (see Chapter 14) and as an employee responsible for carrying out the physician's order (Melia, 1987). Nurses have traditionally occupied a subordinate role to the physician on the multidisciplinary health care team. However, nurses have maintained independent ethical and professional responsibilities, and have the most continuous and intimate contact with clients and their relatives. Thus, the nurse may have gained more information or insight than the physician into the client's or family's needs or wishes, and may, therefore, have identified a problem (Wilson-Barnett, 1986).

Family Members

The role of the family is another potential factor in the development of an ethical problem. The President's Commission (1983, p. 128) has identified that the family is an important source of information and plays a significant role in the health care decision-making process for the following reasons:

1. The family is generally most concerned about the good of the patient.
2. The family will also usually be most knowledgeable about the patient's goals, preferences, and values.
3. The family deserves recognition as an important social unit that ought to be treated, within limits, as a responsible decision maker in matters that intimately affect its members.

4. Especially in a society in which many other traditional forms of community have eroded, participation in a family is often an important dimension of personal fulfillment.

5. Since a protected sphere of privacy and autonomy is required for the flourishing of this interpersonal union, institutions and the state should be reluctant to intrude, particularly regarding matters that are personal and on which there is a wide range of opinion in society.

These presumed benefits of shared family decision making are not indisputable and may be challenged if: the family members have questionable decision-making capacity; there are unresolvable disagreements among the adult family members; there is evidence of abuse or neglect of the older person; there is conflict between the family's interests and the elder's interests; or there is an indication that the family intends to disregard the elder's values, preferences, or previously-stated instructions (President's Commission, 1983).

Thompson, Pender, and Hoffman-Schmitt (1987, p. 22) have identified that concerned families often express "fear, anger, depression, frustration, fatigue, grief, guilt, and financial strain" which compound the difficult decisions which they must make regarding an elderly person. In addition, families have expressed fear of reprisal from nurses and other health care team members when they have chosen not to follow the recommended plan of care (Phillips, 1987). These combined fears create enormous stress for the family and may impede free communication between the family and health care providers.

Presence of Advance Directive or Substitute Decision Maker

One element which may assist in resolving an ethical problem is the presence of an advance directive or the appointment of a substitute decision maker for the elderly client. Individuals who anticipate the need for future health care decisions may communicate their treatment preferences through a variety of means. Verbal comments, a living will, and a durable power of attorney have all been recognized as valid advance directives for future health care treatment decisions.

Verbal comments which indicate a thoughtful and consistent approach to potential or anticipated health care treatment decisions have been recognized as valid declarations of the client's autonomy (In re Storar, 1981). The limitations of verbal comments are readily obvious. Therefore, the use of written advance directives is preferable in health care treatment decisions.

Two forms of written advance directives are important in situations in which the patient is incapable of participating in the specific health care treatment decision: the living will and the durable power of attorney. Living will legislation is specific to each state. However, the general provisions are limited to situations in which *life-sustaining measures* are considered for: an adult, who has a condition which is incurable or irreversible, who is unable to participate in treatment decisions, and who is likely to die soon (Uniform Rights of the Terminally Ill Act, 1987).

The durable power of attorney is a written document which authorizes one person to act in the place of or on behalf of another person (Uniform Durable Power of Attorney Act, 1983). It specifically applies to situations in which the person who conferred the power has become incapacitated or disabled, and in many states it is applicable to health care treatment decision. These legal documents provide a means of extending autonomous decisions into situations where the client is not capable of actively participating in the treatment decision.

The presence of an advance directive does not, however, necessarily simplify an ethical dilemma. In fact, advance directives may generate ethical questions. These questions arise if the directive was drafted with vague language, was signed years before the event, states directives contrary to the family's position, or creates fear by the client or family that the directive would be prematurely invoked (Cohn, 1983; O'Mara, 1987).

The decision of a court-appointed guardian for the client in health care treatment decisions should reflect the best interests of the client. However, the presence of a guardian, as a substitute decision maker, does not assure the resolution of health care treatment problems and may, in fact, create ethical and legal concerns (Weiler & Buckwalter, 1988).

Seriousness of the Consequences of the Decision

The seriousness of the decision has a definite impact upon whether the situation precipitates an ethical problem. Phillips (1987) identified that elderly clients and their caregivers must deal with two types of ethical decisions: (1) the little dilemmas of everyday living; and (2) the big dilemmas, such as the right to die and the right to refuse treatment. For the elderly client, "the underlying issues raised while discussing these concerns included privacy, autonomy, confidentiality, sensitivity, dignity as well as quality of life and death" (Phillips, 1987, p. 38).

For nurses involved in the decision, the everyday questions may in practice be resolved by adopting the principle of paternalism. "Nursing paternalism (or maternalism) is very common, particularly with elderly people who are too weak or confused to refuse all the washing and exercise they are forced to receive" (Wilson-Barnett, 1986, p. 124). For life-threatening decisions, the nurse may be compelled to make an immediate decision, but may be left wondering, "Did I do the right thing?" (Mitchell, 1987; Smurl, 1983).

Phillips (1987) stated that nursing care of the elderly client should minimally include: (1) assurance that basic human needs are met; (2) provision of information in a meaningful and understandable form; (3) protection, nurturance, and support; (4) values clarification and reduction in the fear of isolation and/or retaliation from health care professionals; and (5) maintenance of communication between client, family, and health care providers.

This list appears to include basic elements of nursing care. However, the first factor, the provision of food and water, has created some of the most difficult ethicolegal questions for the elderly and their caregivers. The right of an individual to refuse essential surgical treatment or life-sustaining ventilation has been examined and guidelines have been established in legal and health care environments (Matter of Quinlan, 1976; U.S. Congress, Office of Technology Assessment, 1987). However, another complex and controversial issue has arisen: "Can an individual refuse fluid and nourishment even if it will result in their death?" (O'Neil, 1987). This issue has included controversy concerning whether the administration of food and fluids is: the maintenance of essential human care; the administration of medical interventions; ordinary comfort care; or life-sustaining treatment which may be withheld or withdrawn.

Professional and Personal Philosophy of Care

For nurses, the professional philosophy of care for the elderly has been articulated by the ANA in the *Code for Nurses* (1985) and the *Standards and Scope of Gerontological Nursing Practice* (1987). These written codes were established to provide essential ethical guidance for nursing practice.

As mentioned above, one of the most pressing ethical questions for nurses has become whether food and fluids may be withdrawn or withheld from the elderly client. In order to address this specific concern, the ANA Committee on Ethics issued *Guidelines on Withdrawing or Withholding Food and Fluid* (ANA, 1988). The Committee began the guidelines by asking the question: "Is it morally permissible to withhhold or withdraw food or fluid from sick patients—and should nurses ever be involved in doing so?" The general answer offered by the Committee is "no"; however, circumstances in which the answer is "yes" include: (1) the client who would be harmed by receiving feedings and fluids (e.g., post-surgical patients); (2) the competent and capable client who has refused the food and fluids; (3) the incompetent client who has created a verbal or written advance directive for the refusal of food and fluids;

and (4) when administration would be futile and so burdensome that it would only prolong life so that the client would die of other more painful causes.

These professional codes must impact upon every nurse's practice. However, the individual nurse also has a very personal perspective which is brought to every client encounter. In the care of the elderly, Lueckenotte (1987) has urged the development and implementation of a personal philosophy of care. She suggested that each gerontological nurse ask these questions: "(1) Do you encourage or discourage patient autonomy, within the limits of safety?; (2) Do you include or exclude the patient in the decision-making process?; (3) Do you cultivate or obstruct respectful and dignified treatment of the patient?" (p. 15). Lueckenotte (1987, p. 18) encouraged this personal analysis because she believes that, "making a decision for the patient without having to live with the direct consequences of that decision, as the patient will, requires careful thought within an ethicolegal framework."

Finally, in the development of a personal philosophy of care Fry (1988, p. 150) emphasized that nurses should remember that: "Nurses have a right to remain true to their own conscientious moral and religious beliefs in the face of decisions to forego treatment . . . nurses should realize that they can withdraw from any patient care situation as a matter of conscience, as long as the care of the patient can be transferred to others in an orderly manner and the nurse does not abandon his or her patient."

Carpenter (1988) studied the process by which nurses make ethical decisions in clinical practice. Her findings revealed a ten-stage process that begins with an emotional response upon hearing of an event which affects clinical practice and ends in an aftermath which includes feelings, talking with others, reconsiderations, and change or vows to change. Both affective and cognitive components of the decision-making process are identified. Carpenter's (1988) findings suggest that problems of ethical decision making may be a significant part of the stress in nursing. She also provided evidence that the process of ethical decision making affects nurses' views of themselves and of the nursing profession, and may even have direct bearing on the decision to leave nursing for another career.

OUTCOMES OF WORK-RELATED STRESS

A large body of literature has examined the outcomes of work-related stress. Review of these studies reveals a strong link between stress and adverse physical and psychological consequences (House, et al., 1986;

LaRocco, House, & French, 1980). There is equally compelling evidence, however, that social support serves to mitigate against these adverse effects and reduces burnout among nurses (Constable & Russell, 1986; Turner, 1983). Burnout, a phenomenon characterized by loss of concern for clients, and physical, emotional, and spiritual exhaustion, is a consequence of particular interest to nurses working with the elderly. Burnout may lead to indifference or negative feelings toward elderly clients/residents, overuse of chemical or physical restraints, and heightened potential for elder abuse (Heine, 1986). Nurses who are burned out report feelings of depression, anger, decreased self-esteem, and behavioral and physical problems such as increased alcohol consumption, headaches, fatigue, and ulcers. Burnout also results in administrative difficulties such as high rates of tardiness, absenteeism, and attrition (Goldin, 1985; Morrow-Winn, 1985). Clearly, burnout, depression, job satisfaction, and work involvment are all potentially impacted by work-related stress that can adversely affect the quality of care which nurses provide to their elderly clients.

The outcomes of work-related stress for nurses working with the elderly, according to the Curry model (Figure 16.1), include: *burnout*, defined as a syndrome of emotional exhaustion, depersonalization, and lack of personal accomplishment (Maslach & Jackson, 1981); *depression*, which is the degree of negative affect experienced by the nurse; *job satisfaction*, which is the effective orientation of the nurse toward the work situation; and *work involvement*, defined as the degree to which the nurse identifies with the job (Gray-Toft & Anderson, 1985; House, 1981; Kanungo, 1982; LaRocco, House, & French, 1980; Price & Mueller, 1986).

STRATEGIES TO ENHANCE THE ROLE OF NURSES AS ETHICAL AGENTS

In order for nurses to function more effectively as ethical agents, changes must take place in two basic arenas: nursing education and public policy. Nurses must also be able to understand and implement the process of resolving ethical dilemmas. With regard to changes in nursing education, more nurses need clinical experiences with the elderly in a variety of settings (e.g., acute care, long-term care, community-based clinics, hospice) incorporated into their generic curriculum. However, students should not be forced to care for older adults without proper instruction or role modeling from a competent faculty (Bahr, 1987). At present, this challenging and important nursing specialty (gerontology) is often inadequately taught to students in their formative professional years, contributing to the still-pervasive notion that "anyone can take care of old folks," and that nursing homes remain the "dumping ground" of nurses and clients alike. Much gerontological education simply does not prepare nurses to work with the elderly experiencing ethical dilemmas. Current textbooks and teaching aids are inferior to those developed for other specialties, and the literature contains few successful guidelines or strategies for effectively functioning as ethical agents with the elderly (Taylor & Gallagher, 1988).

As noted by Bahr (1987, p. 6), ". . . nursing students receive little instruction regarding ethics, ethical decision making and legal issues that could enhance their competence in clinical practice when older adults turn to nurses for guidance in serious decisions facing them; or, in cases where nurses are faced with serious situations in nursing practice when caring for older adults." Furthermore, there is compelling evidence in the literature that nursing home personnel in particular are not knowledgeable about the aging process and are especially ill-prepared to deal with the psychological and behavioral problems experienced by more than 75% of geriatric residents (Meunier & Holmes, 1987).

Most undergraduate curricula include a professional development seminar (or something similar) that examines professional issues, and legal and ethical aspects of nursing. These courses must be modified to contain material relevant to working with the elderly, using real-life vignettes, to prepare nurses for the ethical conflicts they will face in the work place. Furthermore, nurses with expertise in the values and principles associated with working with the elderly must be encouraged to publish in the nursing literature and to conduct more workshops and continuing education programs. Administrators of facilities serving the elderly must also promote awareness of ethical issues in their staff through inservice programming and the inclusion of ethical issues and philosophies of care as important components of their policy and procedure manuals. When ethical issues are clearly spelled out in policy and procedure manuals (e.g., how to obtain informed consent from a resident with Alzheimer's disease), nursing staff are more likely to act effectively as ethical agents and with assurance of support for their actions from administration.

Although many changes are needed in nursing education, they must be supported by clear public policy guidelines to be most effective. More than 70% of Americans now die in health care institutions and intensive care units (Thompson, 1984). And yet, prolongation of life without meaningful quality of life is questionable and a significant source of stress for nurses working with the elderly. At present, gerontological nurses have no standardized guidelines from which to answer the question, "What does quality of life, and quality of death, mean?" They are confronted with a variety of views on this issue, including: edicts from the government, which has a moral obligation to ensure human life, and from society, which has a moral responsibility to respect human existence; opinions of legal experts striving to protect human life from abuse by health care professionals; and mandates from religious personnel trying to uphold the sacredness of humanity. Lack of national standards only compounds this problem. For example, some states allow persons with durable power of attorney to make decisions concerning property and health care, and many others have passed living will legislation (Grabenstein-Chandler & Kimbrough, 1986). Considering the many inconsistencies and ambiguities in state legislation, laws need to be established that clearly define conditions under which controversial practices, such as euthanasia, may be conducted, and both nurses and the general public must be educated about their rights and responsibilities under the law. Finally, nurses must also be proactively involved in shaping and defining legislation germane to the health care needs of the elderly.

THE PROCESS OF RESOLVING ETHICAL DILEMMAS

All of the factors described earlier (e.g., the client's level of decision-making ability, stability of capacity, presence of an advance directive or surrogate decision maker) may affect an ethical decision. In some situations the competency of the client may be the central problem, in others the disagreement between the family and the client may create the tension, while in still other situations disagreement between the physician and the client and family may be the source of discord. Examination of all of these factors is essential to the assessment of the ethical problem. A simple solution may evolve through the analysis of the needs of the concerned participants. If a solution is not available, the critical elements and their relationship to each other must be identified and analyzed before resolution is attempted.

Smurl (1983) described the elements of resolving ethical dilemmas as comparable to the steps of the nursing process: observation, judging priorities, and then taking action. By following this familiar path of assessment, planning, and intervention, one potential process for resolving ethical dilemmas may be as familiar as the planning of nursing interventions to meet a client's physiological needs.

Garritson (1988) conducted a study of 177 registered nurses in long-term care facilities in Sweden. She asked these nurses to decide if selected clients, who could not receive oral food and hydration, should be fed by alternative methods or should be allowed to die. The study reported that individual nurses did not consistently select one ethical principle to resolve the problem, but analyzed situational variables described above for resolution of the problem. The ability to resolve ethical dilemmas is one important way to decrease stress associated with working with the elderly.

MANAGING STRESS

How can nurses working with the elderly best manage work-related stress, so as to avoid or diminish the negative psychological and physical consequences of stress, in particular, burnout, depression, decreased job satisfaction, and diminished work involvement? Referring once again to Figure 16.1, it seems logical to examine those antecedent conditions that are amenable to change (that is, not personal characteristics such as age or sex) as appropriate starting points for prophylaxis and intervention.

Looking at organizational and task characteristics that contribute to work-related stress, the most obvious answer would seem to be to correct the situation of nurses working with the elderly who are "underpaid, understaffed, and overworked." Research by Hare and Pratt (1988) has shown that higher levels of nursing burnout in both acute and long-term care facilities may be related to the nature of the physically and emotionally strenuous work tasks, low status in comparison to other positions in the health care system, limited training, poor staff-patient ratios, and low wages and benefits. Further, problems with support in the work environment, especially from peers and supervisors, have repeatedly been shown to be a primary source of stress among nurses (Cronin-Stubbs & Rooks, 1985; Jackson & Maslach, 1982; Vachon, Lyall, & Freeman, 1978). It has also been suggested that nurses who *elect* to work with clients who have a poor prognosis for survival (versus those who do not work with these clients by choice) have reduced vulnerability to burnout because their work provides them with a personal sense of meaning (Hare & Pratt, 1988). Thus, nurses can function as social agents (see Chapter 14) to design interventions such as the following to address organizational sources of stress:

- Improved inservice training, especially in the multidimensional problems of the elderly, emphasizing psychosocial and behavioral problems common in this population. (Nurses should be taught to look for the message or theme being carried out by the disruptive client.)
- Increased variety in job tasks.
- Improved supervision, especially in long-term care settings.
- Implementation of a management style that allows for feedback, flexibility, and sensitivity.
- Clear and realistic objectives for client care. (Nurses need to understand that it is not always their fault if certain clients fail to respond.)

- Higher wages and better benefits for nurses.
- Adequate staffing levels.

Although the latter two recommendations may be considered non-negotiable by some administrators because of increased costs associated with their implementation, it should be noted that the costs related to staff burnout, absenteeism, and turnover far outweigh costs associated with adequate staffing and compensation.

Another source of work-related stress that may be amenable to change has to do with the effect of the physical environment and structural factors. Although very little research has been done in this area, preliminary work by Lyman (1987) suggests that physical and architectural features, such as adequate space, separate activity rooms, staff offices and toilet facilities, client care facilities, barrier-free hallways, visible exits, and amenities such as wide entry doors and ramp emergency exits, may decrease caregiving burden and stress. Thus, nurses should work with administrators to examine carefully and modify institutional and environmental variables that may be contributing to work-related stress.

Enhancing social support networks is another important strategy that can serve as a buffer against the stresses inherent in working with the elderly. Interventions designed to strengthen supportive relationships among staff, staff training on stress management, and work-related counseling have all been shown to reduce vulnerability to burnout, depression, and decreased job satisfaction. For example, support groups are an excellent vehicle for helping nurses to recognize causes of work-related and non-work-related stress, to ventilate feelings, and to examine their own values and belief systems. Standardized instruments, such as the Social Readjustment Rating Scale (Holmes & Rahe, 1967), are helpful for nurses to understand non-work-related sources of stress that may be impinging on their care of the elderly and contributing to the development of adverse physical and psychological symptoms. The Coping Behavior Checklist developed by Leatz (1982) assists nurses to become aware of the various coping techniques they use in response to stressful situations, and can help to suggest alternative coping strategies. In this way counterproductive coping techniques, such as abuse of alcohol and drugs, withdrawal, or "workaholism," can be identified, and more healthful coping mechanisms substituted.

Recognizing causes of work-related stress can also be facilitated in group or individual formats. One useful exercise is for nurses to take a few minutes to think about specific occasions and behaviors of their elderly clients that produce signs of stress in themselves, and then to identify, by writing them down, all such incidents in a column on the left-hand side of a paper. On the right-hand side of the same paper, they are then encouraged to identify some of the factors that contribute to their stress responses, and to examine the underlying reasons why these factors produce stress. Another interesting, educational, and therapeutic group technique involves the discussion of stress-related vignettes. Nurses are asked to bring to the group descriptions of real-life stressful situations with the elderly, and then together to come up with possible interventions. All suggestions are written on a blackboard or flip chart, and the group then selects and prioritizes the best interventions. Group members are encouraged to discuss the advantages and disadvantages of each solution.

Finally, support groups offer an excellent opportunity to encourage nurses working with the elderly to develop a life outside of the work place. Leisure activities, such as non-competitive sports and hobbies, can be cultivated, family, social, and spiritual activities encouraged, and specific relaxation techniques, such as progressive muscle relaxation, taught and practiced. In more severe cases of depression and burnout, mental health consultation and referrals for counseling are appropriate interventions.

CONCLUSION

In this chapter the ethical principles of autonomy, beneficence, distributive justice, and nonmaleficence were examined in relation to ethical decisions which nurses must make in working with the elderly, and as potential sources of stress for the nurse. Several factors contributing to the complexity of ethical decision making in this population were examined, including: the elderly client's level of decision-making ability; the stability of the client's decision-making ability; the physician's suggested course of action; the opinions and concerns of family members; the client's stated wishes regarding treatment or the presence of a legally appointed substitute decision maker for health care decisions; the seriousness of the consequences of the decision; and the individual nurse's professional and personal philosophy of care. The process of ethical decision making has been shown to be a source of stress for nurses, and may even contribute to the decision to leave the profession (Carpenter, 1988).

The chapter also examined the antecedents and outcomes of work stress for gerontological nurses, based upon a conceptual model derived from the work of Curry and colleagues (Curry, et al., 1985; Curry, 1987). Sources of potential stress for nurses working with elderly clients include: objective organizational characteristics; subjective organizational characteristics; social support; personal characteristics; ethical dilemmas; and a lack of a personal philosophy of care. The latter two elements were added by the authors to the original Curry model.

Outcomes of stress were discussed in terms of: burnout; depression; job satisfaction; and work involvement. Educational and public policy strategies for enhancing the role of nurses as ethical agents were set forth, as well as a number of organizational and task characteristics associated with gerontological nursing that may help in the management of stress. Similarly, changes in the physical environment and structural factors were suggested as means to reduce work-related stress. Enhanced social support networks and the use of counseling and support groups were other suggestions to reduce work-related stress.

Nurses who work with the elderly confront many complex, real-life ethical situations that can be extremely stressful. This chapter has attempted to identify some of the more common sources of stress, as well as to suggest some useful strategies for managing stress and developing systems of support to enable nurses to function effectively as ethical agents.

REFERENCES

American Nurses' Association (1985). *Code for nurses with interpretive statements.* Kansas City, MO: Author.

American Nurses' Association (1987). *Standards and scope of gerontological nursing practice.* Kansas City, MO: Author.

American Nurses' Association, Committee on Ethics. (1988). *Guidelines on withdrawing or withholding food and fluid.* Kansas City, MO: Author.

Bahr, Sr. R. T. (1987). Adding to the educational agenda. *Journal of Gerontological Nursing, 13*(3), 6–11.

Beauchamp, T. L., & Childress, J. R. (1983). *Principles of biomedical ethics.* New York: Oxford University Press.

Brennan, T. (1986). Do-not-resuscitate orders for the incompetent patient in the absence of family consent. *Law, Medicine & Health Care, 14,* 13–19.

Carpenter, M. A. (1988). *The process of ethical decision making in psychiatric nursing practice.* Iowa City, IA: University of Iowa, unpublished doctoral dissertation.

Cohn, S. D. (1983). The living will from the nurse's perspective. *Law, Medicine & Health Care, 11,* 121–136.

Constable, J. F. (1983). *The effects of social support and the work environment upon burnout among nurses.* Iowa City, IA: University of Iowa, unpublished doctoral dissertation.

Constable, J. F., & Russell, D. W. (1986). The effect of social support and the work environment upon burnout among nurses. *Journal of Human Stress, 12,* 20–26.

Cronin-Stubbs, D., & Rooks, C. (1985). The stress, social support, and burnout of critical care nurses: The results of research. *Heart-Lung, 14,* 31–39.

Curry, J. P. (1987). Work stress and morale among nursing home employees. NIMH Grant #5R01MH42915-02.

Curry, J. P., Wakefield, D. S., Price, J. L., Mueller, C. W., & McCloskey, J. C.

(1985). Determinants of turnover among nursing department employees. *Research in Nursing and Health, 8,* 397–411.

Fry, S. T. (1988). New ANA guidelines on withdrawing or withholding food and fluid from patients. *Nursing Outlook, 36,* 122, 123, 148–150.

Garritson, S. H. (1988). Ethical decision making patterns. *Journal of Psychosocial Nursing and Mental Health Services, 26,* 22–29.

Goldin, G. J. (1985). The influence of self-image upon the performance of nursing home staff. *Nursing Homes, 34,* 33–38.

Grabenstein-Chandler, J., & Kimbrough, R. (1986). The right to die: Is living will legislation good public policy for the state of Nebraska? Lincoln, NB: Nebraska Legislative Council Legislative Research Division.

Gray-Toft, P. A., & Anderson, J. G. (1985). Organizational stress in the hospital: Development of a model for diagnosis and prediction. *Health Services Research, 19,* 753–774.

Haddad, A. M. (1988). Determining competency. *Journal of Gerontological Nursing, 14*(6), 19–22.

Hare, J., & Pratt, C. C. (1988). Burnout: Differences between professional and paraprofessional nursing staff in acute and long-term care health facilities. *The Journal of Applied Gerontology, 7,* 60–71.

Heine, C. A. (1986). Burnout among nursing home personnel. *Journal of Gerontological Nursing, 12*(3), 14–18.

Holmes, T. H., & Rahe, R. H. (1967). The social readjustment rating scale. *Journal of Psychosomatic Research, 11,* 213–218.

House, J. S. (1981). *Work stress and social support.* Reading, MA: Addison-Wesley.

House, J. S., & Kahn, R. L. (1985). Measures and concepts of social support. In S. Cohen & S. L. Syme (Eds.), *Social support and health* (pp. 83–108). New York: Academic Press.

House, J. S., Strecher, V., Metzner, H. L., & Robbins, C. A. (1986). Occupational stress and health among men and women in the Tecumseh community health survey. *Journal of Health and Social Behavior, 27,* 62–77.

In re Storar, 52 N.Y.2d. 363, 420 N.E.2d 64 (1981).

Institute of Medicine. (1986). *Improving the quality of care in nursing homes.* Washington, DC: National Academy Press.

Jackson, S., & Maslach, C. (1982). After-effects of job related stress. *Journal of Occupational Behavior, 3,* 63–77.

Jacobson, S. P. (1982). Stressful situations for neonatal intensive care nurses. In E. A. McConnel (Ed.), *Burnout in the nursing profession* (pp. 176–184). St. Louis: C. V. Mosby.

Kanungo, R. N. (1982). *Work alienation.* New York: Praeger.

Kapp, M. B. (1987). Interprofessional relationships in geriatrics: Ethical and legal considerations. *The Gerontologist, 27,* 547–552.

Klus, G. W., & Thoreson, E. H. (1980). The nurse's aide: A life of uncertainty. *Nursing Homes, 29,* 42–48.

LaRocco, J. M., House, J. S., & French, J. R. P. Jr. (1980). Social support, occupational stress, and health. *Journal of Health and Social Behavior, 21,* 202–218.

Leatz, C. (1981). *Unwinding: How to turn stress into positive energy.* Englewood Cliffs, NJ: Prentice-Hall.

Lueckenotte, A. G. (1987). Sharpen skills in hospital settings. *Journal of Gerontological Nursing, 13*(3), 12–19.

Lyman, K. A. (1987). Work-related stress for staff in an Alzheimer's day care center: The effects of physical environments. Paper presented to the 40th Annual Scientific Meeting of the Gerontological Society of America, Washington, DC.

Mappes, T. A., & Zembaty, J. S. (1986). *Biomedical ethics* (2nd ed.). New York: McGraw-Hill.

Maslach, C., & Jackson, S. (1981). *Maslach burnout inventory manual*. Palo Alto, CA: Consulting Psychologists Press.

Matter of Quinlan, 70 N.J. 10, 355 A. 2d 647 (1976).

Melia, K. (1987). Everyday ethics for nurses: Whose side are you on? *Nursing Times, 83,* 46–48.

Meunier, G. F., & Holmes, T. R. (1987). Measuring the behavioral knowledge of nursing home employees. *Clinical Gerontologist, 6,* 11–22.

Mitchell, C. (1987). Steadying the hand that feeds. *American Journal of Nursing, 87,* 293–296.

Morrow-Winn, G. (1985). When the pressures mount: Recognizing and coping with stress. *Nursing Homes, 34,* 39–42.

Nelson, L. J. (1986). The law, professional responsibility, and decisions to forego treatment. *Quality Review Bulletin, 12,* 8–15.

Northrop, C. E. (1988). Nursing practice and the legal presumption of competency. *Nursing Outlook, 36,* 112.

O'Mara, R. J. (1987). Ethical dilemmas with advance directives: Living wills and do not resuscitate orders. *Critical Care Nursing Quarterly, 10,* 17–28.

O'Neil, E. A. (1987). Treatment decisions with the terminally ill incompetent patient. *Nursing Economics, 5,* 32–35.

Phillips, L. R. (1987). Respect basic human rights. *Journal of Gerontological Nursing, 13*(3), 36–39.

Pines, A. M., & Kanner, A. D. (1982). Nurses' burnout: Lack of positive conditions and presence of negative conditions as two independent sources of stress. In E. A. McConnel (Ed.), *Burnout in the nursing profession* (pp. 139–145). St. Louis: C. V. Mosby.

President's Commission for the Study of Ethical Problems in Medicine and Biomedical and Behavioral Research. (1982). *Making health care decisions: The ethical and legal implications of informed consent in the patient-practitioner relationship.* Washington, DC: U.S. Government Printing Office.

President's Commission for the Study of Ethical Problems in Medicine and Biomedical and Behavioral Research. (1983). *Deciding to forego life-sustaining treatment: Ethical, medical, and legal issues in treatment decisions.* Washington, DC: U.S. Government Printing Office.

Price, J. L., & Mueller, C. W. (1986). *Absenteeism and turnover of hospital employees.* Greenwich, CT: JAI Press.

Smurl, J. F. (1983). "Did I do the right thing?" Ethical decision making for everyday nursing problems. *Nursing Life, 3*(3), 48–52.

Taylor, C., & Gallagher, L. L. (1988). Structured learning for geriatric consent. *Geriatric Nursing, 9,* 44–45.

Thompson, J., Pender, K., & Hoffman-Schmitt, J. (1987). Retaining rights of impaired elderly. *Journal of Gerontological Nursing, 13*(3), 20–25.

Thompson, L. M. (1984). Cultural and institutional restrictions on dying style in a technological society. *Death Education, 8,* 223–229.

Turner, R. J. (1983). Direct, indirect, and moderating effects of social support on psychological distress and associated conditions. In H. B. Kaplan (Ed.), *Psychosocial stress: Trends in theory and research* (pp. 105–155). New York: Academic Press.

Uniform Durable Power of Attorney Act. 8 A, U. L. A. (1983).

Uniform Rights of the Terminally Ill Act. 9 B, U. L. A. (1987).

U.S. Congress, Office of Technology Assessment. (1987). *Life-sustaining technologies and the elderly.* OTA-BA-306 Washington, DC: U.S. Government Printing Office.

Vachon, M., Lyall, W., & Freeman, S. (1978). Measurement and management of stress in health professionals working with advanced cancer patients. *Death Education, 1,* 365–375.

Veatch, R. M., & Fry, S. T. (1987). *Case studies in nursing ethics.* Philadelphia: Lippincott.

Weiler, K., & Buckwalter, K. C. (1988). Care of the demented patient. *Journal of Gerontological Nursing, 14*(7), 26–31.

Wilson-Barnett, J. (1986). Ethical dilemmas in nursing. *Journal of Medical Ethics, 12,* 123–126, 135.

Index